Thermal Agents in Rehabilitation

Second Edition

Susan L. Michlovitz, M.S., P.T.
Editor
Adjunct Assistant Professor
Department of Orthopedic
Surgery and Rehabilitation
Programs in Physical Therapy
Hahnemann University
Philadelphia, Pennsylvania
and
Director
Physical Therapy Review Services, Inc.
Woodlyn, Pennsylvania

 F. A. DAVIS COMPANY • **Philadelphia**

Last digit indicates print number: 10 9 8 7 6 5 4

The authors and the editors of this book have made every effort to ensure that all heat, cold, and laser agents that are recommended are in accordance with accepted standards at the time of publication. The agents specified within this book may not have specific approval by the Food and Drug Administration (FDA) in regard to the indications and dosages that are recommended by the editors and/or the authors. The manufacturers' product literature and the FDA are the best sources of current usage information. Regarding AIDS precautions, the Centers for Disease Control in Atlanta should be consulted for their most recent recommendations.

Library of Congress Cataloging-in-Publication Data
Thermal agents in rehabilitation / Susan L. Michlovitz [editor] : 2nd ed.
    p. cm. — (Contemporary perspectives in rehabilitation ; v. 6)
    Includes bibliographical references.
    Includes index.
    ISBN 0-8036-6165-7   *1782032 4*
      1. Thermotherapy.   2. Cold — Therapeutic use.   3. Physical therapy.   4. Physical Therapy — methods.   I. Micholvitz, Susan L.
    II. Series.
    [DNLM: 1. Cold — therapeutic use.   2. Heat — therapeutic use.   W1
C0769NS v. 6 / WB 469 T411]
RM865.T47   1990
615.8'32 — dc20
DNLM/DLC
for Library of Congress   90-3286
                                                                          CIP

Dedication for the
Second Edition

To Mary P. Watkins, friend and colleague, for providing encouragement, guidance, and inspiration for my professional growth over the last decade.

Dedication for the First Edition

To Eleanor Jane Carlin for providing me with my first opportunity as a P.T. student and as a faculty member.

Thermal Agents in Rehabilitation

Second Edition

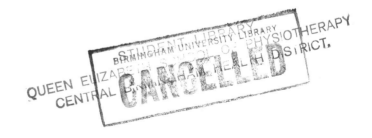

Contemporary Perspectives in Rehabilitation

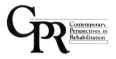

Steven L. Wolf, Ph.D., FAPTA
Editor-in-Chief

PUBLISHED VOLUMES

Thermal Agents in Rehabilitation – Volume 1
Susan L. Michlovitz, M.S., P.T.

Cardiac Rehabilitation: Basic Theory and Application – Volume 2
Frances Brannon, Ph.D., Mary Geyer, M.S., Margaret Foley, R.N.

The Biomechanics of the Foot and Ankle – Volume 3
Robert Donatelli, M.A., P.T.

Pharmacology in Rehabilitation – Volume 4
Charles D. Ciccone, Ph.D., P.T.

Wound Healing: Alternatives in Management – Volume 5
Luther C. Kloth, M.S., P.T., Joseph M. McCulloch, Ph.D., P.T. and
Jeffrey A. Feedar, B.S., P.T.

Thermal Agents in Rehabilitation, 2nd Edition – Volume 6
Susan L. Michlovitz, M.S., P.T.

VOLUMES IN PRODUCTION

Electrotherapy in Rehabilitation (Winter 1990) – Volume 7
Meryl R. Gersh, M.S., P.T.

Foreword

Any textbook that addresses clinical issues must capture the imagination of both students and teacher. To be really worthwhile, such a text must present material that clearly relates to actual practice. *Thermal Agents in Rehabilitation*, ed. 2, does just that.

The first edition of *Thermal Agents* marked the birth of the *Contemporary Perspectives in Rehabilitation* series and shared the purpose of all future volumes—to present relevant, documented information in a problem-solving format. F. A. Davis's allied health editor and I believed that this approach would challenge students, clinicians, and teachers to new insights, lead to treatment based more firmly on scientific reasoning, and therefore result in better quality of care.

Neither F. A. Davis nor I foresaw the enthusiastic reception given to *Thermal Agents* and the series as a whole. With the overwhelming success of the first edition, we soon faced the choice between issuing additional printings or producing a new edition. Sue Michlovitz's persistence in keeping the material up-to-date soon convinced us that the time was ripe for the second edition. I'm sure that the critical acclaim for this version will surpass even the chorus of praise for her first effort. It's clear that not only have the contributors kept abreast of the literature, but Sue has inspired and motivated them with feedback from many readers and users of the first edition.

The Preface to this edition lists specific changes in text and format. I want to stress one important point: We have taken care to provide abundant, appropriate references and documentation for each treatment modality. It was our intent to supply the clinician the information necessary to explain and, if necessary, defend each application. In the decade to come, all clinicians will face increasing pressure to justify their claims for reimbursement for health care; each treatment, each application, must be as scientifically defensible as possible. It is our hope that the scope of this text, its problem-solving approach, and the abundance of reference and documentation will help.

Steven L. Wolf, Ph.D., FAPTA
Series Editor

Preface to the Second Edition

I am pleased with the reception *Thermal Agents in Rehabilitation* has received in the physical therapy community. I have received feedback since publication of the first edition from physical therapy educators and clinicians. I have listened with an open ear to their comments and have incorporated and encouraged the authors to incorporate some of their suggestions into this second edition. Because, it is for my present and future peers that this text is prepared.

Section I, Foundations for the Use of Thermal Agents, provides further elaboration on the stages of inflammation and repair and a clarification of the proliferative and remodeling phases of inflammation. There is more information provided on trigger points and muscle spasm in the chapter on pain.

In Section II, Instrumentation: Methods and Application, additions are made to relevant chapters on documenting treatment procedures and home use of heat and cold. The sections on wound evaluation and care, whirlpool additives, and pool therapy are expanded in Chapter 6 on hydrotherapy. In addition, AIDS precautions now are presented in this chapter. Chapter 7 on ultrasound has been revised to include additional information on ultrasound for tissue healing and more detail on recording and selecting ultrasound intensities. The theoretical foundation for the use of pulsed electromagnetic fields (PEMFs) is now included in Chapter 8. The reader should be advised though that much of this work still needs further investigation to determine the efficacy of PEMFs in managing soft-tissue trauma. Chapter 9 has been retitled to reflect the inclusion of ultraviolet. While PEMFs, low-power laser, and ultraviolet are not considered thermal agents, information on these are often included in introductory courses with thermal agents. Therefore, we have included these agents. At the time of this writing (Spring, 1990), low-power laser is still considered by the Food and Drug Administration as an investigative device.

Section III, Clinical Decision Making, has an expanded discussion of pain and trigger point assessment.

More than 100 new references have been included in this second edition. A Glossary has been added. The Appendix on equipment manufacturers has been deleted because availability of equipment has been changing more rapidly than a textbook can keep it updated.

Susan L. Michlovitz, M.S., P.T.
Editor

Preface to the First Edition

Thermal agents are used in physical therapy and rehabilitation to reduce pain, to enhance healing, and to improve motion. The physical therapist should have a solid foundation in the normal physiological control of the cardiovascular and neuromuscular systems prior to using an agent that can alter the function of these structures. In addition, a background in the physiology of healing mechanisms and of pain serves as a basis for the rationale of using thermal agents.

Often, the decision to include a thermal agent in a therapy plan or to have the thermal agent *be* the sole treatment rendered (as in the case of the frequently used "hot packs and ultrasound combination" for back pain) is based on empirical evidence. The purpose of this book is to provide the reader with the underlying rationale for selection of an agent to be included in a therapy program, based on (1) the known physiologic and physical effects of that agent; (2) the safety and use of the heat/cold agent, given the conditions and limitations of the patient's dysfunction; and (3) the therapeutic goals for that particular patient. The authors have been asked to review critically the literature available that documents efficacy and effectiveness of each thermal agent. A problem-solving approach to the use of thermal agents is stressed throughout the text.

The primary audience for this text is the physical therapist. The student will gain a solid foundation in thermal agents, the clinician will strengthen his or her perspective of thermal agents, and the researcher is given information that will provide ideas for clinical studies on thermal agents. Athletic trainers and other professionals who use thermal agents in their practice should find this text of value.

The text is in three parts. Part I, Foundations for the Use of Thermal Agents, includes information from basic and medical sciences that can serve as a framework for the choice to include thermal agents in a rehabilitation program. A discussion of the proposed mechanisms by which heat and cold can alter inflammation, healing, and pain is included in these chapters.

Part II of the text, Instrumentation: Methods and Application, incorporates concepts of equipment selection, operation and maintenance, and clinical application. The leading chapter in this part is on instrumentation principles and serves to introduce concepts of electrical circuitry and safety as applied to equipment used for thermal therapy. Physical therapists have become responsible for product purchase and making recommendations about products through the expansion of consultation services, private practices, sports medicine clinics, extended care facilities, and home health care. Therefore, we must be prepared to engage in dialogue with manufacturers, product distributors, and other colleagues about the safety and quality of these products. To this end, some practical suggestions are provided in Chapter 3, intended to assist with purchase decisions.

Chapters 4 through 8 discuss the operation and application of heat and cold agents. Numerous principles of clinical decision making are included within each chapter. There are certain principles that are inherent to all agent applications: (1) The patient must be evaluated and treatment goals established; (2) contraindications to treatment must be known; and (3) the safe and effective use of equipment must be understood.

Chapter 9, on low-power laser, deviates somewhat from the overall theme of thermal agents. Low-power laser is not expected to produce an increase in tissue temperature, so its effects could not be attributed to thermal mechanisms. Therefore, this cannot be categorized as a thermal agent. However, I believe this topic is worthy of inclusion in this text because (1) the indications for its use overlap those of thermal agents; (2) laser is a form of non-ionizing radiation as are diathermy and ultrasound, which are used for pain reduction and tissue healing; and (3) laser would most likely be included in a physical therapy student curriculum in the coursework that includes thermal agents. At the time of this writing (summer 1985), low-power laser is still considered by the U.S. Food and Drug Administration as an investigational device. Only carefully designed clinical studies will help determine the laser's clinical efficacy—perhaps contributing to the body of knowledge needed to change the laser's status from an investigational to an accepted therapeutic product.

Part III, Clinical Decision Making, is designed to assist the student and clinician in integrating basic concepts that have been presented throughout the entire book, emphasizing problem solving and evaluation.

Much information has been published in the medical literature on the effects or clinical results of heat and cold application. Oftentimes, the therapist is called upon to justify the use of a certain modality. A careful review of the research literature may be necessary to provide an explanation for treatment.

There are many areas that require further investigation. For example, contrast baths (alternating heat and cold) are often used in sports medicine clinics. But a careful review of the literature reveals that only scanty information supports the use of contrast baths for any patient population. It is important for the clinician to be able to interpret accurately and to apply the methods and results that are presented in the literature. The inclusion of a chapter (Chapter 10) on techniques for reviewing the literature and establishing a paradigm for clinical studies of thermal agents provides the clinician with such a background on which to build.

Chapters 11 and 12 are devoted to specific patient populations in which thermal agents are commonly used. The chapter on sports medicine is representative of a population with a known cause of injury and predictable course of recovery. The majority of these patients are otherwise healthy. On the other hand, the chapter on rheumatic disease presents a model for a patient population that can be expected to have chronic recurrent—sometimes progressive—dysfunction associated with systemic manifestations.

Two appendices are included—temperature conversion scales (this text uses the centigrade scale); and a list of some of the manufacturers of thermotherapy products in the United States.

Susan L. Michlovitz, M.S., P.T.
Editor

Acknowledgments for the Second Edition

The completion of a multiauthored text requires the hard work, dedication, and coordination of many persons. I would like to thank the following people for contributing to this project and assisting me through completion:

Each contributing author.

Laurie Natartez who compiled the Glossary.

Dale R. Fish and Robert Patterson for their feedback on chapters 8 and 9.

My students at Hahnemann University, whose questions and concerns regarding thermal agents I have attempted to address.

Sue Giangrasso and Renada Pasker who typed and retyped the manuscript.

George Widman for the updated photographs for this edition.

The staff at F.A. Davis, including Senior Editor Jean-François Vilain, for their support.

David Clifton and Leslie Buksar Clifton, my business associates, who "tolerated revision well."

Bob Martone who worked with me from the inception of *Thermal Agents* and still has a special place in my life.

Susan L. Michlovitz, M.S., P.T.
Editor

Acknowledgments for the First Edition

The completion of a multiauthor text requires the hard work, dedication, and coordination of many people. I would like to thank the following people for contributing to this project and for assisting me through its completion:

Each of the 10 contributing authors.

Steve Wolf and Mary Watkins for their encouragement, support, and editorial assistance from the conception through the completion of this text.

xiv

The students I have taught at both Hahnemann University and Temple University, whose questions and concerns regarding thermal agents we have addressed. A special thanks to Dorsett Edmunds for her assistance with the literature search for Chapters 4 and 5.

Dean Currier and John Barr for their careful reviews and suggestions of portions of the manuscript.

Wesley L. Nyborg for his corrections and suggestions on therapeutic ultrasound.

Sue Giangrasso for her endless typing and retyping of the manuscript at all hours of the day and night.

Bill McBeth and Bill Holl for photography of some of the clinical pictures in Chapters 3 through 7.

The staff at F. A. Davis for their support. Another special thanks to Phyllis Spagnolo for her careful and precise artwork.

My colleagues at Hahnemann University—especially our Program Director, Risa Granick—for their encouragement during the time I worked on this book.

Susan L. Michlovitz, M.S., P.T.
Editor

Contributors

LUTHER C. KLOTH, M.S., P.T.

Associate Professor
Program in Physical Therapy
Marquette University
Milwaukee, Wisconsin

THERESA McDIARMID, M.Sc., R.P.T., M.C.S.P.

Consultant
Physical Therapy Review Services, Inc.
Woodlyn, Pennsylvania

SUSAN L. MICHLOVITZ, M.S., P.T.—Editor

Adjunct Assistant Professor
Department of Orthopedic
Surgery and Rehabilitation
Programs in Physical Therapy
Hahnemann University
Philadelphia, Pennsylvania
and
Director
Physical Therapy Review Services, Inc.
Woodlyn, Pennsylvania

ROBERTA A. NEWTON, Ph.D., P.T.

Associate Professor
Department of Physical Therapy
College of Allied Health Professions
Temple University
Philadelphia, Pennsylvania

BRIAN REED, Ph.D., P.T.

Associate Professor
Department of Physical Therapy
University of Vermont
Burlington, Vermont

H. T. M. RITTER, III, B.A., C.B.E.T.

Senior Project Engineer
ECRI
Plymouth Meeting, Pennsylvania

LAURENCE M. SEITZ, M.S., P.T.

President
Rehabilitation Performance Center
Elizabeth, New Jersey

WAYNE S. SMITH, M.Ed., P.T., A.T.C.

Arizona Rugby Association, Trainer
Phoenix, Arizona
and
Chief Physical Therapist
U.S. Public Health Service Hospital
Sacaton, Arizona

LYNN SNYDER-MACKLER, Sc.D., P.T., S.C.S.

Assistant Professor
University of Delaware
School of Life and Health Sciences
Physical Therapy Program
Newark, Delaware

MARK T. WALSH, M.S., P.T.

Director
Hand and Orthopedic Rehabilitation Services
"A physical therapy practice"
Levittown, Pennsylvania

MARY P. WATKINS, M.S., P.T.

Associate Professor
Department of Orthopedic Surgery and Rehabilitation
Programs in Physical Therapy
Hahnemann University
Philadelphia, Pennsylvania

STEVEN L. WOLF, Ph.D., FAPTA — Editor-in-Chief

Professor
Department of Rehabilitation Medicine
Emory University School of Medicine
Atlanta, Georgia

VINCENT J. ZARRO, M.D., Ph.D.

Associate Professor of Pharmacology and Medicine
Hahnemann University
Philadelphia, Pennsylvania

MARVIN C. ZISKIN, M.D., M.S., Bm.E.

Professor of Radiology and Medical Physics
Temple University Medical School
Philadelphia, Pennsylvania

CONTENTS

Chapter 5. Biophysical Principles of Heating and Superficial Heat Agents
Susan L. Michlovitz, M.S., P.T.

Chapter 6. Hydrotherapy: The Use of Water as a Therapeutic Agent
Mark T. Walsh, M.S., P.T.

Chapter   7.   Therapeutic Ultrasound 134
Marvin C. Ziskin, M.D., M.S., Bm.E.
Theresa McDiarmid, M.Sc., R.P.T., M.S.C.P.
Susan L. Michlovitz, M.S., P.T.

SECTION I

Foundations for the Use of Thermal Agents

CHAPTER 1

Inflammation and Repair and the Use of Thermal Agents

Brian Reed, Ph.D., P.T.
Vincent Zarro, M.D., Ph.D.

Injury to vascularized tissue initiates a series of responses collectively known as inflammation and repair. These processes serve to control the effects of the injurious agent and return the tissue to a normal state. Inflammation occurs first and is a vascular, hemostatic, cellular, and immune response that serves to dispose of micro-organisms, foreign material, and dead tissue in preparation for the subsequent repair process. Tissue repair is characterized early by proliferation of new blood vessels and by the formation of new connective tissue. This re-establishes tensile strength and makes the repair tissue viable. Later in the repair process, remodeling of the connective tissue takes place, which serves to further increase tissue strength. The exact duration of each of the phases of inflammation and repair is not distinct since the phases overlap and since there is variability from one case to another. It is, however, useful to have a concept of the timing of the phases. A diagram of the approximate timing of these events is presented in Figure 1–1.

Unfortunately, not all repair ends in restoration of normal tissue. Certain human tissues, including epidermis, liver, bone, skeletal muscle, adipose tissue, alimentary tract, epithelium, and tracheobronchial epithelium, can regenerate to varying degrees, but other tissues cannot. To the degree that damaged tissue cannot regenerate, the nonspecific process of scar formation takes place. Scar tissue provides tensile strength, but is otherwise devoid of physiologic function. Because scar tissue tends to become "tight," extensive scarring can be disfiguring and may affect organ function.

It is important to have an understanding of the processes of inflammation and repair and how they can be modified. Physical therapists often must deal with acute inflammatory conditions (e.g., sprains), chronic inflammatory conditions (e.g., rheumatoid arthritis), open wounds (e.g., decubitus ulcers), surgical incisions, or problems secondary to the healing process, such as peripheral edema or limited joint mobility. When appropriate, heat and cold may be used in the course of treatment to modify the

3

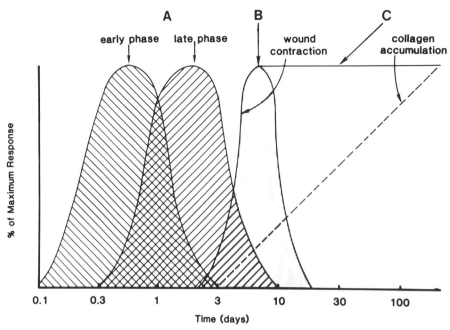

FIGURE 1–1. Phases of wound repair. Healing of a wound has been arbitrarily divided into three phases: (A) inflammation (early and late), (B) granulation tissue formation, and (C) matrix formation and remodeling. These phases overlap considerably with one another and are plotted along the abscissa as a logarithmic function of time. Inflammation is divided into early and late phases denoting neutrophil-rich and mononuclear cell-rich infiltrates, respectively. The magnitude of wound contraction parallels granulation tissue formation, as indicated. Collagen accumulation actually begins shortly after the onset of granulation tissue formation, continuing throughout the phase of matrix formation and remodeling. (From Clark,[2] p 4, with permission.)

inflammatory response. For example, cold is often the first line of defense to minimize the pain and swelling of acute musculoskeletal injuries. Heat, on the other hand, is sometimes used to help resolve subacute sequelae of inflammation and repair, such as hematomas.

The objectives of this chapter are to (1) provide the reader with a basic understanding of the processes of tissue inflammation and repair; (2) describe clinical problems associated with excessive or chronic inflammation and repair; and, (3) review the potential therapeutic role of thermal agents in the processes of inflammation and repair.

INFLAMMATION (DAYS 1–10)

Nearly 2000 years ago, Celsius first described four signs associated with inflammation: swelling, heat, redness, and pain. Later another characteristic, loss of function, was added, and these five signs came to be called the "cardinal signs of inflammation." A boil occurring in the skin as a reaction to invasion by bacteria is a good example of the cardinal signs of inflammation.

Inflammation begins when injury or disease causes a disruption in the normal physiology of a tissue. Table 1–1 lists some common causes of injury that will trigger inflammation. Although the inflammatory reaction follows the same pathway regard-

TABLE 1–1. Some Common Causes of Injury
Producing Inflammation

Trauma (e.g., sprains)	Burns
Bone fractures	Autoimmune diseases:
Foreign bodies	Rheumatoid arthritis
Bacterial invasion	Systemic lupus erythematosus
Decreased blood supply	Polymyositis
Bacteria and fungi	

less of the etiology of the injury, some causes will tend to emphasize certain events. For example, anoxia (such as occurs in peripheral vascular disease) tends to form dry necrotic tissues, whereas bacterial invasion causes pus formation.

The inflammatory process involves a vascular response, a hemostatic response, a cellular response and an immune response. These are controlled by a complex interaction of neural and humoral mediators not yet fully understood.

Vascular Response

The initial stages of inflammation are characterized by vascular changes. Transient vasoconstriction of arterioles occurs, lasting a few minutes. During this time, the vessel walls of the capillaries, and especially the postcapillary venules, become lined with white blood cells (leukocytes), a process known as *margination*. The vasoconstriction is followed by vasodilation, which causes an increase in blood flow and a rise in vessel hydrostatic pressure. Coincident with vasodilation, increased permeability of the microvessels (capillaries, venules) occurs. This is due to the fact that the endothelial cells "round up," creating gaps between the cells. This allows escape of cells, macromolecules, and fluid from the vascular system (Fig. 1–2). Edema occurs because the escaping cells and macromolecules create an osmotic gradient, which causes fluid to move into the interstitial spaces. The lymphatic vessels, which normally clear the interstitium of osmotically active particles, are overwhelmed.

The vascular response to injury probably is caused by local mediators released at the site of injury. Most notable among these are histamine, bradykinin, prostaglandins, and complement fractions. Each of these substances causes vasodilation, and histamine in particular has been implicated in the alteration of microvessel permeability. Histamine is released from mast cells and blood platelets at the injury site.

The type of edema fluid varies with the stage of inflammation. Initially, the permeability of the microvessels is only slightly altered and, therefore, no protein or cells escape. The edema fluid formed is called a *transudate* and consists mainly of water and dissolved electrolytes. It is clear in appearance, contains very few cells, and has a specific gravity under 1.012. As microvessel permeability increases, allowing escape of cells and plasma proteins, the edema fluid, which was at first clear, becomes more viscous (owing to the protein) and cloudy (owing to the leukocytes). The specific gravity rises to more than 1.012, and the fluid is called an *exudate*. When an exudate contains large numbers of leukocytes, it is called pus. A diagrammatic representation of these events is presented in Figure 1–3.

The presence of edema for long periods, especially if it occurs in an area of poor circulation, as in peripheral vascular disease, will interfere with proper oxygenation.

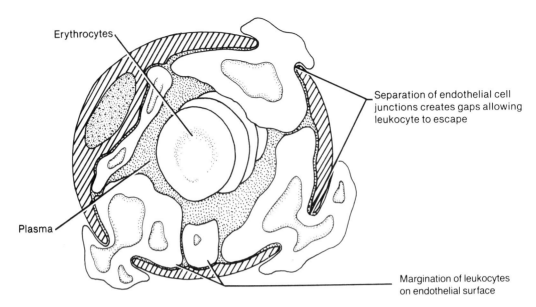

FIGURE 1–2. Vascular response to wound healing. (Adapted from Bryant,[1] p 7.)

So-called *stasis ulcers*, common in peripheral vascular disease, heal poorly in the presence of persistent edema.

The clinical manifestations of inflammation can be explained by the sequence of vascular events. Vasodilation causes the characteristic redness and warmth associated with inflammation. Overexpansion of the interstitial spaces accounts for the observed swelling and accompanying discomfort. Production of bradykinin and prostaglandins augments the pain stimulus.

Hemostatic Response

The hemostatic response functions to control blood loss when blood vessels are ruptured. The small blood vessels retract, helping to seal themselves off. Platelets aggregate and deposit fibrin, which traps red blood cells, creating a blood clot. The fibrin also occludes local lymphatic channels, preventing drainage of fluid from the injured area, thereby localizing the inflammation. When bleeding is internal, confined to a tissue or organ, a mass of clotted blood known as a *hematoma* can develop. Hematomas may cause tenderness and, in muscle tissue, they may limit range of motion or function.

Cellular Response

Leukocytes play a critical role in the inflammatory process, clearing the site of micro-organisms and setting the stage for tissue repair. There are several types of leukocytes, which are listed in Table 1–2. It is useful to note that neutrophils, eosinophils, and basophils are sometimes classified as polymorphonuclear leukocytes, because they have a nucleus consisting of several lobes.

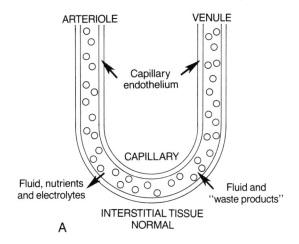

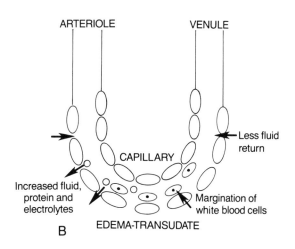

FIGURE 1–3. Diagrammatic representation of the production of edema. *A,*
Normal: The intravascular and extravascular (tissue) pressures are such that
there is an outward movement at the arteriolar end and inward movement at the
venular end. *B, Transudate:* In response
to injury, mediators are produced, arterioles dilate, blood volume and pressure in
the capillaries increase, outward filtration increases, and edema forms. Blood
cells marginate. *C, Exudate:* As inflammation becomes more intense, neutrophils and other blood cells emigrate into
the surrounding tissue to form thick
edema fluid (pus).

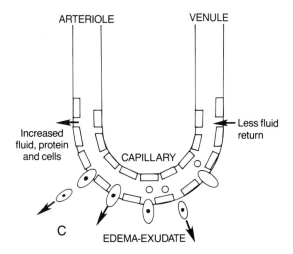

TABLE 1–2. Circulating Blood Cells and Approximate Number
Per Cubic Millimeter*

	Approximate Number of Cells per mm^3	Approximate Percentage
Red blood cells	5,000,000	—
Leukocytes:		
Neutrophils	3,000	55
Lymphocytes	2,100	35
Monocytes	420	7
Basophils	60	1
Eosinophils	120	2
Total leukocytes	6,000	100

The various leukocytes are specialized, thus different types of leukocytes are predominant in the early and late phases of the process. Initially, all types of leukocytes migrate to the site of inflammation in numbers proportionate to their concentration in circulating blood.[1] Since neutrophils are the greatest in number, they characterize early inflammation (see Fig. 1–1). As with all the leukocytes, neutrophils are attracted to the inflamed site by chemotactic agents released at the time of injury. The major function of the neutrophils is to rid the site of contaminating bacteria and debris. They accomplish this by phagocytosis. As some neutrophils disintegrate, their digestive enzymes are released into the tissue. These chemicals perpetuate the inflammatory reaction by acting as irritants and as chemotactic agents, attracting other leukocytes into the area of inflammation.

Late inflammation, which begins shortly after early inflammation, is characterized by the predominance of mononuclear leukocytes (monocytes) and lymphocytes. This is at least partially because these cells live longer than neutrophils and the other polymorphs. In the interstitium, monocytes have the ability to convert into large cells called macrophages, which, like neutrophils, are phagocytic. In fact, they are remarkable for their ability to engulf large amounts of bacteria and cellular debris. In contrast to neutrophils, however, the appearance of monocytes seems to be critical to the initiation of tissue repair.[2] Lymphocytes also are present in the later phase of inflammation. Lymphocytes play a major role in mediating the body's immune reaction, supplying antibodies for specific antigens. It is not surprising, therefore, that they are prominent in chronic inflammatory conditions. An example of this is rheumatoid arthritis, a disease characterized by chronic inflammation in various joints. The characteristic cell types in tissue biopsy of this disease are lymphocytes and monocytes.

For the most part, basophils and eosinophils are involved only in certain types of inflammation and will not be discussed further.

Immune Response

The immune response is both a cell-mediated and a humorally mediated response. The roles of lymphocytes and the phagocytic leukocytes in the immune response have already been described. Another aspect of the immune response, however, is the complement system. Complement is actually a series of enzymatic proteins that are activated by bacterial toxins or immune complexes. Various activated components are involved in many steps in the inflammatory process, including phagocytosis, increasing vascular permeability and providing chemotactic attraction of leukocytes.

In diseases of autoimmunity, the inflammatory response is not beneficial. Because the body perceives certain tissues as foreign, there is an antigen–antibody reaction that results in a chronic inflammatory response against the tissues. Rheumatoid arthritis is one example of an autoimmune disease. In rheumatoid arthritis, chronic synovial inflammation causes destruction of articular cartilage (See Table 1–1 for other autoimmune diseases affecting the musculoskeletal system).

Diseases of autoimmunity or the presence of a foreign body can cause states of chronic inflammation. Chronic inflammation creates unique problems and, therefore, is discussed separately later in this chapter. Chronic inflammation is one indication for intervention in the inflammation and repair process.

TISSUE REPAIR

Proliferative Phase (Days 3–20)

The first phase of tissue repair is a proliferative one involving both epithelial and connective tissues. Epithelium is a covering; it is the layer(s) of cells that form the epidermis of the skin and the surface layer of mucous and serous membranes. Connective tissue, on the other hand, is the cement that connects and supports other tissues. It is relatively acellular, composed of fibrous strands and ground substance, which make up an intercellular matrix. Connective-tissue strength and elasticity varies in tissues such as bone, tendon, ligament, and skin, according to its makeup and degree of organization.

Certain epithelial tissues have a high regenerative capacity and undergo a process known as *re-epithelialization*. In this process, epithelial cells around the periphery of the wound proliferate and migrate across the wound site until the compromised area is covered.

In connective tissue, *fibroplasia* takes place. Fibroblasts arise from undifferentiated mesenchymal cells, migrate into the inflamed area along fibrin strands, and begin to synthesize scar tissue. Scar tissue is a type of connective tissue and, as such, it is composed primarily of the protein *collagen* and mucopolysaccharides. The fibroblast secretes both of these, contributing tensile strength to the repair. Through this process, a *connective-tissue matrix* is re-established.

At the same time, endothelial buds develop from intact capillaries. The endothelial buds eventually connect with other buds forming patent vessels that supply the area. Endothelial buds give the healing wound a characteristic red, granular appearance, hence the term *granulation tissue* is applied to this type of wound tissue. The appearance of granulation tissue is a sign of good progress in a healing wound. Endothelial budding and the other noted events of the proliferative phase are illustrated for skin in Figure 1–4.

Wound contraction is a phenomenon that begins to occur in the connective tissue at this point. Actin-rich fibroblasts known as *myofibroblasts*, which have the ability to contract, accumulate at the margins of the wound. The myofibroblasts move toward the center of the wound, helping to reduce the size of the area to be covered. As previously mentioned, extensive scar contraction can be disfiguring or limit function.

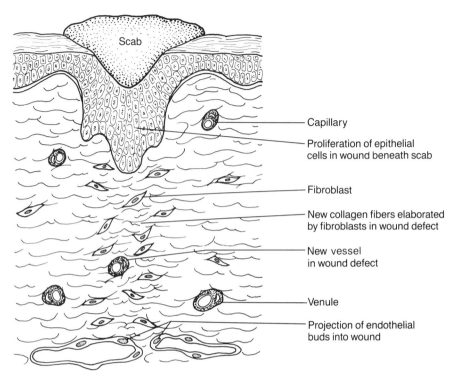

FIGURE 1–4. Proliferative phase of skin wound repair. (Adapted from Bryant,[1] p 14.)

Remodeling Phase (Day 9 Onward)

The second phase of tissue repair is a remodeling of the connective-tissue matrix. This period of scar maturation, which may last for years, is marked by the disappearance of fibroblasts. The collagen fibers initially laid down by fibroblasts are randomly oriented so that the connective-tissue matrix is fragile. During remodeling, the fibers acquire a more organized pattern, parallel to the wound surface, which provides greater tensile strength. It is important to note, however, that despite remodeling scar tissue is never as strong as the tissue it replaces. At maximal strength, scar tissue is only 70 percent as strong as intact tissue.[3] In addition, it is less vascular, creating a diffusion barrier to oxygen and nutrients and making the tissue less able to dissipate applied heat.

The mechanism of remodeling is probably related to collagen turnover. Collagen is taken up and laid down again along strands of fibronectin.[4,5] Abnormal scars may develop when there is an imbalance between collagen production and uptake. Overproduction of collagen can result in a *hypertrophic scar* or a *keloid scar*. The biologic differences between these two types of scars are still being defined, but the clinical distinction is that a hypertrophic scar is contained within the boundaries of the original wound, while a keloid scar extends beyond the borders of the original wound.[6] Treatment of hypertrophic scars and keloid scars with surgery, pressure, radiation, corticosteroids, and other drugs has had limited success.[7] An example of keloid scarring is illustrated in Figure 1–5.

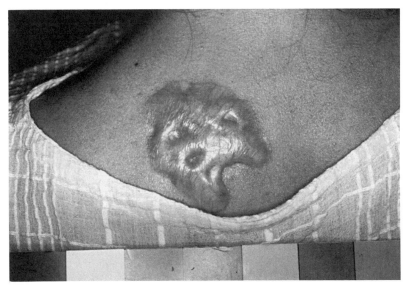

FIGURE 1-5. This keloid of the left posterior scapular area is a result of thermal injury to the back. This thermal injury occurred as the result of carbon dioxide laser treatment of a decorative tattoo. (Courtesy of David B. Apfelberg, M.D., Palo Alto, CA.)

INFLAMMATION AND REPAIR IN SPECIAL TISSUES

The general processes of inflammation and repair are similar in all tissues, although in some tissues unique cell types are involved. In bone, for example, osteoblasts and osteoclasts carry out remodeling to create new haversian systems. In injured peripheral nerves, Schwann cells act to phagocytize nonviable nerve axons and form a neurilemmal tube to receive new axon buds. In skeletal muscle, satellite cells are involved in the regeneration of damaged tissue.[8] A detailed discussion of inflammation and repair in these special tissues is beyond the scope of this chapter. For such information, the reader should consult texts that deal specifically with bone, nerve, or muscle.

CHRONIC INFLAMMATION

Normally, the acute inflammation reaction is virtually complete in 2 weeks. If the reaction continues for 1 month, it is called *subacute inflammation*. If it continues for months or years, it is called *chronic inflammation*. Chronic inflammation may occur as an autoimmune response or as an extension of acute inflammation, as may occur if a joint is repeatedly traumatized. Sometimes, however, chronic inflammation represents a reaction to a specific stimulus. In all cases, the chronic inflammatory response differs considerably from acute inflammation. Invasion of lung tissue, for example, by the tuberculosis organism does not cause the characteristic signs of inflammation. Instead, the body reacts to the hard coating of the organism by surrounding it with lymphocytes and monocytes. Macrophages are formed, and these cells with ingested debris attempt to seal off the organism and confine it to one area. Unlike acute inflammation, in which the major cell type is the neutrophil, the predominant cells involved in chronic inflammation are the lymphocytes, the monocytes, and the macrophages.

Another major difference between acute inflammation and chronic inflammation is the extent of fibroblastic proliferation. As the chronic process continues, more fibroblasts are formed, more collagen is produced, and scar formation becomes extensive. In chronic inflammation, therefore, the usual result is replacement of normal tissue with scar, even in organs that have the ability to regenerate. In the musculoskeletal system, this can mean the development of *adhesions*. Adhesions are simply scar tissues, especially internal scar tissues, that limit mobility. These may occur in or around joint capsules, tendons, or muscles. For optimal function of healed articulating and gliding tissues, a delicate balance between adequate tensile strength and adequate mobility is required, and chronic inflammation does not lend itself to such a balance. Lack of movement within the available range of motion promotes the development of adhesions, therefore, active and passive range-of-motion exercises are important for maintaining motion in patients with chronic inflammatory diseases of the musculoskeletal system.

FACTORS THAT MODIFY INFLAMMATION AND REPAIR

A number of factors may modify all or some of the steps in the inflammation and repair processes. Factors such as advanced age, malnutrition, anemia, and peripheral vascular disease hinder inflammation and repair. Metabolic disorders may also interfere with wound healing. This is especially true for diabetes mellitus. Diabetics are prone to peripheral vascular disease in both macrovessels and microvessels. In addition, peripheral neuropathies are common in diabetics, increasing the probability of traumatic injury to the limbs. Finally, diabetics have a dampened immune response, which compromises their ability to combat infection. For all these reasons, diabetics are prone to soft-tissue ulcers that are slow to heal.

Certain drugs can inhibit inflammation. Corticosteroids, such as prednisone and cortisol, are powerful anti-inflammatory drugs that stabilize cell membranes, thereby inhibiting production of prostaglandins and related thromboxanes and leukotrienes. These drugs are sometimes used for chronic inflammatory conditions, but they are not always the first choice because of their strong side effects. Nonsteroidal anti-inflammatory drugs (NSAIDs), such as aspirin and ibuprofin, also inhibit inflammation by interrupting the production of prostaglandins but, in this case, the mechanism is interruption of the pathway by which prostaglandins are synthesized from arachidonic acid. NSAIDs have fewer side effects than corticosteroids and are often used to reduce inflammation. A schematic of prostaglandin synthesis and the site of action of the corticosteroids and of the NSAIDs is presented in Figure 1–6.

Prolonged immobilization promotes the development of adhesions and limited motion, even after normal healing.[9] There is little doubt that immobilization aids early inflammation and repair. The need to apply a limb cast to immobilize a bone fracture or to suture a gaping soft-tissue wound seems self evident, and there is good experimental evidence that immobilization produces faster healing.[10,11] Immobility, however, is necessarily accompanied by adhesions and stiffness. Studies of animal models have demonstrated that immobilization for up to 9 weeks has caused adhesions in all areas of synovial joints and that the connective tissue has been biochemically altered, having abnormal collagen cross-linking and decreased elasticity.[9] Remobilization is critical to recovery of function after inflammation and repair. For this reason, *continuous passive*

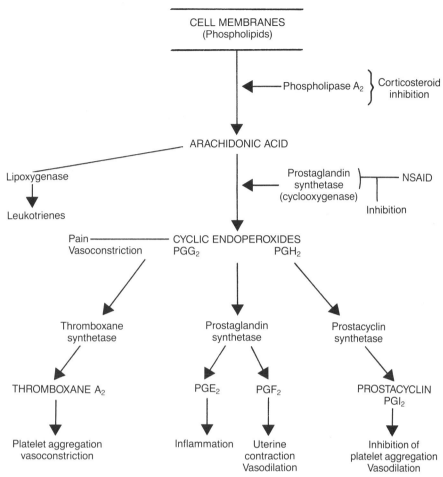

FIGURE 1–6. Pathway of synthesis of prostaglandins and site of NSAID inhibition of cyclo-oxygenase. (Adapted from Nikander, McMahoon, and Ridolfo: Nonsteroidal anti-inflammatory agents. Ann Rev Pharmacol Toxicol 19:469, 1979.)

motion (CPM) by machine is often employed as soon as possible after the injured area is stable. This is usually supplemented with active and passive range-of-motion exercises. Studies on dogs with tendon lacerations have demonstrated superior functional outcome with immobilization and early CPM, compared to immobilization only.[9,12]

Some physical agents can also affect inflammation. These include electrical stimulation, total-contact casting, hyperbaric oxygen, and thermal agents, including therapeutic ultrasound. The role of thermal agents in inflammation and repair will be considered here.

EFFECTS OF THERMAL AGENTS ON INFLAMMATION AND REPAIR

In general, physical therapists use cold applications (cryotherapy) to treat acute inflammatory conditions, such as sprains, and heat therapy for subacute or chronic inflammatory conditions, such as chronic tendonitis. The rationale for these tenets has been that cold minimizes acute edema and hemorrhage and provides a good analgesic effect, whereas heat increases blood flow and thereby assists in the reabsorption of late inflammatory exudates and debris.

There is some experimental data to justify this approach to treatment. The effects of heat and cold in experimentally induced inflammation were studied by Schmidt and coworkers and were summarized in a review article.[13] Edema was induced by injecting various noxious substances into rat paws and measuring the degree of swelling. Models of both acute arthritis and chronic arthritis involving antigen–antibody reaction were studied. Heat was either administered as whole-body hyperthermia or was applied to the paws and tail only. Cold was applied as whole-body hypothermia. The results are summarized in Table 1–3. It can be seen that the effects of heat or cold varied according to the stage of inflammation. Heat inhibited inflammation in the model of chronic inflammation. Cold inhibited the more acute types of inflammation.

The premise that cold is beneficial for acute inflammation is supported by other basic research. Rippe and Grega[14] demonstrated that cooling decreased the effects of histamine on capillary permeability, presenting a rationale for the use of cold with edema. Recent studies of postburn edema in rodents demonstrated that immediate cooling did, indeed, minimize edema formation.[15,16] Dorwart and colleagues[17] reported that in dogs, synovial fluid leukocytes exposed to cold had reduced phagocytic activity, another indication of dampened inflammation.

The basic research findings on cold are complemented by clinical-research findings. Application of cold in acute inflammatory conditions has been associated with reduced edema,[18–20] lowered leukocyte counts,[18,21] reduced analgesic intake,[18,22] increased pain threshold,[23,24] and reduced indices of muscle spasm and soreness.[25]

Although deep heat, such as diathermy, has traditionally been used to aid in the reabsorption of subacute hematomas, evidence for the efficacy of this treatment is equivocal. Fenn[26] induced hematomas in rabbit ears and treated them with daily short-wave diathermy for 30 minutes. The area of the treated hematomas was significantly reduced by the sixth day of treatment. Lehmann, Dundore, and Esselman,[27] on the other hand, studied the clearance of radioactively labeled red cells injected into pigs treated with microwave diathermy. No difference in the clearance of the red cells was observed between the treated and the nontreated sides of the animals.

A different rationale for the use of heat modalities in chronic inflammatory conditions comes from in vitro observations that heat combined with stretch can alter the viscoelastic properties of connective tissue, making it more extensible.[28–31] Thus, "heat and stretch" is a logical strategy for helping to overcome adhesions. Proof for the clinical efficacy of this strategy is presently lacking.

Heat may be beneficial in chronic inflammatory conditions, but it exacerbates acute inflammation.[13,32] In skin and soft-tissue infections such as furuncles and carbuncles, superficial heat in the form of hot compresses or soaks is a time-honored treatment. These treatments localize the inflammation and accelerate abcess formation so the

TABLE 1–3. The Effects of Heat and Cold on Inflammation

	Heat	Cold
Acute inflammation	Aggravated	Depressed
Chronic inflammation	Depressed	—
Prostaglandin production	—	Aggravated

abcess can be drained. For acute musculoskeletal inflammations, however, there is a general concensus that heat applications should be avoided for fear they will exacerbate hemorrhage and edema.[32] The presumed mechanism for this is that heat will produce increased blood flow and thereby increase microvascular hydrostatic pressure. Indeed, in clinical studies, investigators found that heat aggravated edema formation and pro-longed recovery time in acute orthopedic injuries.[33,34]

The generalization about the effects of heat on chronic inflammation may not apply with deep heats in rheumatoid arthritis. Harris and McCroskery[35] studied the effect of temperature on degradation of cartilage by rheumatoid synovium. They demonstrated a fourfold increase in enzymatic lysis of human cartilage in vitro with a temperature increase of 5°C. This marked increase in damage might be due to an elevated metabolic rate of the macrophages and the destructive enzymes in this autoimmune disease.[35,36] An increase in joint temperature might increase cartilage destruction in patients with rheumatoid arthritis, and since the deep-heat modalities (ultrasound, diathermies) would be most likely to elevate joint temperature, it may be best to avoid the deep-heat treatments in patients with rheumatoid arthritis.[32,36] Superficial heats (such as hot packs or infrared radiation), by contrast, have not been associated with rheumatoid cartilage destruction. Horvath and Hollander[37] made intra-articular temperature measurements in normals and arthritics and found that joint temperature actually fell in response to hot packs. It has been postulated that this was due to a reflex shunting of blood flow away from the joint to the more superficial tissues.[36,37]

It is interesting to note that ultrasound, usually considered a deep-heating agent, has been associated with improved wound healing. The work of Dyson and associates[38-40] has demonstrated accelerated inflammation and repair processes in vitro, as well as improved healing of venous stasis ulcers with ultrasound. These results, however, have been achieved at low levels of ultrasound intensity; therefore, they may be due to nonthermal effects of ultrasound rather than thermal effects.

ADDITIONAL CLINICAL CONSIDERATIONS

It is well to remember that inflammation and repair are natural and desirable processes. Intervention in these processes with thermal agents or other modalities is appropriate only when the intervention will facilitate or accelerate the process, or when undesirable effects of the processes must be controlled. Take, for example, the case of an acute second-degree ankle sprain. Left untreated, the patient will suffer marked pain and edema and will keep the ankle immobilized for a prolonged period. Initial treatment with cold, compression wrap, elevation, and rest will control pain and edema and will allow early remobilization. An example of an appropriate heat intervention would be the case of a patient who has suffered a fractured femur and, as a result, has been in traction for 6 weeks. Upon removal from traction, range of motion of the knee is likely to be limited. Application of hot packs and ultrasound, followed by exercise using techniques such as proprioceptive neuromuscular facilitation (PNF), will help to remo-bilize the joint and strengthen the surrounding musculature. Continuous passive motion (CPM) at bedside also would be helpful in such a case.

It should be apparent that thermal agents are not best used in isolation of other forms of therapy. Rather, they should be but one part of the treatment plan. The therapist must assess the state of inflammation and repair, decide upon the appropriate thermal agent, and then incorporate it into the overall treatment plan, continually monitoring the clinical outcome.

SUMMARY

The processes of inflammation and repair are normal responses to injury, serving to restore tissue integrity. The inflammatory process is a complex event involving vascular, hemostatic, cellular, and immune responses that are controlled by numerous neural and humoral mediators. Tissue repair involves proliferation of new connective tissue and blood vessels and, over time, remodeling of the scar.

When the inflammation or repair processes become excessive or chronic, therapy is directed at attenuating the process. Several physical agents can affect inflammation and repair, including the thermal agents. In general, cryotherapy is used in acute inflammatory conditions, and heats are used in chronic inflammatory conditions. The various heat and cold applications are reviewed in subsequent chapters of this text.

REFERENCES

1. Bryant, WM: Wound Healing. Clinical Symposia (Ciba) 29(3):9, 1977.
2. Clark, RAF: Overview and general considerations of wound repair. In Clark, RAF and Henson, PM (eds): The Molecular and Cellular Biology of Wound Repair. Plenum Press, New York, 1988, p 4.
3. Levenson, SM, et al: The healing of rat skin wounds. Ann Surg 161:293, 1965.
4. Bryant, WM: Wound Healing. Clinical Symposia (Ciba) 29(3):15, 1977.
5. Clark, RAF: Overview and general considerations of wound repair In Clark, RAF and Henson, PM (eds): The Molecular and Cellular Biology of Wound Repair. Plenum Press, New York, 1988, p 17.
6. Peacock, EE, Madden, JW and Triea, WC: Biologic basis for treatment of keloids and hypertrophic scars. South Med J 63:755, 1970.
7. McPherson, JM and Piez, KA: Collagen in dermal wound repair. In Clark, RAF and Henson, PM (eds): The Molecular and Cellular Biology of Wound Repair. Plenum Press, New York, 1988, p 488.
8. Allbrook, D: Skeletal muscle regeneration. Muscle & Nerve 4:234–245, 1981.
9. Wood, SL, et al: The importance of controlled passive mobilization on flexor tendon healing: A biochemical study. Acta Orthop Scand 52:615, 1981.
10. Frank, C, Amiel, D, and Akeson, WH: Healing of the medial collateral ligament of the knee: A morphological and biochemical assessment in rabbits. Acta Orthop Scand 54:1917, 1983.
11. Nystrom, B and Holmlund, D: Experimental evaluation of immobilization in operative and nonoperative treatment of Achilles tendon rupture: A radiographic study in the rabbit. Acta Chir Scand 149:669, 1983.
12. Gelberman, RH, et al: Effects of early intermittent passive immobilization on healing canine flexor tendons. J Hand Surg 7:170, 1982.
13. Schmidt, KL, et al: Heat, cold and inflammation. Rheumatology 38:391, 1979.
14. Rippe, B, Grega, GJ: Effects of 150 prenaline and cooling on histamine-induced changes of capillary permeability in the rat hindquarter bed. Acta Physiol Scand 103:252, 1978.
15. Biomgren, I, et al: The effect of different cooling temperatures and immersion fluids on post-burn oedema and survival of the partially scalded hairy mouse ear. Burns 11(3):161, 1985.
16. Jakobsson, OP and Arturson, G: The effect of prompt local cooling on oedema formation in scalded rat paws. Burns 12(1):8, 1985.
17. Dorwart, BB, et al: Effects of heat, cold and mechanical agitation on crystal-induced arthritis in the dog. Arth Rheum 16:540, 1973.
18. Schaubel, HH: Local use of ice after orthopedic procedures. Am J Surg 72:711, 1946.
19. Basur, R, Shepard, E, and Mouzos, G: A cooling method in the treatment of ankle sprains. Practitioner 216:708, 1976.
20. Cote, DJ, et al: Comparison of three treatment procedures for minimizing ankle sprain swelling. Phys Ther 68(7):1072, 1988.
21. Farry, PJ, et al: Ice treatment of injured ligaments: An experimental model. New Zealand Med J 12:12, 1980.
22. Conolly, WB, Paltos, N, and Tooth, RM: Cold therapy: An improved method. Med J Aust 2:424, 1972.
23. Benson, TB and Copp, EP: The effects of therapeutic forms of heat and ice on the pain threshold of the normal shoulder. Rheumatol Rehabil 13:101, 1974.
24. Gammon, GD and Starr, I: Studies on the relief of pain by counterirritation. J Clin Invest 20:13, 1941.
25. Prentice, WE: An electromyographic analysis of the effectiveness of heat or cold and stretching for inducing relaxation in injured muscle. Journal of Orthopedic and Sports Physical Therapy 3:133, 1982.
26. Fenn, JE: Effect of pulsed electromagnetic energy (Diapulse) on experimental hematomas. Canad Med Assoc J 100:251, 1969.

27. Lehmann, JF, Dundore, DE, and Esselman, PC: Microwave diathermy: Effects on experimental hematoma resolution. Arch Phys Med Rehabil 64:127–129, 1983.
28. LeBan, MM: Collagen tissue: Implications of its response to stress in vitro. Arch Phys Med Rehabil 43:461, 1962.
29. Lehmann, JF: Effect of therapeutic temperatures on tendon extensibility. Arch Phys Med Rehabil 51:481–487, 1970.
30. Warren, CG, Lehmann, JF, and Koblanski, JN: Heat and stretch procedures: An evaluation using rat tail tendon. Arch Phys Med Rehabil 57:122, 1976.
31. Gersten, JW: Effect of ultrasound on tendon extensibility. Am J Phys Med 34:362, 1955.
32. Feibel, A and Fast, A: Deep heating of joints: A reconsideration. Arch Phys Med Rehabil 57:513, 1976.
33. Barnes, L: Cryotherapy: Putting injury on ice. The Physician and Sports Medicine 7(6):130, 1979.
34. Wallace, L, et al: Immediate care of ankle injuries. Journal of Orthopedic and Sports Physical Therapy 1:46, 1979.
35. Harris, ED and McCroskery, PA: The influence of temperature and fibril stability on degradation of cartilage collagen by rheumatoid synovial collagenase. N Engl J Med 290:1, 1974.
36. Hollander, JL: Collagenase, cartilage and cortisol. N Engl J Med 290:50, 1974.
37. Horvath, SM and Hollander, JL: Intra-articular temperature as a measure of joint reaction. J Clin Invest 28(3):469, 1949.
38. Dyson, M and Suckling, J: Stimulation of tissue repair by ultrasound: A survey of the mechanisms involved. Physiotherapy 64(4):105, 1978.
39. Dyson, M: Therapeutic applications of ultrasound. In Nyborg, WL and Ziskin, MC (eds): Biological Effects of Ultrasound. Churchill Livingstone, New York, 1985, p 121.
40. Dyson, M: Mechanisms involved in therapeutic ultrasound. Physiotherapy 73:116, 1987.

CHAPTER 2

Contemporary Views on Pain and the Role Played by Thermal Agents in Managing Pain Symptoms

Roberta A. Newton, Ph.D., P.T.

Pain is a protective mechanism that alerts the individual to make an appropriate response to prevent further tissue damage. Pain is defined as an unpleasant sensory and emotional experience that is associated with actual or potential tissue damage; or pain may be described in terms of such tissue damage.[1] Pain is a sensory experience described in quite different terms than other sensory modalities. Touch, for example, is a peripheral stimulus perceived as a particular touch sensation, whereas pain is a complex phenomenon described in terms of a pluridimensional theory encompassing sensory, emotional, motor, and cultural components.

One of every four people in the United States is affected by pain each year. When the pain state outlasts the initial trauma and subsequent recovery period, the pluridimensional aspect of the pain experience is quite evident. The chronic pain state not only affects the individual experiencing pain, but it is also physiologically and psychologically draining to the individual's family and close associates. Total cost for treatment of the chronic pain patient and work days lost is tremendous.[2] Estimates in dollars and day loss at work pertain only to those individuals with chronic pain conditions and do not include the acute pain state—that is, headaches, injuries, or the postoperative period. With the increasing cost to remediate pain and the gap in the understanding of normal and chronic pain mechanisms, an Interagency Committee of the United States Government was established to address these issues. Since 1978, the interdisciplinary investigation of pain mechanisms and its remediation has proliferated.

The ability of the clinician to treat appropriately a painful condition is dependent upon a sound clinical problem-solving approach. Such an approach includes an understanding of the normal neurophysiologic mechanisms of pain; knowledge of mechanisms associated with acute, chronic, and referred pain; appropriate assessment techniques; and rationale for the selection of a particular therapy. Furthermore, the clinician needs to analyze critically the literature and use only those reports that have appropriate research design, which includes good documentation of methodology and results. Caution should be taken when extrapolating data from laboratory research to direct patient care.

The purposes of this chapter are to (1) present the current concepts of pain theory; (2) present theories relating to acute, chronic, and referred pain; (3) discuss methods for assessing pain; and (4) provide an overview of the role of thermal agents in pain management. The theories on pain will provide the student and clinician with the basic foundation necessary to pursue the literature further. Both review articles and original research articles are included in the reference list.

PAIN THEORIES: SPECIFICITY, PATTERN, AND GATE CONTROL

Pain theories to date are pluridimensional and multidisciplinary. They can be categorized into three major areas. The sensory–discriminative component serves to analyze the noxious stimulus in terms of its location and intensity. The affective–motivational component includes the emotional responses, goals, desires, and expectations of the individual. The cognitive–evaluative component refers to the process by which the noxious sensation is examined, is compared with past experiences, and is given meaning in relation to the present and future implications of the pain experience. An individual's reaction to the noxious stimulus also is influenced by cultural connotations. Thus, the response to a noxious stimulus may range from a simple flexion response to more complex escape plans to a very complex psychophysiologic behavior pattern seen in the chronic pain patient.[3]

Early pain theories were based upon simple neuroanatomic circuitry or a single neurophysiologic concept. As technology advanced, pain theory became more sophisticated. The impetus to examine the pain mechanism was a new theory, the gate control theory of Melzack and Wall.[4] Since that time (1965), neurophysiologic, neuroanatomic, and neurochemical approaches have begun to delineate the peripheral and central mechanisms of pain. Furthermore, the mechanisms involved in the centrifugal (descending) control of pain are being identified. New hypotheses are being developed and tested. Successful testing of these hypotheses adds new pieces to the puzzle or revises already established pieces. Many gaps in the pain puzzle still exist. As a result, pain theories are dynamic and constantly changing. This section provides the reader with a historic perspective of pain theories and the theories currently used.

Specificity and Pattern Theories

Two traditional and opposing theories for pain evolved during the late 1800s.[5,6] These theories are the specificity theory and the pattern theory, respectively. The specificity theory proposed that a specific pain system existed. When pain receptors located in the skin are stimulated, the impulses are transmitted via a direct pathway to the pain center located in the brain. Von Frey[5] used the Müller doctrine of specific nerve

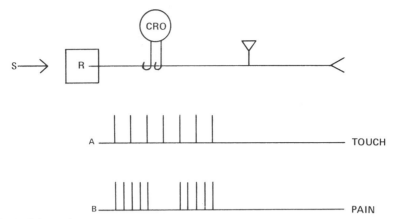

FIGURE 2–1. Schematic representation of the pattern theory. (*A*) Action potentials resulting from a touch stimulus (stimuli) and recorded on a cathode ray oscilloscope (CRO). The resultant sensation is touch. (*B*) Action potentials resulting from a noxious stimulus and recorded on a cathode ray oscilloscope. The resultant sensation is pain. Key: S = stimulus; R = receptor; CRO = cathode ray oscilloscope.

energies, anatomic evidence, and scientific deductive reasoning to develop his theory. The Müller principle states that a stimulus applied to a receptor produces the same sensation in the brain center regardless of the type of stimulus. Since free nerve endings are located in skin throughout the entire body, and an intense stimulus applied anywhere on the skin results in a pain sensation, he logically reasoned that free nerve endings are pain receptors. Thus, the specificity theory states that any noxious or potentially tissue-damaging stimulus applied to the surface of the skin results in a pain sensation.

The pattern theory denotes that the pattern or coding of sensory information is the key element. The coding is temporal, and spatial sequencing of action potentials are generated in the periphery. This theory negates the idea of a specific pain receptor, but rather considers the intense stimulation of nonspecific receptors as the adequate stimulus for eliciting the pain sensation. Figure 2–1 demonstrates this principle. A touch stimulus applied to a receptor produces a particular pattern of action potentials. The resultant sensation is touch. A potentially damaging touch stimulus applied to the receptor produces a different pattern of action potentials, and the resultant sensation is pain. One fallacy of this principle is that specific specialized receptors have been documented histologically.

Gate Control Theory

In 1965, Melzack and Wall[4] proposed a new theory relating to the pain experience. This theory represents a cornerstone in the development of neurophysiologic mechanisms that addresses the concept of peripheral and central gating. The gate theory incorporates the feature of receptor specialization from the specificity theory with spatiotemporal coding of action potentials from the pattern theory. To these two concepts, Melzack and Wall[7] added the interaction of peripheral afferents with a modulation system located in the substantia gelatinosa of the spinal gray matter. Furthermore,

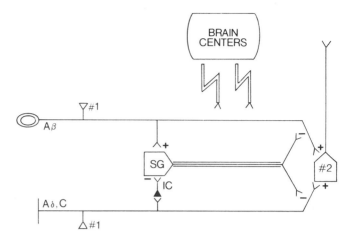

FIGURE 2–2. Schematic representation of the revised Melzack and Wall gate control theory. Key: #1 = first-order neuron, either Aβ, Aδ, or C primary afferent; #2 = second-order neuron (T cell); SG = substantia gelatinosa; IC = inhibitory interneuron.

they proposed a descending modulatory system. Figure 2–2 is a schematic representation of the gate control theory.

The neuroanatomic features of this circuit include large-diameter sensory neurons (Aβ); small-diameter sensory neurons (Aδ,C); the substantia gelatinosa that corresponds to Rexed's laminae II and III of the dorsal horn of the spinal gray matter; and a transmission cell (T cell), also known as a tract cell or second-order neuron. The A-beta, A-delta, and C neurons are also termed first-order neurons, or primary afferents. Both the large- and small-diameter primary afferents impinge upon the substantia gelatinosa cells and upon the second-order neuron. The substantia gelatinosa acts as a modulator (gate control) by terminating presynaptically upon the large- and small-diameter afferent neurons just before their termination upon the second-order neuron. The control is postulated to occur by the neurophysiologic mechanism termed *inhibition*.

When the substantia gelatinosa is active, an increase in presynaptic control on the first-order axons occurs and the "gate" is in the relatively closed position; that is, a decrease in the amount of sensory input to the second-order neuron cell occurs. On the other hand, a reduction in substantia gelatinosa activity results in a decrease in the amount of presynaptic control on the first-order neuron, and the "gate" is considered to be in a relatively open position; that is, the amount of sensory information reaching the second-order neuron is relatively unaltered. The balance of activity in the large- and small-diameter sensory neurons determines the relative position of the "gate."

If large-diameter afferents are activated, an initial increase in the second-order neuron activity occurs and is followed by a reduction of activity. The initial increase is due to direct activation of the second-order neuron by primary afferents. The reduction is an indirect result due to large-diameter afferents also activating substantia gelatinosa cells, which in turn leads to presynaptic inhibition of the primary afferents. This causes the gate to close.

If, however, the small-diameter afferents are activated, the initial increase in T-cell activity is caused by the primary afferents. The small-diameter primary afferents also activate inhibitory interneurons that inhibit activity of the substantia gelatinosa cells. This results in a decrease in the amount of presynaptic control on the large- and small-diameter sensory neurons and opens the gate.

Melzack and Wall[4] proposed that when the balance of small- to large-diameter neuronal input is no longer maintained and reaches a critical value, the second-order neurons are activated. The activation of this ascending system leads to the perception of pain and behavioral responses.

One component of the system that was briefly, but not fully, described was the descending control system. Melzack and Wall[7] proposed that central events such as emotion and past experience evoke descending input, which impinges upon the gating mechanism to block pain sensation at the spinal level.

As various hypotheses were tested, the theory was revised.[8,9] Revisions of the gate control theory led to the realization that a more complex neural circuitry exists in the dorsal horn. For example, postsynaptic connections play a modulatory role in the gating mechanism; and the idea that non-nociceptive ($A\beta$) and nociceptive ($A\delta,C$) neurons are the large- and small-diameter afferents, respectively. Furthermore, successful testing of the hypothesis that A-beta afferents "close the gate" led to the use of transcutaneous electrical nerve stimulation (TENS) for pain modulation in humans.[10]

Extensive clinical testing of externally applied electrical stimulators for pain relief in the chronic-pain patient began in the early 1970s.[11] The Melzack and Wall gate control theory of pain, provides a partial neurophysiologic explanation for the use of TENS to relieve acute and chronic pain.

PERIPHERAL AND CENTRAL NERVOUS SYSTEM MECHANISMS SUBSERVING PAIN

When examining current concepts of pain, neurophysiologic and neurochemical relationships need to be examined. The amount of knowledge gained in this area within the past two decades far exceeds knowledge accumulated in other areas of neuroscience. As a result, theories are rapidly revised. Students and clinicians should be aware that no pain theory is engraved in stone. This is witnessed by continuing changes in the current pain literature and in applications of pain theories to justify clinical procedures.

Peripheral Mechanisms

NOCICEPTORS

Receptors responsible for the transmission of pain impulses are described morphologically as free nerve endings. The best-studied nociceptors are the nociceptors located in the skin.[12-15] Nociceptors found in the viscera and in the cardiac and skeletal muscles are less well understood.[16] Stimuli adequate for excitation of nociceptors include intense heat, intense cold, strong mechanical deformation, and chemical substances. Those receptors that respond to only one noxious stimulant are termed *specific nociceptors*, whereas those nociceptors that respond to several noxious stimuli are termed *polymodal nociceptors*. How the nociceptor changes the stimulus to action potentials is not completely understood.

Antidromic activation of the primary afferents by an electrical stimulus results in the release of a substance at the receptor ending. This substance is assumed to be substance P.[17] If this hypothesis were successfully tested, it would support the existence of a peripheral hyperalgesic mechanism. Furthermore, chemical substances such as prostaglandin E, bradykinin, and serotonin are released in the skin near nociceptors when trauma or inflammation occur.[18] These or similar substances may be released in muscle upon injury to the muscle.[19] The role of these substances to alter the responsiveness (i.e., increased sensitivity or sensitization) of the nociceptor is currently being investigated.

PRIMARY AFFERENT NEURONS

The use of electrical stimulation with preferential blockade of peripheral nerves in man has revealed two distinct populations of primary afferent neurons subserving pain.[15,20,21] One group, when preferentially stimulated, evokes a sharp and pricking pain sensation of short duration. This group of afferents is the myelinated A-delta (Aδ), or group III, primary neurons. Conduction velocities of these afferents range between 4 and 30 m per second. The second group, when activated, produces a longer-lasting burning sensation, which is dull and more diffusely localized. These primary afferents are the unmyelinated C, or group IV, afferents. Conduction velocities of C afferents range between 0.5 and 2 meters per second. (These two pain sensations are also termed first and second pain, respectively.)

Primary afferent neurons are also classified according to the type of stimulus that activates the nociceptor or its associate neurons, or both. Three types of nociceptive afferents have been identified: noxious mechanical, mechanothermal, and polymodal. One type is the A-delta high-threshold mechanoreceptor afferent, which responds exclusively to noxious mechanical stimulation. A second type is the A-delta heat nociceptive afferent, which is currently termed the *mechanothermal nociceptor*.[22] This afferent responds to both noxious mechanical and intense thermal stimuli. The third major type of afferent is the C polymodal nociceptive afferent, which responds to noxious heat in the 45°C to 51°C range, to noxious mechanical stimulation, and to noxious chemical stimulation. Approximately one third of the C afferents respond to intense cold; however, their activation does not contribute to the perception of pain.[23] Approximately 85 to 90 percent of the C nociceptor afferents identified in primates are C polymodal afferents. To date, all identified C neurons in humans are C polymodal afferents. In humans, the relationships between activation of A-delta mechanothermal afferents and perception of first pain and activation of C-polymodal afferents and perception of second pain have been established.[24]

Electrophysiologic studies on the cat saphenous nerve demonstrate that the A-delta afferents exhibit excitation failure when stimulated at 10 to 30 Hz.[25] On the other hand, C afferents exhibit excitation failure at stimulation rates of 5 to 10 Hz. Excitation failure is the process by which an action potential is not generated each time the nerve fiber is externally stimulated.

TERMINATION OF NOCICEPTIVE AFFERENTS IN THE DORSAL HORN

The majority of the primary afferents course through the dorsal root and terminate on cells located in the dorsal horn of the spinal gray matter. Just before entry into the spinal cord, similar types of afferents begin to group together. Those signaling pain (Aδ,C) travel through the lateral division of the dorsal root and may travel several spinal segments within Lissauer's tract before entering the spinal gray matter. The large primary afferents travel through the medial division of the dorsal horn and penetrate directly into the dorsal horn.[26] Although the majority of the afferents enter the spinal cord through the dorsal root, a significant population (20 percent of the unmyelinated neurons) enters the spinal cord through the ventral root.[27,28] This latter population is of particular clinical interest when considering reasons for the return of pain in those patients having undergone dorsal rhizotomies for pain relief.

Both histochemical and electrophysiologic studies demonstrate termination of C afferents in lamina I (marginal layer) and lamina II of the spinal cord. Termination of C afferents in lamina III is questionable.[7] A-delta mechanonociceptive afferents have been identified in lamina I, lamina III, and layers IV to VI. Large-diameter A-beta afferents have a few direct connections in laminae I and II, and most extensively terminate in laminae III, IV, and V. Termination of these afferents in lamina V is questionable.

Central Mechanisms of Pain

SECOND ORDER NEURONS

The details of the neuronal circuitry of those cells that lie within the confines of the dorsal horn are complex and not within the scope of this chapter. Such detailed descriptions may be found elsewhere.[7,27] Two categories of second-order neurons that form ascending-projection systems are the spinothalamic and trigeminothalamic tracts. These neurons are also called wide-dynamic-range neurons and nociceptive-specific neurons.

The wide-dynamic-range neuron is considered to be the T cell described in the gate control theory. The cell body of this neuron is located in lamina V of the dorsal horn of the spinal gray matter. These neurons are termed *wide-dynamic range* because they receive input from multiple sources (Fig. 2–3A). A-beta mechanoreceptive, A-delta, and C nociceptive afferents impinge upon the wide-dynamic-range neurons. Each neuron receives input from a large number of primary afferents. These second-order neurons code action potentials so that a low frequency of action potentials represents a touch stimulus. A higher frequency of action potentials represents a noxious pinch.[29]

The second class of second-order neurons is the nociceptive-specific neurons, which respond exclusively to noxious mechanical or thermal stimuli, or both (Fig. 2–3B). In contrast to the wide-dynamic-range neuron, these neurons receive input from a small number of primary afferents. These cells are concentrated in lamina I, but some neurons have been found in lamina V. As evidenced by their name, these neurons receive input from high-threshold A-delta mechanosensitive afferents and C polymodal nociceptive afferents. The nociceptive-specific neurons are further subdivided into a group that responds only to noxious mechanical stimulation carried exclusively by the A-delta high-threshold mechanosensitive afferents. The second subclass of nociceptive-specific neurons responds to intense, nonpainful pressure and to noxious stimuli.

The contributions of these second-order neurons to the perception of pain are well substantiated. The wide-dynamic-range neurons contribute to the localization aspect of pain, as well as modality discrimination (i.e., touch vs. mechanical pinch). Furthermore, activation of these neurons in humans leads to reports of burning or needlelike sensations that are confined to a specific area of the body.[30] On the other hand, the nociceptive-specific neurons are more modality specific; that is, they provide information to the central nervous system about the specific type and location of the noxious stimulus.

Both the nociceptive-specific and wide-dynamic-range neurons signal intensity of pain. Furthermore, a prolonged activation lasting several hundred milliseconds occurs in the cells.[16] The activation could be due to the release of substance P from the endings of

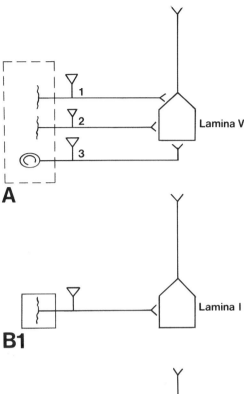

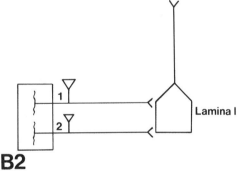

FIGURE 2–3. Schematic representation of categories of second-order neurons. (*A*) Wide-dynamic range neuron with convergent input from primary neurons: #1 = C polymodal afferent; #2 A = Aδ nociceptive afferent; #3 = Aβ mechanoreceptive afferent. (*B1*) Nociceptive-specific neuron with input exclusively from Aδ high-threshold mechanoreceptive afferent. (*B2*) Nociceptive-specific neuron with convergent input from primary neurons: #1 = C polymodal afferent; #2 = Aδ nociceptive afferent.

the wide-dynamic-range neurons.[31] This finding, when substantiated, will provide one possible mechanism for second pain and one possible mechanism for continued pain perception in various painful conditions.

This discussion of the second-order neuron is limited to a brief description of the neuronal characteristics and the primary afferent input. Convergence of known and postulated input from other sources will be described elsewhere (centrifugal control of pain). These two neuronal classes comply with other theories to fit the role of ascending neurons subserving pain. The nociceptive-specific neurons fit the specificity theory for permitting a pain input to reach higher centers in a relatively unaltered fashion. On the other hand, the wide-dynamic-range nociceptors fit the category of the T cell as described by the Melzack and Wall gate control theory.

Ascending Projections and Higher Centers Subserving Pain

Both laboratory and clinical evidence support the hypothesis that the wide-dynamic-range neurons and the specific-nociceptive neurons are only two classes of neurons that compose the spinothalamic tract. Some second-order neurons activated by mechanical stimulation need to be considered in a modulatory role for pain control.[29] Thus, the spinothalamic tract participates in many of the components of pain; that is, affective, arousal, sensory-discriminative, as well as other functions. To classify this tract in the old terminology, paleospinothalamic and neospinothalamic, is an oversimplification.[32] This classical pain pathway, located in the ventrolateral quadrant of the spinal cord, not only terminates in the ventroposterolateralis nucleus (VPL) of the thalamus, but it also sends collaterals to the medial brainstem region.[33]

Many levels of the neuraxis have a role in the pain process. Data implicating higher center processing of pain are derived from a variety of techniques performed upon a variety of species, including humans.

MEDULLA AND PONS

Ascending fibers from the ventrolateral quadrant of the spinal cord send projections to: (1) the medial portion of the reticular formation, particularly the nucleus gigantocellularis; (2) the lateral pons; and (3) the central gray area. These collaterals are termed the *spinoreticular projection*.

White and Sweet[34] noted that stimulation of structures in the medulla of conscious humans produce both the sensory–discriminative and the affective–motivational components of the pain response. The sensory component corresponds to observations of animals that show many neurons in this area respond to noxious stimuli.[35] The affective–motivational component corresponds to the observation that electrical stimulation within the nucleus gigantocellularis (NGC) in animals produced escape behavior in cats,[36] whereas destruction of the NGC resulted in a deficit in escape behavior.[37]

The NGC is a relay in the spinoreticulothalamic system for pain transmission. Furthermore, the NGC connects with autonomic nuclei, which are also located in the reticular formation. These connections play a role in autonomic responses to intense and noxious stimuli.[27] Since reticular formation has connections with autonomic centers, the limbic forebrain structures, and the hypothalamus, this area is more involved in the autonomic and affective components of pain than in subserving a discriminatory function.

MESENCEPHALON

Mesencephalic structures receive projections from a variety of areas, including the spinoreticular projection. Electrical stimulation of the medial periaqueductal gray region in humans elicits emotional responses such as unpleasantness and fear. The pain tends to be deep and confined to midline structures.[38] Destruction of these mesencephalic structures does not alter localization of acute noxious stimuli.[39] The midline structures are more allied with the emotional aspects of the pain process, whereas the lateral structures are more closely associated with the sensory–discriminative aspect; however, this is not a mutually exclusive relationship.

THALAMUS

Considerable evidence demonstrates that wide-dynamic-range neurons and nociceptive-specific neurons of the spinal cord project to three main nuclei of the thalamus: the ventrobasal nuclei, the posterior nuclei, and the medial intralaminar nuclei. Few neurons in these groups respond exclusively to the nociceptive input.[40]

Noxious input to the ventrobasal complex (nucleus ventralis posterior, nucleus ventralis lateralis) projects to discrete areas of the contralateral side of the body. Approximately 6 to 10 percent of the cells in this region respond to noxious stimuli.[41] In humans, lesions in the ventrobasal complex produce deficits in somatosensory discrimination. Tingling in a specific location typically is described when these nuclei are stimulated.[38] This observation suggests a sensory–discriminative component of painful stimuli that is supported by studies in the cat. This observation is further supported by anatomic evidence that these neurons project to both the primary (SI) and secondary (SII) areas of the somatosensory cortex.[27]

The role of the posterior thalamic nuclei in pain is conflicting. This region lacks somatotopic organization, and receives input from a wide sensory area.[40] The majority of somatosensory input arises from the contralateral side of the body. In humans, stimulation of this area elicits a pain sensation.

Cells of the medial and intralaminal thalamic nuclei have large receptive fields, lack somatotopic organization, and receive bilateral input. Nuclei forming the intralaminar complex include the nuclei paracentralis, centralis medialis, centralis lateralis, centromedian, and parafascicularis (Cm–Pf).[27] These nuclei respond to auditory, visual, and intense mechanical stimuli. They receive input from the ventrolateral quadrant of the spinal cord as well as indirect input from the nucleus gigantocellularis.

Electrical stimulation of the Cm–PF complex in humans produces a burning or aching sensation referred primarily from contralateral regions of the body. Recordings from some neurons in these regions demonstrate that these cells respond to pinprick.[42] Lesions in this area are marginally effective in relieving intractable pain. The nondiscriminative quality of pain is removed while preserving the sensory–discriminative aspect. This observation provides a clue that these diffuse thalamic nuclei are involved in the affective quality of pain. Further evidence is that these neurons project not only to the cerebral cortex, but also, to the limbic cortex and amygdala.

CORTEX

The role of the primary somatosensory area in pain perception is not clearly understood. Lesions in this area do not affect acute or chronic pain, and electrical stimulation does not produce pain.[34] The SI cortex, therefore, while serving an important function for spatiotemporal discrimination of sensation, is not an important region for perception of pain.

The secondary somatosensory area of the cerebral cortex has been more extensively studied. This area receives an extensive projection from the posterior thalamic nuclei. Furthermore, these neurons receive multisensory input. Although some researchers have reported no alteration in pain perception with lesions in this area,[34] others have reported hypalgesia.[30]

Researchers have recorded neuronal activity in this region following electrical stimulation of tooth-pulp afferents.[27,43] An increase in stimulus intensity produces an increase in activity recorded in the SII region.

The cortex, then, is involved with the pain mechanisms at two levels. The first level is sensory discrimination, such as localization. A second level is a more complex system associated with complex behavioral responses that include affective and motivational responses and comparisons of pain sensation with past experiences.

In summary, the rostrad projections for pain involved many levels of the neuraxis. The interconnections of these various systems are complex and not completely understood. The use of electrical stimulation or lesioning studies provides some information about the function of a particular system, but these studies may not be a true representation of what actually occurs in the intact, awake animal.

Centrifugal Control of Pain

Although the ascending control system for regulation of sensory input is well established, the descending control system for modulation of pain has only been examined extensively since the late 1960s. The major impetus occurred in 1969 when Reynolds[44] noted that electrical stimulation of the periaqueductal gray (PAG) area produced analgesia in unanesthetized rats. Since that study, modulation of noxious input at the spinal level has been identified,[45] as well as descending control of pain at various levels of the neuraxis. A second major impetus was the isolation of an endogenous substance in neural tissue by Hughes[46] in 1974. This substance, enkephalin, fits the criteria for an endogenous substance that, when released, inhibits pain.

Correlative evidence for centrifugal control of pain is based on studies using stimulation-produced analgesia (SPA) and microinjections of exogenous opiates. Naloxone is used extensively in these studies. Naloxone is a morphine antagonist that competes for the same receptor site as the opiates (such as morphine), the enkephalins, and beta-endorphine (β-endorphin). A receptor site is a specialized region of the neuronal membrane. A neurochemical substance has a specific molecular configuration that matches a particular receptor site (Fig. 2–4). When the neurochemical substance attaches to the receptor, physiologic responses mediated by the chemical transmitter occur. For example, depolarization or hyperpolarization of the nerve membrane occurs. An antagonist has a similar molecular configuration that permits the antagonist to attach to the receptor site and "tie up" spaces available for the neurochemical substance to attach. As a result, the effects of the neurochemical substance are reduced or blocked. In many instances, the antagonist has a greater affinity for the receptor site and can even reverse the effects of the agonist.[47] For example, naloxone is an antidote for morphine overdose and can be used to examine the effects of a thermal agent in pain reduction.

Location and density of the opiates varies among species. The highest concentrations occur in the limbic cortex (most specifically, the anterior amygdala), the periaqueductal gray, the hypothalamus, the thalamus, and to a lesser degree the cortex, caudate nucleus, other midbrain structures, and the gray matter of the spinal cord.[48] Although many brain structures have opiate receptor areas, the question arises as to the importance of the opiate receptor in a particular region subserving pain inhibition.

The two most-studied endogenous opiates are β-endorphin and methionine enkephalin (met-enkephalin). β-endorphin is a 31-amino-acid chain with a half-life of approximately 4 hours. Half-life refers to the time needed for inactivation of the substance by enzymes located in the tissue. β-endorphin has potent effects, including catatonia with corresponding inhibition of neuronal cell activity in the caudate nucleus, cortex, brainstem, and thalamus; analgesia; and behavior disturbances. Since β-endorphin is found in the pituitary and is long-lasting, it is involved with whole animal responses associated with severe stress.[49]

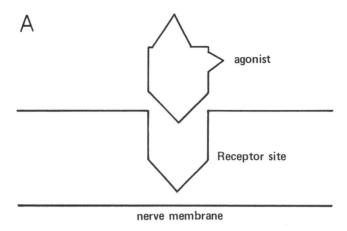

FIGURE 2–4. (*A*) An agonist (e.g. morphine) approaching a receptor site located on the neuronal nerve membrane. (*B*) An antagonist (e.g., naloxone) approaching the same receptor site.

The enkephalins—met-enkephalin and leucine enkephalin—are 5-amino-acid molecules with a half-life of 2 minutes. These peptides have been identified in many regions of the brain and in different concentrations. Areas that have a high concentration of enkephalin also have an increased density of neurons containing substance P or serotonin (5-HT). The postulated role of these neuropeptides in pain regulation will be discussed subsequently.

SPINAL LEVEL

The neuronal activity for pain regulation at the spinal level is not completely understood. Wall[27] noted that electrical stimulation of cells in the substantia gelatinosa decreases primary afferent activity and inhibits neurons in lamina V that were activated by noxious stimuli. The neurochemical transmitter that mediates inhibition is gamma-aminobutyric acid (GABA). Microinjection of opiates into the spinal cord also inhibits activity of dorsal-horn neurons elicited by noxious stimuli.[50] This observation is supported by the finding that neurons containing enkephalin exist in the substantia gelatinosa (Fig. 2–5).[51] These neurons are prominent in laminae I and II, but are also found in laminae III and V. These neurons serve functions other than inhibitory functions and are activated independent of descending pain modulatory systems.

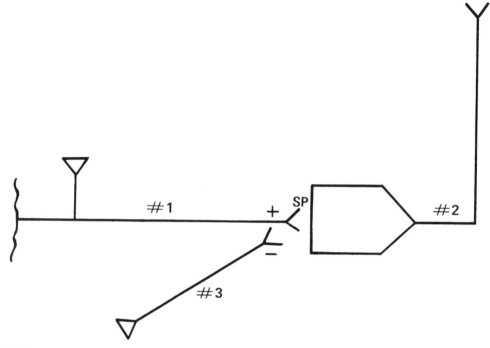

FIGURE 2–5. Schematic representation of presynaptic inhibition of an enkephalinergic neuron (#3) upon a primary afferent neuron (#1) containing substance P (SP). The primary afferent neuron is synapsing with a second-order neuron (#2).

PAIN INHIBITION FROM SUPRASPINAL LEVELS

This modulatory control not only occurs at the spinal level, but also at supraspinal sites. These systems include both neural opiate and nonopiate projections. Furthermore, humoral opiate and nonopiate pain modulatory systems exist.[45] These latter systems are activated in response to very stressful situations and are involved in systemic responses.

Pain regulation by the periaqueductal gray (PAG) area is mediated via indirect pathways. The PAG projects to the nucleus raphe magnus, nucleus reticularis magno-cellularis, and nucleus reticularis gigantocellularis (NRGC) (Fig. 2–6), which in turn projects to the dorsal horn of the spinal cord.[52] The nucleus raphe magnus, when stimulated, inhibits the A-delta afferent input more than A-beta input. This nucleus also contains serotonin-carrying neurons.

Studies indicate that descending serotonergic neurons are heavily concentrated in lamina I and have a direct monosynaptic inhibitory effect on the second-order neuron (ascending tract neuron).[53] Although a serotonin-mediated descending pathway has been identified for pain inhibition, it may not be essential for the opiate or SPA pain mechanisms.[22] Furthermore, the raphe nucleus may use additional and yet unidentified pathways.

A second system, originating in the pons, produces dorsal-horn inhibition and analgesia. This system is a norepinephrine (NE)-mediated system that originates in the region of the ventral locus ceruleus, nucleus subceruleus, and medial and lateral para-brachial nuclei. The descending inhibitory system terminates directly by second-order neurons, or indirectly by an enkephalinergic interneuron.

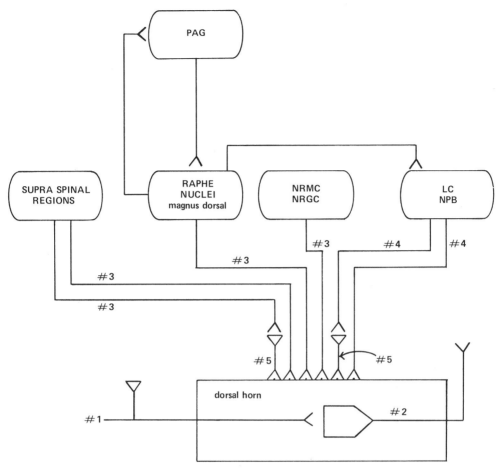

FIGURE 2–6. Schematic representation of centrifugal control of pain. Known and postulated pathways are drawn. Key: PAG = periaqueductal gray; NRMC = nucleus reticularis magnocellularis; NRGC = nucleus reticularis gigantocellularis; LC = locus ceruleus; NPB = medial and lateral parabrachial nuclei; #1 = primary afferent neuron; #2 = second-order neuron; #3 = serotonin neuron; #4 = norepinephrine neuron; #5 = enkephalin neuron.

Neuropharmacologic studies further complicate the puzzle by demonstrating the coexistence of several neurotransmitters in the same cell; for example, serotonin (5-HT) and substance P are found in cells in the spinal cord,[54] and enkephalin and substance P are found in the descending brainstem neurons.[55] The functional significance of this coexistence is not known.

To summarize, at least two distinct descending systems for pain inhibition exist. One system, the opiate pathways using the enkephalin interneuron, is dependent upon the norepinephrine system. A second system does not use an opiate mediator interneuron. Advances in the area of descending systems and dorsal-horn circuitry have proliferated in recent years. Owing to the complexity of the system, many details are lacking and numerous hypotheses exist. The approach taken by researchers is to identify connections by neuroanatomic, neurophysiologic, and neurochemical means. By examining the interactions of the various components, a more sophisticated explanation of the system will be provided, rather than just considering the descending systems as filters for noxious input. Furthermore, the various motor and behavioral responses will be delineated.

PAIN CONDITIONS: ACUTE, CHRONIC, AND REFERRED

The underlying neurophysiologic mechanisms to explain acute, chronic, and referred pain are also incomplete. Complexity arises in the chronic pain condition, since the pain state outlasts the initial experience and involves complex psychologic and physiologic responses. Each pain state and proposed mechanisms associated with each will be explained.

Acute Pain

The acute pain experience may last a few minutes or several days. It is defined as "pain of recent and sudden onset, usually, but not always, with demonstrable etiology and limited course."[56] Usually, the unpleasant experience is associated with autonomic and emotional responses. The primary function of acute pain is to alert the individual of potential tissue damage so that appropriate measures may be taken—that is, withdraw from the stimulus or seek medical assistance.

Generally, a noxious or potentially tissue-damaging stimulus activates nociceptors, and the information is carried via A-delta or C afferents to the spinal cord. Upon reaching the spinal cord, several routes are available. The information is transmitted to the sympathetic preganglionic neuronal pool, whereby reflex responses in the peripheral vascular system and other visceral organs are elicited. Connections to the ventral horn upon the alpha and gamma motoneuronal pool evoke reflex responses, including skeletal-muscle contraction to escape the stimulus or muscle spasm. Nociceptive information transmitted to higher centers results in autonomic and emotional responses, as well as pain perception.

Several mechanisms are proposed to explain the prolonged after-discharge noted with acute pain. Sensitization of nociceptors is a decrease in the threshold value of the receptor to additional stimuli or enhancement of the response. The increase in sensitivity at the site of injury is termed *primary hyperalgesia*. The area surrounding the injury may also be sensitized, in which case the patient experiences secondary hyperalgesia. Secondary hyperalgesia is believed to be due to antidromic activation of C primary afferents and release of substance P in the region.[22] A second postulate for after-discharge is the release of substance P from small primary afferents upon the second-order neuron.

Similar mechanisms can explain the pain–spasm–pain cycle in skeletal muscle. The initial injury produces an initial contraction for splinting or immobilization of the injured part. Continued muscle contraction leads to muscle ischemia and release of chemical substances that sensitize A-delta and C pain afferents in the muscle. By-products of metabolism alone do not produce nociceptive activation,[57] but factors such as bradykinin, serotonin, and histamine are implicated.[58] The heightened sensitivity of the nociceptors leads to additional reflexive contraction in the muscle; the result is a positive feedback loop. A similar loop can be established in the sympathetic reflex arc. Re-establishment of inhibitory mechanisms stops the pain–spasm–pain cycle.

Chronic Pain

Chronic pain is defined as "pain of long duration, often associated with anguish, apprehension, depression, or hopelessness,"[56] and extends months to years beyond the recovery period or recurs intermittently for years. Some clinicians use 6 months post-trauma or post-disease as a basis to consider pain as chronic; others designate the length of time in accordance with a particular condition. Both environmental and psychologic factors are important considerations in the evolution of this type of pain.[59] Emotional, physiologic, and behavioral responses differ from acute pain.

Underlying neurophysiologic mechanisms include positive-feedback loops, as described earlier; that is, an increase in the sensitivity of the nociceptors leads to a maintained pain–spasm–pain cycle. This results in semipermanent, or permanent, changes at the spinal level to maintain these loops. A second mechanism involves long-lasting peripheral nerve compression.[27] Compression results in the destruction of large primary afferent neurons. As a result, an imbalance of large (tactile) and small (pain) fiber input occurs, thereby keeping the gate open.

Chronic pain, however, extends beyond the neurophysiologic model, as is evidenced by Loser's schema.[60] The first level, nociception, is the application of a stimulus that activates A-delta and C primary afferents. The second level, pain, is the perception of the noxious stimulus. Suffering, the third level, is described as negative affective responses. This last level is activated by pain perception, stress, or anxiety. Suffering leads to the fourth level, pain behavior. The responses elicited by this level are evident in both verbal and nonverbal communication (i.e., posture, fascial expressions, drug intake, continued seeking of medical attention, and becoming a non-functioning member of society). When treating these patients, observational analysis should be used to measure pain relief rather than relying exclusively on verbal reports. Although chronic pain has a physiologic component, a multidimensional view is needed to elucidate all components of this condition.

Referred Pain and Trigger Points

Referred pain is "pain felt at a site in the body elsewhere from the source of disease or injury."[56] It is considered an error in localization. Referred pain from the viscera to the body surface is projected upon the same dermatome. For example, myocardial pain afferents arise from T-1 to T-5, and pain associated with a myocardial infarction is felt at the T-1 to T-2 dermatomes, radiating down the arm. Furthermore, referred pain is not exclusively unique to visceral afferents.[61]

Two theories explain the concept of referred pain. Both are based on convergence of visceral and somatic terminations on higher-order neurons. Evidence is available for convergence on the same neuron in the deep layers of the dorsal horn.[62] The convergence-facilitation theory states that visceral afferents lower the threshold of the second-order neuron to incoming cutaneous input. Thus, only the cutaneous information reaches the higher centers of the nervous system.

The second theory, the convergence-projection theory, considers that the pain experienced at a particular site is learned by the association of multiple cues. This site, then, does not necessarily correspond to the site of injury.

Travell[63] identified irritable points in the muscle (trigger points) that referred pain. The term *trigger point* refers to a small hypersensitive area in muscle or fascia. When a trigger point is stimulated by intense heat, cold, or pressure, pain is referred to a remote site. Other terms used to describe this hypersensitive area are fibrositis, myositis, myalgia, or myofascial pain. The etiology of trigger points is unknown. Some researchers believe inflammation is a factor.[64] Others examined fibrositic nodules taken from muscles and noted an increase in acid mucopolysaccharides in connective tissue.[65] More recently, researchers believe that prolonged muscle contraction results in local ischemia, which causes chemical and morphologic changes in the muscle.[66,67] Morphologic changes include swelling of mitochondria and destruction of myofilaments in the I-bands. In severe cases, contractile elements are destroyed. Further research is needed to determine the morphologic and neurophysiologic changes of trigger points.

Clinically, trigger points are identified primarily by palpation. Specific referred patterns elicited from trigger points are evidenced for each muscle. References are available that diagram muscles of the trunk and extremities with their referred pain profile.[68,69] In order to evaluate and select appropriate treatment for the pain patient, therefore, an understanding of the known and theorized mechanisms underlying various painful states is needed.

ASSESSMENT OF PAIN

A comprehensive assessment of the pain experience provides the clinician with an indication of the source(s) of pain, so that the cause of the pain is treated and not just the symptomatology. Furthermore, the assessment helps in the selection of the appropriate thermal agent(s) and provides a baseline to document improvement. Not only verbal descriptions of pain, but nonverbal clues (including facial expressions and posture) also should be recorded. Components of pain assessment also should include the use of pain scales (to determine quantity), body diagrams (to delineate location), and word descriptors (to describe quality).

Pain Scales

The most commonly used pain assessment is a rating scale. A 10-centimeter scale is marked in several ways: (1) a series of numbers from 0 to 10 marked on the scale; (2) verbal rating scale (VRS), with a series of descriptors; or (3) a visual analog scale (VAS), with only the ends of the scale marked.[70] Depending upon the word choice of the latter two scales, the intensity or the affective quality of pain is assessed. For example, the word choice of "strong" or "intense" is used to evaluate the intensity of pain, whereas phrases such as "bad as it can be" or "as unpleasant as it can be" are used to assess the affective quality.

When designing such a test, the following points should be considered. The scale should be drawn accurately. For example, if the horizontal line becomes thicker, then a cue concerning the intensity of pain is given to the patient. Only one pain scale is drawn on the page, so that an as-accurate-as-possible measure is obtained, not biased by previously marked pain scales. Another manipulation of the pain scale is the reversal of the scale so that the most intense measure is on the left, or so that the scale is presented vertically. Whether these reversals of scale provide a better documentation of pain has not been studied. Scott and Huskisson[71] examined a vertical versus horizontal VAS and noted that, although patients scored slightly lower using the horizontal scale, a significant difference was not noted between the two.

Both the VRS and VAS can be converted to a numerical format so that arithmetic manipulations can be performed. The scales correlate for pain measurement ($r = 0.84$, $p < 0.01$) and pain relief ($r = 0.81$, $p < 0.001$).[72] Many researchers believe the VAS is a more sensitive indicator.[73]

These scales are simple and quick to use, but they have limitations. First is the assumption that the categories of descriptors on the VRS or the numerical scale can be partitioned into equal psychologic units. Second is the assumption that a simple linear scale can assess one component in a very complex pain experience, and that the patient can accurately remember pain intensity. These scales also are influenced by personal experience, culture, and expectations, including what the patient considers is expected of him or her by the therapist.

McGill Pain Questionnaire

In an attempt to assess the multidimensional aspects of pain, the McGill Pain Questionnaire (MPQ) was developed.[74,75] The researchers developed a pain assessment that included three classes of word choices to evaluate the sensory, evaluative, and affective components of pain. These descriptors were obtained with a high degree of agreement from subjects with different educational, socioeconomic, and cultural backgrounds. The questionnaire is also designed to quantitate pain. The measures are the total number of words chosen (NWC), the pain-rating index (PRI), and the present-pain intensity (PPI).

The word descriptors are divided into three categories and 20 subcategories. Each subcategory contains up to six words that are qualitatively similar and are ranked in descending order according to intensity. Each word is assigned a numerical value. The sensory category contains 13 subcategories to describe the pain in terms of the spatio-temporal, pressure, thermal, and sharp–dull aspects of pain. Words such as "flickering" and "beating" describe the temporal aspect; "jumping" and "shooting" describe the spatial aspect; "stabbing," "cramping," and "tugging," describe the pressure aspect; and "burning" and "scalding," describe the thermal aspect of the pain experience. The affective category, divided into six subcategories, describes pain in terms of autonomic responses, fear, and tension. Pain descriptors such as "terrifying," "sickening," and "vicious" are included. The third category, evaluative, is a single category used to describe the intensity of the total pain experience. Words such as "annoying," "unbearable," and "troublesome" are used.

The patient is instructed to circle one word from each category that best describes his or her pain. If a category does not apply, it is left unmarked. Values for NWC and PRI are obtained from this list. NWC is the number of words (or categories) chosen. The PRI is obtained by assigning a numerical value to each word choice, then determining the mean. This value is an average measure of the pain experience and is a sensitive indicator in pain assessment.

Melzack[74,75] determined that the PRI correlated significantly with NWC ($p < 0.01$). Both the reliability and validity of the PRI scale have been tested on patients with a variety of painful conditions.[76–78] Unique profiles have been identified for chronic pain conditions, including, for instance, low back pain and arthritis.[79]

Another part of the pain questionnaire is the body diagram. A front and back view of a human is presented, and the patient marks the location of the pain on the diagram. The patient also marks "E" or "I" by the area where the pain is — "E" for external pain and "I" for internal pain.

Part three addresses pain in relation to duration and activities that influence the intensity. The patient describes the pain as being continuous, intermittent, or momentary, and then lists those activities that increase or decrease pain. The patient notes the time of day when the pain is better or worse, which can be correlated with the type of activities that cause or reduce pain.

The fourth part of the evaluation relates to pain intensity. A five-point scale is marked with the terms mild, discomforting, distressing, horrible, and excruciating. The patient is asked to describe pain intensity at that moment — at the time when the pain is at its worst, and at the time when the pain is at its least. This test is the present pain index (PPI), which gives an indication of pain during the administration of the questionnaire.

Additional information gathered on the MPQ includes a medical history, drug intake, and present treatments. (If further information is needed, the patient is given a standardized home recording card.) The original questionnaire has been adapted to a shorter version (Fig. 2–7). The advantage of the MPQ is that it provides a greater sensitivity in assessing pain than the analog scale does.

1. Where is your Pain?

Please mark, on the drawings below, the areas where you feel pain.
Put E if external, or I if internal, near the areas which you mark.
Put EI if both external and internal.

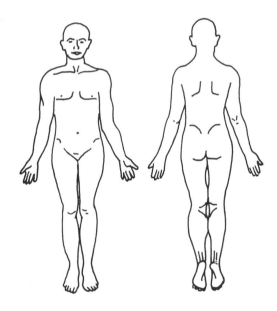

2. Please mark on the scale how much pain you have.

VISUAL ANALOGUE SCALE

PAIN AS
BAD AS IT _____ NO PAIN
COULD BE

FIGURE 2–7. Adapted from parts 1, 2, and 3 of the McGill Pain Questionnaire.

Other Assessments

Other testing methods have been used in the acute[80] and, most particularly, in the chronic-pain-patient population. Two assessments deserve brief mention, but to provide details is beyond the scope of this text. The Sensory Decision, or Signal Detection Theory (SDT) is designed to discriminate among sensory stimuli (pain sensations) and is not a measure of the intensity of pain experienced. Controversy exists as to the use of this test in pain measure. Another commonly used test to assess the chronic pain patient is the Minnesota Multiphasic Personality Inventory (MMPI). Specific chronic-pain-personality profiles have been determined from the MMPI. Additional information on assessment of pain is presented in Chapter 10.

3. <u>Pain Rating Index</u>

There are many words that describe pain. From the list below, select only those words that describe your pain as it feels right now. Only select one word in each column, and only if it applies to your pain. YOU DO NOT NEED TO MARK A WORD IN EVERY COLUMN—ONLY MARK THOSE WORDS THAT DESCRIBE YOUR PAIN!

1.	2.	3.	4.
Flickering Quivering Pulsing Throbbing Beating Pounding	Jumping Flashing Shooting	Pricking Boring Drilling Stabbing	Sharp Cutting Lacerating

5.	6.	7.	8.
Pinching Pressing Gnawing Cramping Crushing	Tugging Pulling Wrenching	Hot Burning Scalding Searing	Tingling Itchy Smarting Stinging

9.	10.	11.	12.
Dull Sore Hurting Aching Heavy	Tender Taut Rasping	Tiring Exhausting	Sickening Suffocating

13.	14.	15.	16.
Fearful Frightful Terrifying	Punishing Grueling Cruel Vicious Killing	Wretched Blinding	Annoying Troublesome Miserable Intense Unbearable

17.	18.	19.	20.
Spreading Radiating Penetrating Piercing	Tight Numb Drawing Squeezing Tearing	Cool Cold Freezing	Nagging Nauseating Agonizing Dreadful Torturing

FIGURE 2–7. *Continued.*

APPLICATION OF THERMAL AGENTS FOR PAIN RELIEF

Clinical rationale for pain relief is based primarily upon empiric observation and integration of information from basic and applied sciences. Although heat and cold are known to relieve pain in a variety of conditions, including tissue injuries and arthritis, the underlying mechanisms are unknown. Local neurologic and vascular changes in response to the thermal agent and the mechanisms accounting for such changes await systematic testing and evaluation.

Heat

Muscle spasm secondary to some type of muscle, joint, or neurologic trauma is relieved by heat. To review, a pain–spasm–pain cycle arising from trauma excites nociceptors located in the skin or muscle. An increase in their activity causes pain perception and reflex muscle activation. With prolonged muscle activity, ischemia results, which activates muscle nociceptors and causes self-sustained muscle spasm. Trauma to the area releases algesic chemicals, such as substance P or bradykinin, in the area of the nociceptors. These chemicals sensitize the nociceptors. The sympathetic reflex arc also contributes to the pain–spasm cycle. For example, if vasoconstriction occurs, contraction of smooth muscle activates surrounding nociceptors. Inhibition of pain may result from nervous system changes or vascular changes (Fig. 2–8).

Cosentino and colleagues[81] reported a decrease in sensory nerve conduction velocity following the application of ultrasound. The decrease is similar to that reported for motor nerve conduction velocity. This observed phenomenon may be related to the frequency component of ultrasound and not the thermal effects. This mechanism, however, has yet to be elucidated.

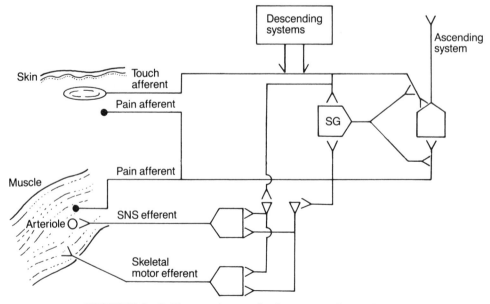

FIGURE 2–8. Figure schema of pain-spasm-pain mechanism.

Mense[82] noted that direct warming of the cat muscle spindle decreases neuronal activity of the secondary endings and increases the neuronal activity of the primary endings. Increases in primary afferent activity of the spindle closes the gate. Mense also observed increased Golgi tendon organ (GTO) activity upon warming. GTOs inhibit the homonymous motoneuronal pool, which provides an inhibitory input to break up the pain–spasm–pain cycle. Caution should be used when extrapolating the data to clinical procedures, since the thermal agent in Mense's study was applied directly to exposed nerves of the cat.

The counterirritation theory is based on a gating mechanism[83] and can be used to explain thermal effects on the pain–spasm–pain cycle. Application of an external heat source produces a bombardment of activity from thermoreceptors. This increase in action potentials blocks pain input. Melzack and Wall's[84] gate theory provides the necessary circuitry for such blockage. Another central nervous system phenomenon is generalized, or whole body, relaxation. Relaxation produces pain relief, particularly if pain results from tension or skeletal muscle spasm. Activation of the descending pain inhibitory systems during thermal heating awaits justification.

Vascular changes in response to application of heat also can reduce pain. Vasodilatation and increase in blood flow up to 30 ml per 100 g of tissue have been observed.[85] A greater blood flow increases the supply of nutrients to the area for repair process and removes byproducts from the injured tissue. Byproducts include prostaglandins, bradykinin, and histamine, all implicated in receptor and afferent fiber sensitization that can cause a pain–spasm–pain cycle. Local heating also activates somatovisceral reflex arcs. Stimulation of cutaneous thermoreceptors decreases activity of the sympathetic nervous system and produces a vasodilatation in deeper blood vessels.

Cold

The use of cold to decrease pain is through brief intense or prolonged cold. Both local and central nervous system mechanisms are used to explain pain reduction.

Travell[86] identified three possible mechanisms underlying the effects of brief intense cold: receptor adaptation; a counterirritant effect; and a neurogenic effect. A decrease in skin temperature following the application of a vapocoolant spray produces cooling sufficient to cause receptor adaptation.[6] This idea was referenced to the findings of Cattell,[87] whereby tactile receptors adapt to an intermittent stream of air. Whether or not the effects produced by these two dissimilar types of stimuli are equivalent is unknown at this time.

The counterirritant effect is based on the research by Gammon and Starr.[88] They observed that a 4°C to 10°C cold application to the skin relieves pain induced by a topical application of capsaicin. This observation and the neurogenic effect can be based on the gate theory; that is, an irritant can block pain fibers by activation of receptors to close the gate. Furthermore, Iggo[27] noted that any intense stimuli that are noxious to the individual activate inhibitory processes, by a yet undefined mechanism. He does not advocate the use of noxious stimuli as a therapeutic means for pain reduction.

When cold is applied for a longer period of time, both local and central changes occur. One central nervous system model, the gate mechanism, has been described. Cooling of the skin (35°C to 24°C during a 7-second to 10-second period) results in a rapid increase in the frequency of the action potentials recorded on the afferent fiber.[89] This activity blocks pain input. To date, no evidence supports activation of the endorphin system by cold thermal agents.

Metabolic changes occur in both the receptor and afferent axons. Nerve conduction velocities have been examined in response to cooling longer than 5 minutes. For every 1°C decrease in intramuscular temperature, a decrease of 1.2 m per second in motor conduction occurs,[85] and a corresponding 2 m per second decrease is noted for sensory nerve conduction velocities.[90] Smaller-diameter afferents are more sensitive to cold than larger-diameter afferents. These observations, then, would decrease the probability of pain input to continue.

The local vasomotor response to cold is immediate vasoconstriction. This would result in an initial decrease in the amount of vasodilator substances released into the surrounding tissue, which would decrease the degree of sensitization of nociceptors.

SUMMARY

As is shown in this chapter, pain theories are dynamic and changing. What is postulated to date will be successfully defended or refuted. Current review articles are available to keep the clinician abreast of these changes. As the theories advance, so must the rationale for clinical treatment using thermal modalities.

REFERENCES

1. Merskey, H and Able-Fessard, DG: Pain terms: A list with definitions and notes on usage. Pain 6:249, 1979.
2. Bonica, JJ: Pain research and therapy: Past and current status and future needs. In Ng, KY and Bonica, JJ (eds): Pain, Discomfort and Humanitarian Care. Elsevier, New York, 1979, pp 1–48.
3. Mayer, DJ and Price, DD: A physiological and psychological analysis of pain: A potential model of motivation. In Pfaff, D: Physiological Mechanisms of Motivation. Springer-Verlag, New York, 1982, pp 433–471.
4. Melzack, R and Wall, PD: Pain mechanisms: A new theory. Science 150:971, 1965.
5. von Frey, J: Beitrage zur physiologica des schmerzsinns. Ber kgl sachs Ges Wiss 46:185, 1894.
6. Goldscheider, A: Veber den Schmertz in Physiologischer und Klinischer Hensicht. Berlin, Hirschwald, 1894.
7. Wall, PD: The role of substantia gelatinosa as a gate control. In Bonica, JJ (ed): Pain. Raven Press, New York, 1980, pp 205–231.
8. Nathan, PW: The gate-control theory of pain: A critical review, Brain 99:123, 1976.
9. Wall, PD: The gate control theory of pain mechanisms: A re-examination and re-statement. Brain 101:1, 1978.
10. Wall, PD and Sweet, WH: Temporary abolition of pain in man. Science 155–108, 1967.
11. Long, DM: External electrical stimulation as a treatment of chronic pain. Minnesota Medicine 57:195, 1974.
12. Georgopoulos, AP: Functional properties of primary afferent units probably related to pain mechanisms in primate glabrous skin. J Neurophysiol 39:79, 1976.
13. Burgess, PR and Perl, ER: Myelinated afferent fibers responding specifically to noxious stimulation of the skin. J Physiol (Lond) 190:541, 1967.
14. LaMotte, RH and Campbell, JN: Comparison of responses of warm and nociceptive C-fiber afferents in monkey with human judgments of thermal pain. J Neurophysiol 41:509, 1978.
15. Van Hees, J: Human C-fiber input during painful and nonpainful skin stimulation with radiant heat. In Bonica, JJ and Able-Fessard, D (eds): Advances in Pain Research and Therapy, Vol 1. Raven Press, New York, 1976, pp 35–40.
16. Zimmermann, M: Peripheral and central nervous mechanisms of nociception, pain, and pain therapy: Facts and hypotheses. In Bonica, JJ, et al (eds): Advances in Pain Research and Therapy, Vol. 3. Raven Press, New York, 1979, pp 3–32.
17. Lynn, B: The detection of injury and tissue damage. In Wall, PD and Melzack, R (eds): Textbook of Pain. Churchill-Livingstone, New York, 1984, pp 19–33.
18. Beck, PW, et al: Nervous outflow from the cat's foot during noxious radiant heat stimulation. Brain Res 67:373, 1974.
19. Mense, S and Schmidt, RF: Muscle pain: Which receptors are responsible for the transmission of noxious

stimuli? In Rose, FC (ed): Psychological Aspects of Clinical Neurology. Blackwell Scientific Publications, Oxford, 1977, pp 265–278.

20. Torebjork, HE and Hallin, RG: Perceptual changes accompanying controlled preferential blocking of A and C fibre responses in intact human skin nerves. Exp Brain Res 16:321, 1973.

21. Kerr, FWL: An overview of neural mechanisms of pain. Neurosci Res Program Bull 16:30, 1978.

22. Dubner, R and Bennett, GJ: Spinal and trigeminal mechanisms of nociception. Ann Rev Neurosci 6:381, 1983.

23. LaMotte, RH, et al: Peripheral neural mechanisms of cutaneous hyperalgesia following mild injury by heat. J Neurosci 2:765, 1982.

24. Price, DD, et al: Peripheral suppression of first pain and central summation of second pain evoked by noxious heat pulses. Pain 3:57, 1977.

25. Torebjork, HE and Hallin, RG: Excitation failure in thin nerve fiber structure and accompanying hypalgesia during repetitive electrical skin stimulation. In Bonica, JJ (ed): Advances in Neurology, Vol 4. Raven Press, New York, 1974, p 733.

26. Kerr, FWL: Neuroanatomical substrates of nociception in the spinal cord. Pain 1:325, 1975.

27. Yaksh, TL and Hammond, DL: Peripheral and central substances involved in rostrad (ascending) transmission of nociceptive information. Pain 13:1, 1982.

28. Kerr, FWL and Wilson, PR: Pain. Ann Rev Neurosci 1:83, 1978.

29. Price, DD and Dubner, R: Neurons that subserve the sensory-discriminative aspects of pain. Pain 3:307, 1977.

30. Mayer, DJ, Price, DD and Becker, DP: Neurophysiological characterization of the anterolateral spinal cord neurons contributing to pain perception in man. Pain 1:59, 1975.

31. Hokfelt, T, et al: Experimental immunohistochemical studies on the localization and distribution of substance P in cat primary sensory neurons. Brain Res 100:235, 1975.

32. Melzack, R: The Puzzle of Pain. Basic Books, New York, 1973.

33. Price, DD, et al: Spatial and temporal transformation of input to spinothalamic tract neurons and their relation to somatic sensation. J Neurophysiol 41:933, 1978.

34. White, JC and Sweet, WH: Pain and the Neurosurgeon: A Forty-Year Experience. Charles C. Thomas, Springfield, 1969.

35. Pearl, GS and Anderson, KV: Response patterns of cells in the feline caudal nucleus reticularis gigantocellularis after noxious trigeminal and spinal stimulation. Exp Neurol 58:231, 1978.

36. Casey, KL: Somatosensory responses of bulboreticular units in awake cat: Relation to escape-producing stimuli. Science 173:77, 1971.

37. Anderson, KV and Pearl, GS: Long term increases in nociceptive thresholds following lesions in feline nucleus reticularis gigantocellularis (abstr). 1st World Congress on Pain 1:70, 1975.

38. Nashold, BS, Jr., Wilson, WP, and Slaughter, G: The midbrain and pain. In Bonica, JJ (ed): Advances in Neurology, Vol 4. Raven Press, New York, 1979, pp 69–169.

39. Schuarcz, Jr: Periaqueductal mesencephalotomy for facial central pain. In Sweet, HW, Labrador, R, and Martin-Rodriguez, JG (eds): Neurosurgical Treatment in Psychiatry, Pain and Epilepsy. University Park Press, Baltimore, 1977, pp 661–667.

40. Casey, KL and Jones, EG: Suprasegmental mechanisms: An overview of ascending pathways: Brain-stem and thalamus. Neurosci Res Program Bull 16:103, 1978.

41. Nyquist, JK: Somatosensory properties of neurons of thalamic nucleus ventralis lateralis. Exp Neurol 48:123, 1975.

42. Inshijima, B, et al: Nociceptive neurons in the human thalamus. Confin Neurol 37:99, 1975.

43. Andersson, SA, Keller, O, and Vyklicky, I: Cortical activity evoked from tooth pulp afferents. Brain Res 50:473, 1973.

44. Reynolds, DV: Surgery in the rat during electrical analgesia induced by focal brain stimulation. Science 164:444, 1969.

45. Mayer, DJ: The centrifugal control of pain. In Ng, L and Bonica, JJ (eds): Pain, Discomfort, and Humanitarian Care. Elsevier, Amsterdam, 1980, pp 83–105.

46. Hughes, J: Search for the endogenous legend of the opiate receptor. Neurosci Res Program Bull 13:55, 1975.

47. Pert, C: Opiate receptors and pain pathways. Neurosci Res Program Bull 16:133, 1978.

48. Basbaum, A and Fields, HL: Endogenous pain control systems: Brainstem spinal pathways and endorphin circuitry. Annual Review Neuroscience 7:309–338, 1984.

49. Hughes, J: Intrinsic factors and the opiate receptor system. Neurosci Res Program Bull 16:141, 1978.

50. Duggan, AW: The differential sensitivity to L-glutamate and L-aspartate of spinal interneurons and Renshaw cells. Exp Brain Res 19:522, 1974.

51. Elde, R, et al: Immunohistochemical studies using antibodies to leucine–enkephalin: Initial observations on the nervous system of the rat. Neuroscience 1:349, 1976.

52. Basbaum, AI, Clanton, CH, and Fields, HL: Three bulbospinal pathways form the rostral medulla of the cat. J Comp Neurol 178:209, 1978.

53. Hoffert, MS, et al: Immunocytochemical identification of serotonergic axonal contacts on characterized neurons in cat spinal dorsal horn. Anat Rec 202:83A, 1982.

54. Pelletier, G, et al: Immunoreactive substance P and serotonin present in the same dense-core vesicles. Nature 293:71, 1981.

55. Hokfelt, T, et al: Evidence for enkephalin immunoreactive neurons in the medulla oblongata projecting to the spinal cord. Neurosci Lett 14:55, 1979.
56. Report of the Panel on Pain to the National Advisory Neurological and Communicative Disorders and Stroke Council. HEW, NIH Pub #79-1912, Bethesda, MD, 1979, p 201.
57. Kniffki, KD, et al: Responses of group IV afferent units from skeletal muscle to stretch, contraction, and chemical stimulation. Exp Brain Res 31:511, 1978.
58. Fock, S and Mense, S: Excitatory effects of 5-hydroxytryptamine, histamine and potassium ions on muscular IV afferent units: A comparison with bradykinin. Brain Res 105:459, 1976.
59. Fordyce, WE: Behavioral Methods for Chronic Pain and Illness. CV Mosby, St. Louis, 1976.
60. Fordyce, WE: A behavioral perspective on chronic pain. In Ng, LKY and Bonica, JJ (eds): Pain, Discomfort, and Humanitarian Care. Elsevier, New York, 1980, pp 233–252.
61. Procacci, P and Zoppi, M: Pathophysiology and clinical aspects of visceral and referred pain. In Bonica, JJ, et al: Advances in Pain Research and Therapy, Vol 5. Raven Press, New York, pp 643–658.
62. Hancock, MD, et al: Convergence of visceral and cutaneous input onto spinothalamic tract cells in the thoracic spinal cord of the cat. Exp Neurol 47:240, 1975.
63. Travell, J: Temporomandibular joint dysfunction. J Prosthet Dent 10:745, 1960.
64. Frost, A: Diclofenac versus lidocaine as injection therapy in myofascial pain. Scandinavian Journal of Rheumatology 15:153, 1986.
65. Brendstrip, P, Jespersen, K, and Asboe-Hansen, G: Morphological and chemical connective tissue changes in fibrositic muscles. Annals of Rheumatology 16:438, 1957.
66. Bengtsson, A, Henriksson, K-G, and Larsson, J: Muscle biopsy in primary fibromyalgia. Light microscope and histochemical findings. Scandinavian Journal of Rheumatology 15:1, 1986.
67. Lund, N, Begtsson, A, and Thornborg, P: Muscle tissue oxygen pressure in primary fibromyalgia. Scandinavian Journal of Rheumatology 15:165, 1986.
68. Travell, JG and Simons, DG: Myofascial Trigger Point Manual. Williams & Wilkins, Baltimore, 1982.
69. Simons, DG and Travell, JG: Myofascial origins of low back pain. Postgrad Med 73:66, 1983.
70. Cracely, RH: Psychophysical assessment of human pain. In Bonica, JJ (ed): Advances in Pain Research and Therapy, Vol 3. Raven Press, New York, 1979, pp 805–824.
71. Scott, J and Huskisson, EC: Vertical and horizontal analogue scales. Ann Rheum Dis 38:560, 1979.
72. Ohnhaus, EE and Adler, R: Methodological problems in the measurement of pain: A comparison between the verbal rating scale and the visual analogue scale. Pain 1:379, 1975.
73. Price, DD and Harkins, SW: Combined use of experimental pain and visual analogue scales in providing standardized measurements of clinical pain. The Clinical Journal of Pain 3:1, 1987.
74. Melzack, R and Torgerson, WS: On the language of pain. Anesthesiology 34:50, 1971.
75. Melzack, R: The McGill Pain Questionnaire: Major properties and scoring methods. Pain 1:277, 1975.
76. Klepac, RK, et al: Sensitivity of the McGill Pain Questionnaire to intensity and quality of laboratory pain. Pain 10:199, 1981.
77. Byrne, M, et al: Cross validation of the factor structure of MPQ. Pain 13:193, 1982.
78. Reading, AE: A comparison of MPQ in chronic and acute pain. Pain 13:185, 1982.
79. Gracely, RH: Pain measurement in man. In Ng, LKY and Bonica, JJ (eds): Pain, Discomfort and Humanitarian Care. Elsevier, New York, 1980, pp 111–137.
80. Reeves, JL, Jaeger, B, and Graff-Radford, SB: Reliability of the pressure algometer as a measure to trigger point sensitivity. Pain 24:313–321, 1986.
81. Cosentino, AB, et al: Ultrasound effects on electroneuromyographic measures in sensory fibers of the median nerve. Phys Ther 63:1789, 1983.
82. Mense, S: Effects of temperature on the discharges of muscle spindles and tendon organs. Pflugers Arch 374:159, 1978.
83. Parsons, CM and Goetzl, FR: Effect of induced pain on pain threshold. Proc Soc Exp Bio Med 60:327, 1945.
84. Melzack, R and Wall, P: The Challenge of Pain. Penguin Books, New York, 1982.
85. Lehmann, JF and DeLateur, BJ: Therapeutic heat. In Lehmann, JF (ed): Therapeutic Heat and Cold, ed 4. Williams & Wilkins, Baltimore, 1990, pp 429–432.
86. Travell, J: Myofascial trigger points: Clinical view. In Bonica, JJ, Able-Fessard, DG (eds): Advances in Pain Research and Therapy, Vol 1. Raven Press, New York, 1976, pp 919–926.
87. Cattell, M and Hoagland, H: Response of tactile receptors to intermittent stimulation. J Physiol 72:392, 1931.
88. Gammon, GD and Starr, I: Studies on the relief of pain by counter-irritation. J Clin Invest 20:13, 1941.
89. Hensel, H: Thermoreception and Temperature Regulation. Academic Press, New York, 1981.
90. Buchthal, F and Rosenfalck, A: Evoked action potentials and conduction velocity in human sensory nerves. Brain Res 3:1, 1966.

Instrumentation: Methods and Application

CHAPTER 3

Instrumentation Considerations: Operating Principles, Purchase, Management, and Safety

H.T.M. Ritter, III, B.A., C.B.E.T.

In opening this chapter, it is significant to note that most of the earliest applications of electricity in medicine were intended as physical therapy devices. Experiments with electrotherapy are on record from the 18th century.[1] Diathermy was first described late in the 19th century, and ultrasound was under investigation shortly thereafter.[2] Today, there is perhaps a greater variety of instrumentation to be found in hospital physical therapy departments than in any other patient care area. Outpatient physical therapy centers also can have a large variety of equipment.

A basic knowledge of electrical principles is essential for safety in the physical therapy clinic and for an understanding of devices such as ground fault circuit interrupters, diathermy units, and ultrasound generators. The author assumes that the reader has had previous exposure to these basic principles, including electron flow, Ohm's law, capacitance, and inductance. For a comprehensive review of electrical terminology and theory, the reader may refer either to Cromwell[3] or to Spooner.[4]

The objectives of this chapter are to (1) present the basic principles and physiologic effects of 60 Hz alternating current; (2) discuss the reasons for grounding electrical devices and for installing ground fault circuit interrupters in hydrotherapy areas; (3) offer guidelines for prepurchase evaluation, acquisition, and knowledgeable management of equipment; and (4) review general and device-specific inspection procedures, including calibration methods and appropriate standards.

ELECTROMAGNETIC ENERGY

The entire range of radiation, or electromagnetic spectrum, includes heat, radio, and light waves, as well as ultraviolet, x-rays, and cosmic rays. It is important to know, however, that ultrasound energy is not electromagnetic, but rather a mechanical/pressure waveform that cannot be transmitted by air. Notice from careful study of Figure 3–1 that shortwave (SWD) and microwave (MWD) diathermy are both safely in the nonionizing section. This means that radiation effects are thought to be purely thermal. These energies are not capable of stripping electrons from atoms.

The electromagnetic spectrum also reveals that each form of radiation can be described by a frequency (f) and a wavelength (λ). All forms of radiant energy are self-propagating and travel in a vacuum at the speed of light (c), which is 300 million meters per second. The reader should be aware of the formula that interrelates these three quantities: $c = f\lambda$. Since c is a constant, frequency or wavelength can be derived even when just one of them is known. For instance, given that the wavelength of shortwave diathermy is 11.062 meters, calculate its frequency.

$$f = c/\lambda = \frac{3 \times 10^8 \text{ m/sec}}{11.062 \text{ m}} = 27.12 \times 10^6 \text{ cycles/sec} = 27.12 \text{ mHz}$$

Radiation energy is directly proportional to frequency. Therefore, cosmic rays are far more penetrating than is infrared radiation. Within the infrared spectrum, the higher-frequency radiation, near visible light, is more penetrating than "far" infrared. The biologic effects of electromagnetic radiation depend on frequency, exposure duration, tissue characteristics, and power density.

In dealing with instrumentation for thermal therapy, there is no need to be concerned with direct current (DC). The domain of relevant alternating current (AC)

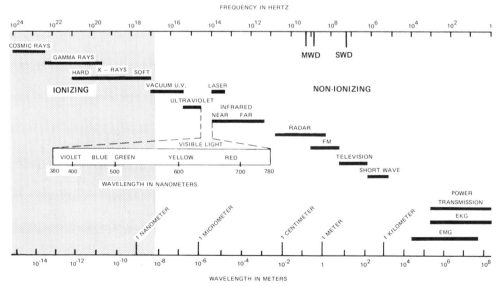

FIGURE 3–1. A graphic representation of the electromagnetic system. (Adapted from IES Lighting Handbook, ed 5, 1972).

frequencies ranges from the 60-Hz power-line supply through the megahertz region for diathermy up to infrared radiation.

POWER SUPPLY: 115 VAC–60 Hz

Conventional power-line voltage in North America alternates at the very regulated frequency of 60 Hertz (abbreviated Hz and denoting cycles per second). The accuracy of electric clocks, for instance, depends on this constant, since "line" voltage frequently varies between 110 and 125 volts. Every electrical device intended for operation on line voltage will bear a label that typically lists 110, 115, 117 or 120 volts—alternating current (VAC), as distinguished from direct-current voltage (VDC). (Some heavy-duty devices, such as treadmills, may require a 230-volt source.) The label will also indicate the line frequency (60 Hz) and either a current or a power rating. For instance, a new solid state ultrasound unit specifies "120 VAC 60 Hz, 0.5 amp maximum." The same information could have been conveyed by indicating 60 watts instead of listing current:

$$\text{Power} = \text{Voltage (E)} \times \text{Current (I)} = 120 \times 0.5.$$

Voltages and their frequencies can be seen and measured with an oscilloscope. A comparison of symbols and waveforms for DC and AC is illustrated in Figure 3–2.

TRANSFORMERS

Electricity is transmitted from generating stations over long distances at very high voltages (e.g., 230,000 volts). Before commercial distribution, voltage must be dropped to the 115-volt range. While whirlpool motors, paraffin baths, and infrared lamps operate directly off this line voltage, some instruments have power supplies that require a lower AC voltage. Others may require a boosting of voltage at some point.

Transformers accomplish these necessary voltage manipulations. Typically, they are composed of two adjacent coils on an iron core and operate on the principle of electrical induction. When alternating current flows through the input or primary

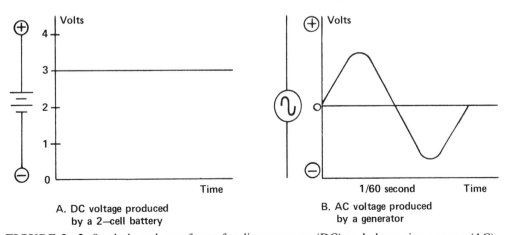

FIGURE 3–2. Symbols and waveforms for direct current (DC) and alternating current (AC).

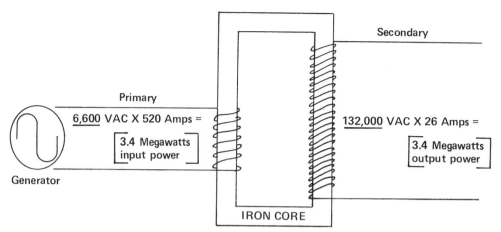

FIGURE 3–3. A step-up transformer used for electrical power transmission. Lowered secondary current greatly reduces losses due to heating of the power distribution wires. (Note: "Step-up" or "step-down" refers to secondary *voltage.*)

winding of a transformer, it creates a surrounding magnetic field. This field, in turn, cuts through the secondary winding and induces an output current. Note that there is no electron flow between primary and secondary windings. Output voltage and current are determined by the ratio of primary to secondary winding turns. When transformer windings have approximately the same number of turns, output voltage will equal input voltage, and the unit is referred to as an isolation transformer. This type of transformer, which can be used as a safety device, will be discussed later.

The concept of input power equaling output power (assuming no coupling losses) is fundamental to understanding step-up and step-down transformers. Again reviewing the power formula $P = E \times I$, it can be seen that, for a given input power to the primary, a stepped-up voltage is associated with a proportional reduction in secondary current (Fig. 3–3).

If a transformer secondary has fewer turns than its primary winding, output voltage will be reduced. For example, an ultrasound generator has a step-down transformer that drops line voltage to approximately 24 volts, which is then fed to the unit's power supply.

POWER DISTRIBUTION AT THE USER'S END

Figure 3–4 illustrates the terminology and mechanism of power distribution to the familiar point of an electrical receptacle. It also depicts a simplified current flow to, from, and within a representative ultrasound unit.

As previously described, electrical power is commercially supplied in a range of 110 to 125 volts, alternating at the frequency of 60 Hz. Although only two conductors are actually required for a voltage source, a third conductor can be employed to enhance electrical safety. This line is referred to as "ground" and, most often, is actually connected to a rod in the earth either in, or just outside, a building. As a rule, the plumbing system of a building is also considered to be "grounded." Ground is a universal electrical reference point that is at a zero-voltage potential.

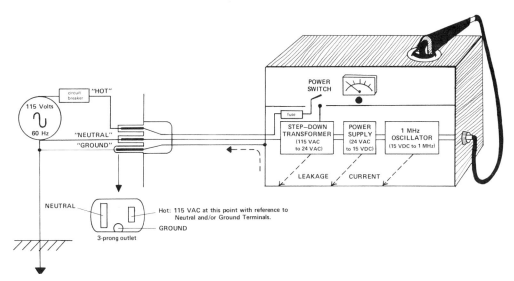

FIGURE 3–4. A device is powered by the voltage between the hot and neutral conductors. Normal leakage current is conducted away from metal housing (chassis) by the ground wire.

Current circulates to and from the ultrasound unit through wires designated as hot and neutral. In spite of careful design and proper insulation, minute currents will nevertheless stray (much of it capacitively) from the hot/neutral circuit to adjacent conductive surfaces. Then, if a path exists, these so-called leakage currents will flow to any object that is grounded, completing their return back into the power system. (Note carefully in Fig. 3–4 that the neutral side of the electrical service is also connected to ground.)

If an electrical device loses its line cord/receptacle grounding, a patient or therapist, or both, can become a substitute path for leakage current from its conductive exterior, for instance, to any grounded surface, as illustrated in Figure 3–5. Most people have experienced leakage current as a mild tingling or buzzing sensation in touching certain electrical devices that are powered by two-wire line cords. Since resistance of the human body is in a range of 100 to 1,000,000 ohms (depending, for instance, on how much tissue is between the contact sites, and if they are damp or dry), the normally intact ground wire in three-wire line cords, with resistance less than 1 ohm, will divert any nontherapeutic current before it can cause electrical shock. Such current is simply dumped into the receptacle's ground terminal.

Users of line-powered instruments should know that leakage current is a normal phenomenon. Widely recognized standards[5,6] recommend a maximum of 100 microamperes for exterior surface (chassis) leakage. This amount is approximately one-tenth the current believed necessary to stimulate sensory perception. Leakage from an applicator (or electrode) intended for direct patient connection should not exceed 50 microamperes.

In the event of a major degradation of electrical insulation (for example, water seepage into the unit's electronic circuits), an unintended path to ground, or "ground fault," is likely to result. This would produce excessive leakage current, commonly termed "fault current." As with normal leakage current, the fault current would be conducted away from the unit by its ground wire. The fuse, with a typical current rating of 1 to 2 amperes, should then melt open when fault current exceeds that limit.

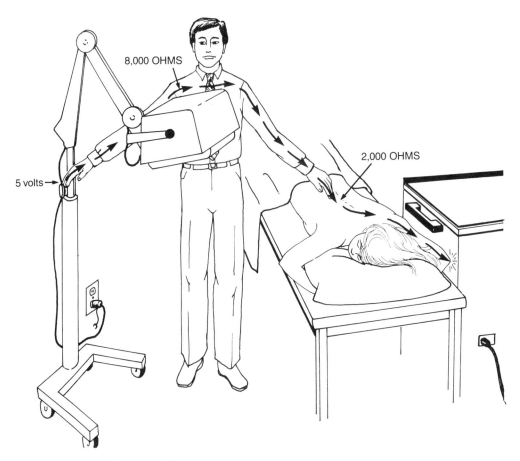

FIGURE 3–5. A realistic leakage current hazard. Three-wire line cord is plugged into a two-blade outlet using a "cheater" plug. Cold pack unit completes circuit to ground.

$$\text{Leakage current} = \frac{\text{Voltage}}{\text{Resistance}} = \frac{5 \text{ volts}}{10,000 \text{ ohms}} = 500 \text{ microamperes}$$

At this point, visualize the hazard that would exist in the absence of a low-resistance grounding connection. The 1 to 2 amperes could end up flowing to ground through someone's body, with possibly fatal consequences. Ground-wire integrity, therefore, must be inspected routinely to verify low resistance between conductive chassis surfaces and the grounding pin of the power plug.

Double insulation is a design technique that introduces a second layer of insulation between the "live" internal components of a device and the operator. Many manufacturers are turning to plastic and other nonconductive materials for chassis fabrication as an alternative method of minimizing risks from stray currents. This usually makes chassis grounding unnecessary, and a two-wire line cord would therefore be acceptable. The device should be labeled, preferably on its nameplate, as being double-insulated. Hydrotherapy devices, however, are an exception; these always require grounding.

Ground Fault Circuit Interrupters

Equipment used in hydrotherapy areas presents a major potential for electrical hazards arising from ground faults. Installation of ground fault circuit interrupter (GFCI) protection for all receptacles that serve these locations can effectively eliminate such hazards. In general, GFCIs are required for all receptacles within 1.5 meters of therapeutic tubs.[7]

Note that the name for this device is nearly descriptive: The (power) circuit is interrupted when a ground fault is sensed. The same device is frequently referred to as a ground fault interrupter or GFI. This terminology is misleading, because it suggests that the fault itself is eliminated.

A sensor within the GFCI constantly monitors the currents in the hot and neutral lines that feed a given receptacle. The assumption is that input current in the hot line of a device should very nearly equal current in its neutral line. A substantial difference of 5 milliamperes between hot and neutral suggests that a ground fault exists and is diverting current return from neutral to ground (Fig. 3–6). Since the maximum safe transthoracic current (through intact skin) is deemed to be 5 milliamperes, GFCI activation is set to occur at this level.

Tripping time is almost instantaneous; a button labeled RESET extends out of its channel when the circuit is interrupted. Once the ground fault is identified and eliminated, this same button is depressed to reactivate the GFCI. Depressing the TEST button generates a low-level internal ground fault, causing the unit to trip. This test should be exercised monthly to verify operation. Annual inspection of GFCIs, using a calibrated external test device, is also advocated.[6]

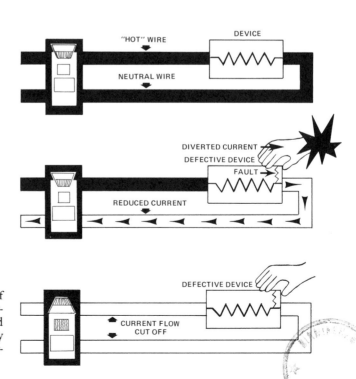

FIGURE 3–6. Operation of a ground fault circuit interrupter (GFCI). (Adapted from Square D Company product information literature.)

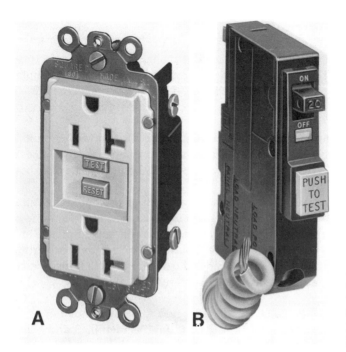

FIGURE 3–7. Ground fault circuit interrupters: (*A*) Receptacle style; (*B*) Circuit breaker style. (From Square D Company, Lexington, KY, with permission.)

A GFCI can be integrated within a power receptacle or as part of the circuit breaker for that receptacle. Figure 3–7 illustrates both configurations.

Isolation Transformers

External isolation transformers are fading into history, as older equipment is being replaced. Isolation transformers are used to lower the leakage current of some older devices that generate chassis leakage far in excess of 100 microamperes, but that are otherwise safe and functional.

As previously discussed, output voltage of an isolation transformer is of the same magnitude as line voltage. The difference is that the secondary voltage is not referenced to ground. Therefore, the leakage current from a device plugged into the transformer will not seek or flow to ground.

One to Six Thousand Milliamperes

The effects of 1-second exposures to 60-Hz currents are summarized in Table 3–1. The current levels listed are average figures; actual effects would vary as a function of many factors, including body size, physical condition, and age. Wet skin also would greatly increase resultant risk current. For perspective in reviewing Table 3–1, it is helpful to know that the current that flows through a 100-watt bulb is almost 1 ampere.

As current frequency increases, its physiologic shock hazards diminish. At frequencies greater than 10 kHz, current of sufficient intensity produces tissue heating with no other apparent effect on the neuromuscular system. High-frequency electromagnetic

TABLE 3–1. Effects of 60-Hz AC Current Flowing Arm to Arm
through the Chest*

Current in Milliamperes	Physiologic Effect
1	Threshold of perception; tingling
5	Maximum current considered to be harmless (Typical GFCI tripping level is 4–6 mA)
10–20	Sustained muscular contractions
50	Pain, exhaustion; possible fainting
100–300	Ventricular fibrillation
1000–6000 (1–6 amps)	Body muscle system contracts violently; probable respiratory paralysis and burns

*Adapted from Bruner, JMR: Hazards of electrical apparatus. Anesthesiology 28:400, 1967.

current is the active mechanism of shortwave diathermy and is most commonly delivered with capacitive air-gap applicators or inductance drum applicators.

Oscillators

As is commonly known, AC signals in radio frequency range can be directed and
transmitted through air. A shortwave diathermy unit, for instance, with a frequency of
27.12 MHz, is just a step removed from a citizens' band (CB) radio transmitter. An
electronic circuit known as an oscillator is used to develop an alternating or oscillating
output from a DC source. Any specific (resonant) frequency can be obtained as a
function of the associated timing circuit's capacitance and inductance. Waveforms
produced can be sinusoidal, square, sawtoothed, or unidirectional pulses, as illustrated
in Figure 3–8.

In physical therapy instrumentation, oscillators are integral to ultrasound, shortwave diathermy, and electric stimulator units. For patient treatment, the waveform can
be either continuous or cyclically interrupted (pulsed).

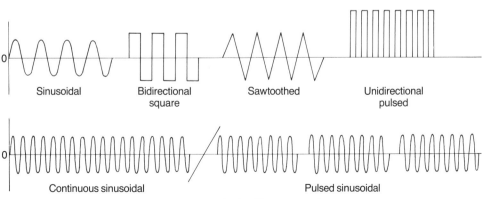

FIGURE 3–8. Oscillator waveforms.

PREPURCHASE EVALUATION
AND ACQUISITION OF EQUIPMENT

Considering equipment costs, and the fact that most devices have a reasonable life expectancy of 8 to 10 years, it is vital that a thorough prepurchase investigation be conducted. Information should be sought and assembled from every possible source. ECRI (formerly, Emergency Care Research Institute) is an independent nonprofit organization devoted to improving health-care technology, facilities, and procedures. It offers three publications that should be consulted in the preliminary stage of equipment acquisition. *Health Devices* is a monthly journal that features brand-name evaluations and ratings based on ECRI's testing. *Hospital Product Comparison System* presents background information on a large number of device categories coupled with a listing of manufacturers and a tabulation of specifications and features by model number. *The Health Devices Sourcebook* is a directory of medical devices, trade names, and manufacturers that is updated annually.

It would be additionally advisable to solicit the experiences of therapist colleagues who have used specific devices in various clinics and departments. Review the following questions:

1. Have there been any major defects or failures? (If so, was warranty service readily available?)
2. Have there been any problems in obtaining accessories or product support?
3. Does the device have any operational difficulties?
4. Can clinical effectiveness be assessed?
5. Is operation of the equipment adequately described for you and your staff members to refer to, if necessary?

After limiting the field to perhaps three models, the next step is to arrange for a minimum 1-week trial period for each unit under a normal patient load. The salesperson or a technical representative should perform an in-service presentation for all staff members who will be evaluating the equipment.

During the test period, difficulties are likely to arise under the varying circumstances of patient treatment. A log should be maintained to record all such problems and relevant patient comments so that they can be reviewed with the representative. Careful documentation will help to distinguish genuine deficiencies in the equipment or accessories from operator error.

When available, consult with the biomedical instrumentation department (may also be referred to as biomedical or clinical engineering), a biomedical equipment technician (BMET), or whoever is responsible for maintaining existing equipment. They should be asked to perform an electrical safety inspection on the loaned equipment and to examine its service manual. Review their experience with the product and manufacturer, and establish whether any specialized test equipment would be required for inspection, repair, or calibration. Consider together whether there would be any unusual assembly or installation requirements and estimate associated costs. If accessories are needed for routine operation of the device, their annual cost should be estimated.

Finally, analyze the terms of the warranty; most are for 1 year. Verify that the warranty will not start until the equipment is installed and functional. Ascertain how this service would be performed: Is it available locally or must the user package and ship the defective unit back to the manufacturer?

The end result of the decision process will be a purchase order (P.O.) for the selected device. In addition to quantity, description, and shipping address, a P.O. should specify:

1. Operator and service manuals (two each: one for the physical therapy department, and one for the biomedical instrumentation department).
2. All applicators and accessories agreed upon.
3. An introductory in-service presentation.
4. How and where warranty service will be performed and, possibly, a maximum "down" time limit.
5. Payment will be made after successful completion of an acceptance inspection.

It may be desirable to notify the sales representative upon delivery of the equipment so that this person can do the unpacking and assembly. If shipping damage has occurred, their representative can handle any necessary adjustments. Otherwise, an in-service orientation can be performed for the entire staff.

In an institution with a biomedical instrumentation department, the new equipment generally will be tagged with a control number to facilitate documentation of inspection and repair. Manufacturer performance specifications should be selectively verified. (For instance, ultrasound and diathermy output frequencies would not normally be checked.) When the unit passes its acceptance inspection, final authorization for payment can be made.

Operator Manuals

Under ideal circumstances, a therapist should be very familiar with a newly acquired device by the time it is put into service. Many manufacturers provide a checklist in their operator or service manuals (Table 3–2) for troubleshooting anticipated problems.

TABLE 3–2. A Checklist for Troubleshooting for a Hot Pack Unit (Hydrocollator M-2)*

Problem	Cause	Remedy
Unit plugged in, water does not get hot with switch on	Breaker for electric circuit off	Turn breaker on
	Thermostat not functioning	Replace thermostat
	Heating element burned out	Replace element
	On–off switch broken	Replace switch
Cloudiness of water	Seepage from packs (worn out)	Replace packs
	Too long a period between cleanings	Drain and clean
Packs too hot	Thermostat set too high	Adjust thermostat
	Thermostat failure	Replace thermostat
Unit boils	Thermostat failure	Replace thermostat
Packs too cool	Thermostat set too low	Adjust thermostat
	Power failure	Check electric circuit

*From Chattanooga Corporation, Chattanooga, TN, with permission.

In addition, operator manuals typically include the following information: indications, contraindications, and precautions for using the device; function and location of controls; serial procedures for treatment. Accessories and methods of application are generally illustrated and described. The stocking of certain spare items may also be recommended. A careful review of all operator manuals, therefore, should be a definite part of orientation for employees new to a clinic.

Equipment Care and Service

Instrumentation service personnel generally estimate that 30 to 60 percent of reported equipment problems turn out to be attributable to operator error of some sort. Before initiating a request for service, therefore, recheck the entire setup and, if necessary, review the operator manual.

In the absence of a pilot light or output power, first test the electrical receptacle with another device. When either the circuit breaker for the receptacle or the breaker on the instrument is tripped (and the institution does not have a policy requiring an electrician or equipment technician to reset breakers), the therapist can attempt the reset. Circuit breakers do occasionally trip for no apparent reason. If, however, a reset breaker immediately trips again, do not attempt to reset it a second time. Remember also to check for a tripped GFCI in situations of interrupted power.

There are three cases of equipment malfunction that should cause a device to be instantly removed from operation. Whenever anyone experiences an electrical shock, smells an unusual odor (chemical or burning), or actually sees smoke, the device in question should be unplugged and prominently labeled "DEFECTIVE—DO NOT USE." Request an immediate investigation by the biomedical instrumentation department. Decide whether an incident report is necessary. Communicate the experience to ECRI directly by phone or with a copy of the ECRI Problem Reporting Form (Fig. 3–9).

Accidental damage will occur: transducers are inevitably bumped and dropped, and fluids have a way of finding chassis ventilation openings. Repeated operator abuse, on the other hand, is inexcusable. Never roll a device over its line cord or pull a power plug by yanking the cord. Avoid wrapping cables and cords too tightly; it is likely to make them intermittent or degrade their insulation. Do not force controls that are stuck, or connectors improperly mated. Significantly, the experience of biomedical instrumentation personnel indicates that the majority of legitimate equipment defects are mechanical rather than electrical. Loose knobs and hardware, broken casters, and damaged strain reliefs are very common defects.

Whenever a nonemergency problem cannot be resolved by the user, it should be reported with ample detail to the appropriate service group. Unless this happens to be the manufacturer, it may be necessary for the therapist first to explain the function or demonstrate the operation of the equipment to the service individual. In most cases, the training of biomedical equipment technicians and even clinical engineers tends to focus on operating room and intensive care unit instrumentation. As a result, their inspections of physical therapy equipment are frequently limited to electrical safety checks, with little or no attention to actual performance. Be prepared, therefore, to review jointly each device in the department and to develop protocols for functional inspections. The next section of this chapter offers suggestions relevant to this task.

ECRI Problem Reporting Form

Use this form to report a hazard or problem related to the use of medical devices or equipment. Telephone, fax, or telex reports are also acceptable.

Your personal and institutional identities will not be revealed in any way without your permission.

Your Name: _____ **Date:** _____
Please type or write legibly

Title: _____

Department: _____

Institution: _____

Address: _____

_____

Phone: _____ **Ext.:** _____

May we identify you to the manufacturer and/or supplier of the device(s) involved? **Yes** ☐   **No** ☐

DEVICE IDENTIFICATION

Please be as specific as possible in identifying the devices involved. Please add any other information that might be helpful and omit any items that are not known or that appear to be irrelevant to this particular problem.

Type of Device(s) Involved: _____

_____

Manufacturer:_____ Model: _____

Serial/Lot No.:_____ Expiration/Use Before Date: _____

How Long in Use?_____ Condition: _____

Date Last Inspected or Serviced: _____Date Problem Occurred:_____

If requested, will you send the affected device to ECRI for examination? **Yes** ☐   **No** ☐

Were other devices involved? **Yes** ☐   **No** ☐ If yes, please identify all other units on the reverse side of this form, including the information listed above.

Are other units of the same model similarly affected? **Yes** ☐ **No** ☐

PROBLEM DESCRIPTION

Could (or did) the described problem result in injury? **Yes** ☐   **No** ☐   **Unknown** ☐

Please use the **reverse side of this form or separate sheets** to describe the hazard or problem in detail. Include how it was discovered, any action you took, and the response of any vendors or manufacturers. Attach copies of any related correspondence, where possible. Sketches, photographs, or copies of portions of operating manuals are often helpful in describing the problem, especially if the affected device is not available for examination at ECRI. Retain all disposable accessories involved in an incident. Please do not send any device to ECRI until requested.

SIGNATURE:

Please mail completed form to:

A NONPROFIT AGENCY

5200 Butler Pike, Plymouth Meeting, PA 19462 · 215-825-6000 · TWX 510-660-8023 · Fax 215-834-1275
This form may be reproduced without prior permission.

ECRI-02-1188 Rev.

FIGURE 3–9. Problem Reporting Form.

DEVICE-SPECIFIC INSPECTIONS

Superficial Heat and Cold

Most devices employed to deliver superficial heat or cold therapy incorporate thermostats to maintain defined temperature ranges. For instance, paraffin bath temperatures are usually maintained between 51°C and 54°C.

Thermostats are mechanical switches that may actually turn on and off many times an hour to achieve temperature regulation. They do fail periodically and require replacement. More commonly, however, control settings are tampered with, both inadvertently and intentionally. Calibration, therefore, may be required at any time. The internal thermometers of therapy appliances must also be monitored during inspections.

Some units may have integral timers for terminating treatment after a prescribed interval. Timer accuracy and actual power deactivation or alarm functions must be verified on such devices.

Hydrotherapy

Again, with whirlpool baths and Hubbard tanks, thermometer precision must be routinely checked. In fact, it is probably advisable that a therapy department or clinic have its own calibrated electronic thermometer with both air and submersible sensors. This will prove useful for occasional spot-checking of any of its device thermometers.

A whirlpool turbine must never be operated without water fully covering its impeller. Impellers should be checked to ensure free rotation: They are often partially wrapped with bandage material that restricts flow and turbulence.

Experience of some therapists suggests the wisdom of securing a turbine to its bath tank with an additional set screw or bolt.[8] This precaution eliminates the hazard of an energized motor falling into a filled tank during adjustment of turbine ejector height.

Inspections of hydrotherapy locations should additionally test the secureness of hand rails, stools, and overhead patient lifts. If a tank is mobile, the condition of its casters and drain hose should be assessed.

Ultrasound

To date, of all physical therapy devices, Federal Performance Standards exist only for ultrasonic products.[9] (A 1980 proposed standard for microwave diathermy[10] was withdrawn in 1983.) Specifically, in terms of performance, ultrasound units sold since 1979 are required to:

1. Indicate the magnitudes of ultrasonic power and intensity with an accuracy of ±20 percent (both for continuous and amplitude-modulated waveform operation).
2. Control treatment time: 0 to 5 minutes, ±0.5 minutes; 5 to 10 minutes, ±percent; >10 minutes, ±1 minute.

Although some generators manufactured before 1979 are still in use, most, with proper calibration, should be able to meet these specifications.

An ultrasound power meter, pictured in Figure 3–10, should be a standard piece of test equipment in a biomedical instrumentation department. Transducer output power is

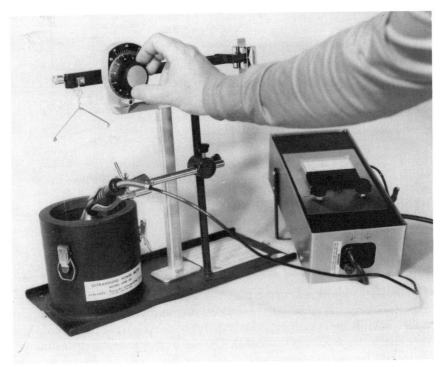

FIGURE 3-10. Testing of an ultrasound unit using a power meter. (From Ohmic Instruments, with permission.)

radiated into distilled, degassed water at 30°C. Verification of output power accuracy is advisable on a semi-annual basis, and recalibration is always necessary when a transducer is replaced.

For more detailed information about transducer beam patterns and intensities, a device known as a hydrophone would be required. Principles of hydrophone operation are illustrated in Figure 3-11. The use of this test instrument by therapists is generally limited to ultrasound research applications. A manufacturer uses a hydrophone to establish and specify the beam nonuniformity ratio (BNR) of a transducer. BNR is the ratio of the maximum intensity on the transducer to the average intensity of the transducer's effective radiating area (refer to the discussion of BNR in Chapter 7).

Most problems with ultrasound units are traceable to either the transducer itself or the cable assembly. A therapist can quickly check for ultrasonic output by wrapping a ring of 1-inch tape around the front edge of the transducer and pouring a half inch of water into this cavity. At a power setting of 10 to 15 watts, boiling agitation and possibly a cone will be observed.

During this test, the transducer cable should be flexed, especially at the transducer and chassis connector strain reliefs. If an intermittency exists, it will be manifested by a sudden decrease or interruption of output power, causing the water agitation to diminish or disappear. Defective transducer assemblies are usually returned to the manufacturer for rebuilding.

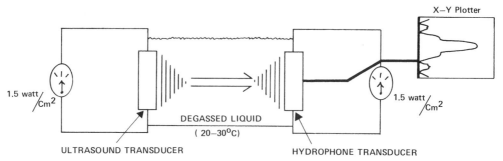

FIGURE 3-11. Piezoelectric materials can convert AC voltage to mechanical vibrations, which can then be converted back to voltage of the original frequency. Using a hydrophone and recorder, a transducer's spatial characteristics can be dipicted.

Diathermy

An accurate, standardized method for verifying output power actually delivered to a patient has not been developed for shortwave diathermy.[11] One microwave unit (TAG MED Model TDS-2450-2) purports this capability. (TAG MED has been acquired by DynaWave Corporation, Geneva, Illinois). The electromagnetic energy actually coupled to a patient and the resultant amount of heating produced are functions of operator technique, exposure time, the anatomy and electrical properties of the treatment location, as well as spatial distribution and temporal characteristics (continuous versus pulsed output) of the radiated energy. At present, commercially available diathermy power meters are of little use other than for gathering baseline data on output, beginning with the acceptance inspection. They merely indicate power delivered to a fixed resistance in a test device.

A simple and inexpensive neon light bulb taped to a tongue blade is generally sufficient to indicate the presence of diathermy output. The bulb will have an orange glow if held near the applicator(s), or next to their cables (unless they are shielded).

Cables should always be kept spaced apart and several inches away from anything that is conductive (mattress covers of springs) or that may be grounded (including other energized devices and their line cords and plumbing fixtures). Also be cautious of some plastics and synthetics (for example, nylon) which, although nonconductive, possibly may be heated by electromagnetic diathermy.[12]

Timers can be tested against manufacturer's specifications. Observe that output power is, in fact, deactivated when a set time expires. Operation of patient emergency cut-off switches and their pull ropes should also be verified.

ELECTRICAL SAFETY

As discussed earlier, electrical safety depends greatly on maintaining the integrity of device grounding, and periodically verifying that chassis leakage currents do not exceed 100 microamperes. For equipment in general care areas of hospitals, a minimal testing interval of 12 months is stipulated by the National Fire Protection Association (NFPA). The NFPA, along with organizations such as AAMI, ANSI, ECRI, and JCAHO (Table 3-3), have developed a variety of guidelines, protocols, and standards for an extensive range of medical instrumentation and facilities.[5,6,13,14] In some cases, legislative

TABLE 3–3. Organizations Dealing with Medical Device
Information, Standards, and Regulations

AAMI	Association for the Advancement of Medical Instrumentation 1901 North Fort Myer Drive, Suite 602 Arlington, VA 22209 (703) 525-4890
ANSI	American National Standards Institute 1430 Broadway New York, NY 10018 (212) 354-3300
ECRI	5200 Butler Pike Plymouth Meeting, PA 19462 (215) 825-6000
FDA	Center for Devices and Radiological Health Food and Drug Administration 8757 Georgia Avenue Silver Spring, MD 20910 (301) 427-8200 or (800) 638-6725
JCAHO	Joint Commission on Accreditation of Healthcare Organizations 875 North Michigan Avenue Chicago, IL 60611 (312) 642-6061
NFPA	National Fire Protection Association Batterymarch Park Quincy, MA 02269 (617) 770-3000

bodies have adopted certain standards and made them binding regulations. Hospitals generally comply with standards, however, to reduce potential equipment-related liabilities and to obtain institutional accreditations.

Appropriate documentation for every inspection (and repair) must be generated and kept for each piece of equipment. An inspection interval of less than 12 months may be indicated if a device has an extensive repair history or if use is especially heavy.

Equipment that is either portable or mobile tends to be repeatedly plugged in and out of receptacles. For this reason, all AC power receptacles and plugs should be hospital-grade quality (usually signified by a green dot). Annual testing of receptacles is also recommended.[6] Such inspections verify physical integrity of the outlet, as well as grounding continuity ($\geq$4 oz).

Generally, documented inspection of devices, receptacles, and GFCIs is performed by the hospital's biomedical instrumentation department or an outside service contractor. Although standards do not specifically apply to private clinics or offices, these locations should nevertheless have grounded power receptacles throughout and GFCIs in hydrotherapy areas. So-called cheater plugs, which adapt three-blade power plugs to two-blade receptacles (thus defeating grounding), and extension cords are never to be used.

SUMMARY

Effective and safe use of thermal instrumentation requires a thorough familiarity with each device, as well as a general understanding of electrical principles. A therapy department or clinic should establish and maintain a file of clinical and technical information for every piece of equipment in use.

Therapists should develop a close working relationship with biomedical instrumentation personnel, using their resources to help evaluate new devices and to perform regular inspection and preventive maintenance of existing equipment. Inspections should verify both electrical safety and performance. Appropriate documentation of all inspection and repair activities must be kept for each device. Electrical receptacles and ground fault circuit interrupters require annual testing.

REFERENCES

1. Licht, SH: History of electrotherapy. In Stillwell, GK (ed): Therapeutic Electricity and Ultraviolet Radiation, ed 4. Williams & Wilkins, Baltimore, 1983.
2. Licht, SH: History of therapeutic heat. In Lehmann, JF (ed): Therapeutic Heat and Cold, ed 3. Williams & Wilkins, Baltimore, 1982.
3. Cromwell, L, et al: Medical Instrumentation for Health Care. Prentice-Hall, Englewood Cliffs, NJ, 1976.
4. Spooner, RB: Hospital Electrical Safety Simplified. Instrument Society of America/Prentice-Hall, Englewood Cliffs, NJ, 1983.
5. Safe Current Limits for Electromedical Apparatus. ANSI/AAMI:ES1, 1985.
6. Safe use of electricity in patient care areas of hospitals. In Standard for Health Care Facilities. National Fire Protection Association 99, Quincy, MA, 1990.
7. Therapeutic pools and tubs in health care facilities. In National Electrical Code. National Fire Protection Association 70, Quincy, MA, 1990.
8. Gieck, JH: Precautions for hydrotherapeutic devices. Clinical Management 3:44, 1983.
9. Performance Standards for Sonic, Infrasonic, and Ultrasonic Radiation Emitting Products: 21 CFR 1050:10. Federal Register 43:7166, 1978.
10. Performance Standard for Microwave Diathermy Products: 21 CFR 1030. Federal Register 45:50359, 1980.
11. Evaluation: Shortwave diathermy units. Health Devices 8:175, 1979.
12. Shortwave or microwave diathermy: A fire hazard? Health Devices 12:197, 1983.
13. Health Devices Inspection and Preventive Maintenance System. ECRI, Plymouth Meeting, PA, 1990.
14. Accreditation Manual for Hospitals. Joint Commission on Accreditation of Healthcare Organizations, Chicago, 1989.

CHAPTER 4

Cryotherapy: The Use of Cold as a Therapeutic Agent

Susan L. Michlovitz, M.S., P.T.

Cold agents are used as first-aid measures after trauma and as adjunctive tools in rehabilitation of musculoskeletal and neuromuscular dysfunctions. *Cryotherapy* is an age-old remedy for pain relief, fever reduction, and control of bleeding and, more recently, has been applied to prevent or reduce edema of traumatic origin and inflammation, decrease muscle-guarding spasms, and temporarily diminish spasticity before exercise.

A number of agents are available to achieve the common goal of reducing tissue temperature. These agents include cold or ice packs, ice cubes for ice massage, ice-soaked towels, vapocoolant sprays, cold baths, and controlled cold-compression units.

The objectives of this chapter are to (1) discuss the physical principles underlying energy transfer with cooling agents; (2) explain the biophysical effects resulting from cold application; (3) discuss the clinical conditions for which cold can be of benefit; (4) discuss the techniques used for the administration of cryotherapy; and (5) discuss precautions to be taken to ensure the safety of the patient during cryotherapy.

PHYSICAL PRINCIPLES

Heat removed or lost from an object is referred to as *heat abstraction*, or *cooling*. When cold is applied, therefore, it lowers the temperature of the skin and underlying tissues by abstracting, or removing, heat from the body. The two modes of energy transfer used for therapeutic cooling include conduction and evaporation.

Conduction

The most common methods of cooling are placing ice or cold packs over an area or immersing a distal extremity in cool or cold water. The body part comes in direct contact with the cold agent. Energy transfer in these cases is by conduction. *Conduction* is the transfer of heat by the direct interaction of the molecules in the hot area with those in the cooler area. Internal energy is gained by the slower moving, cooler particles from the more rapidly moving hotter particles.[1]

The magnitude of the temperature change and secondary biophysical alterations will depend on several factors, including: (1) the temperature difference between the cold object and the tissue; (2) the time of exposure; (3) the thermal conductivity of the area being cooled; and (4) the type of cooling agent (for example, ice versus water).

The rate of heat transfer by conduction can be summarized by the following equation:

$$D = \frac{\text{area} \cdot k \cdot (T_1 - T_2)}{\text{thickness of tissue}}$$

where D equals rate of heat loss (cal/sec); area equals amount of body surface area cooled or heated (cm²); k equals thermal conductivity of tissues (cal/sec/cm² × °C/cm²) (Table 4–1); and T_1 and T_2 equal temperatures of warm and cool surfaces (°C).

The greater the temperature gradient between the skin and the cooling source, the greater will be the resulting tissue temperature change. For example, following a 15-minute immersion of the forearm in a water bath of 1°C, subcutaneous tissue temperature dropped by 24°C.[2] With the same duration and area of exposure at 17°C, the decrease in temperature in the subcutaneous tissue was only 6°C.[3]

When considering the ability of cold to lower the temperature of subcutaneous tissues, muscles, and joints, the time of exposure is important. The deeper the tissue, the longer the time required to lower the temperature (Fig. 4–1). Changes in skin temperature will occur very rapidly (within a minute or less) upon exposure to cold. Subcutaneous tissue and muscle temperature can also be reduced by topical cold application, but additional time is required to allow for conduction of energy. Muscle temperature at a depth of 4.3 cm can be lowered by an average of 1.2°C when cooled with an agent at 10°C.[4] It can take as long as 30 minutes, though, to lower muscle temperature at a depth of 4 cm by 3.5°C using ice packs.[5]

TABLE 4–1. Thermal Conductivities
(cal/sec)/(cm² × °C/cm)

Material/Tissue	Thermal Conductivity (k)
Silver	1.01
Aluminum	0.50
Ice	0.005
Water at 20°C	0.0014
Bone	0.0011
Muscle	0.0011
Fat	0.0005
Air at 0°C	0.000057

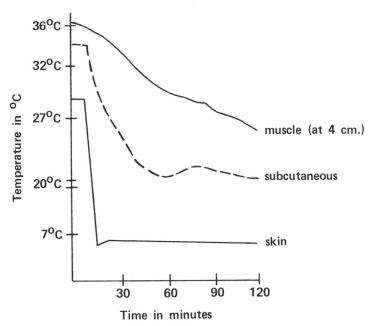

FIGURE 4–1. Temperature changes during ice pack application to the calf. (Adapted from Bierman and Friedlander.[5])

Thermal conductivity (Table 4–1) is a measure of the efficiency of a material or tissue to conduct heat. For example, metals are better heat conductors than are nonmetals. Tissues with a high water content, such as muscle, have better thermal conductivity than does adipose tissue. Adipose acts as an insulator, providing resistance to heat flow (for example, gain or loss). The amount of fat may influence the degree and rate at which muscle can be cooled[6,7] and, conversely, can be returned back to its precooled temperature.

In addition to the consideration of thermal conductivity, the effects of cold on blood flow to the area are important in order to understand why a cooled area can take such a long time to return to the precooled temperature. It can take a cooled area, in fact, longer than a heated area to return to resting values. Arterial blood coming from the body core is warmer than the cooler venous blood returning from the periphery. Arteries and veins course through the body in juxtaposition to each other. Normally, as warm blood flows toward the periphery, it passes by the cooler blood in veins, which are in juxtaposition to the arteries. There is a countercurrent heat exchange between the warmer arterial blood and the cooler venous blood. After an area is heated, the vasodilation of arterioles allows cooler blood to rush into the area and carry away the heat. Cold causes a vasoconstriction of arterioles, decreasing the amount of warm blood flowing into the area. Thus, countercurrent heat exchange is reduced, and the area may not rewarm very rapidly. When ice packs were applied around the knee of a dog for 1 hour, it took longer than 60 minutes after removal of the cold source before tissue temperature returned to resting values.[8] When hot packs were applied for the same duration, temperature rose to peak within 15 minutes, and then began to decline. The hot packs caused a vasodilation allowing cooler blood to flow into the area, dissipating heat. As long as the heat being added was greater than that being carried away, the temperature remained elevated. After the heat source was removed, heat was rapidly lost by convection and radiation.

Intramuscular temperature of the gastrocnemius remained lowered for at least 3 hours following 20 minutes of cold baths at 10°C[9] for at least 4 hours following a 30-minute cold bath at 10°C[10] and for at least 1½ hours following 20 minutes of ice packs.[11] The level of activity can also influence the return of temperature to precooling levels. If exercise is performed following cooling, this will facilitate an increase of blood flow to the area, resulting in a faster rate of rewarming.

The form in which cold therapy is applied (for example, ice or cold-water baths) may contribute to the degree of cooling. The magnitude of temperature change would be expected to be greater when ice packs are used, compared with cold-water baths or frozen gel packs. Quadriceps muscle temperature in dogs was reduced by 11.3°C following 1 hour of chipped ice compared with a decrease of 8.4°C when gel packs were applied for the same time.[12] The ice may be more effective in cooling an area because of the amount of internal energy required to melt the ice; that is, to break apart the solid bonding forces of the ice molecules. The internal energy is used first to change the ice to water before raising its temperature.[1]

Evaporation

Vapocoolant sprays use evaporation as a means of energy transfer. Vapocoolant sprays, such as Fluori-Methane (Gebauer Chemical Company, Cleveland, OH), are volatile liquids that are bottled under pressure and are emitted in fine sprays when the bottles are inverted. As the liquid comes out of the bottle, it begins to evaporate. When this transition occurs, the steam cools and, upon contact with the skin, extracts heat. The vapocoolant spray feels colder than room-temperature water sprayed on the skin because, like alcohol, it evaporates more quickly than water. (The fluorocarbon mixture has a lower boiling point than water.) The spray is applied for only a few sweeps across the skin. Skin temperature can drop to about 15°C, with negligible changes in subcutaneous tissue and muscle temperatures.[13]

BIOPHYSICAL EFFECTS

Many of the clinical uses of cold are predicated on the physiologic changes resulting from tissue-temperature reduction. Cold is used in the management of acute trauma, because: (1) The resulting arteriolar vasoconstriction reduces bleeding; (2) the decrease in metabolism and vasoactive agents (e.g., histamine) reduces inflammation and outward fluid filtration; and (3) elevation of the pain threshold affords the patient more comfort. A reduction in skeletal muscle spasm can be postulated to be an interplay of factors, including a decrease in pain and a decrease in sensitivity of muscle-spindle-afferent fibers to discharge. Spasticity can be temporarily diminished owing to a decrease in the sensitivity of the muscle spindle to stretch. Muscle performance may be temporarily enhanced following short-duration cold. Pain, and perhaps joint inflammation in certain inflammatory rheumatic diseases, can be decreased. But some patients may experience an increase in joint stiffness secondary to the effect of cold on increasing tissue viscosity and decreasing tissue elasticity. When tissue viscosity is increased, and elasticity is decreased, the resistance to motion increases.

Hemodynamic Effects

When cold is applied, the immediate response is vasoconstriction of cutaneous blood vessels and reduction in blood flow. The amount of blood flow to an area is inversely proportional to the resistance factors impeding flow. Vessel diameter is the most significant factor relating to blood flow. Any influence that will cause vascular smooth muscle to contract will reduce vessel diameter (i.e., vasoconstriction). Conversely, when smooth muscle tone decreases, as happens with heating, vessel diameter increases (i.e., vasodilation).

Generally, exposure to cold for a short time (15 minutes or less) results in vasoconstriction of arterioles and venules. The mechanisms of action causing vasoconstriction involve an interplay of factors, including the direct action of cold on smooth muscle[14] and a reflex cutaneous vasoconstriction.[15]

The blood flow to skin is primarily under neural control and plays an important role in thermoregulation.[15] Vasoconstriction of cutaneous vessels occurs as part of the heat-retention mechanisms of the body. When skin temperature is lowered, cold thermal sensors (free nerve endings) in the skin are stimulated, causing a reflex excitation of sympathetic adrenergic fibers. Increased activity of these fibers causes vasoconstriction. This reflex vasoconstriction can also result in a generalized cutaneous vasoconstriction. The blood-flow decrease is greatest in the area that is directly cooled. For example, blood flow in a hand cooled in ice water changed from a resting value of 16 ml per 100 ml per minute down to 2 ml per 100 ml per minute (Fig. 4–2).[16] Contralateral changes resulting from generalized cutaneous vasoconstriction were less pronounced.

As cooled blood returns to the general circulation, it stimulates the heat-conservation area in the preoptic region of the anterior hypothalamus. Stimulation of this area will result in further reflex cutaneous vasoconstriction. If a large area of the body is cooled, shivering will occur as a heat-retention mechanism.

Decreases in joint blood flow have also been demonstrated following cold application.[17] Ten minutes of ice packs at 0°C to the knee joints of dogs resulted in decreases in resting blood flow averaging 56 percent. The flow returned to precooled values approximately 25 minutes after the cold was removed.

The viscosity of blood, in part, determines resistance to blood flow. If viscosity increases, so does resistance to blood flow. The increase in blood viscosity resulting from cold exposure contributes to the decrease in blood flow. Figure 4–3 summarizes the

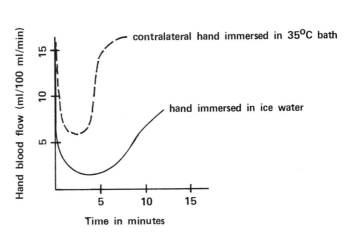

FIGURE 4–2. Blood flow to the hands following ice water immersion of one hand (Adapted from Folkow, et al.[16])

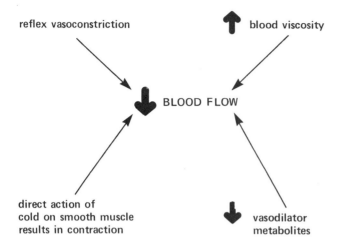

FIGURE 4–3. Action of cold stimulus on local blood flow.

mechanisms of action contributing to the reduction in local blood flow caused by cold application.

When tissue temperature reduction is maintained for a long time, or when temperature is reduced below 10°C, a cold-induced vasodilation can follow the initial period of vasoconstriction. This phenomenon was first recognized and reported by Lewis[18] in 1930. He found that when fingers were immersed in an ice bath, skin temperature decreased during the first 15 minutes. This reduction was followed by cyclic periods of increasing and decreasing temperature, which Lewis correlated with vasodilation and vasoconstriction, respectively. During the cycling periods, temperatures never returned to near-preimmersion values. This cycling was termed the "hunting response," and was felt by Lewis to be mediated by activity within an axon reflex. As skin was cooled to less than 10°C, pain would result, causing afferent sensory impulses to be carried antidromically toward skin arterioles. An unidentified neurotransmitter, termed substance "H," similar in action to histamine, was hypothesized to be released, resulting in arteriolar vasodilation. As warm blood came in and elevated temperature above 10°C, the ice bath was again effective in causing a vasoconstriction.

The "hunting response" appears to occur predominantly in apical areas, where arteriovenous (A–V) anastomoses are located in the skin.[18,19]

There has been much speculation and investigation over the ensuing years to clarify the causes of cold vasodilation. In addition to activation of an axon reflex, some researchers feel that cooling to less than 10°C can inhibit myogenic activity of smooth muscle[2,20] or reduce the sensitivity of blood vessels to catecholamines,[15] thus causing vasodilation.

Cold vasodilation can also occur without the hunting (cycling) component. Clarke and associates[2] cooled human forearms at a temperature of 1°C. A marked increase in blood flow to 3 to 4 times the precooled values occurred after 15 minutes of immersion. Only a slight increase in blood flow was noted with temperatures at 10°C. This cold vasodilation was thought to be a deep response, probably in skeletal muscles, and was assumed to be local, because no reflex changes were noted in the contralateral extremity.

Post-traumatic Edema and Inflammation

For the first 24 to 48 hours following injury, cold is usually the thermal agent of choice. The rationale for its use includes: (1) less fluid filtration into the interstitium, owing to vasoconstriction; (2) less inflammation and less pain; and, (3) a decrease in metabolic rate. Knight[21] hypothesizes that the efficacy of cold for the care of acute injuries is due to the reduction in metabolism and, thus, a decrease in secondary hypoxic injury. The choice of cold has largely been based on empiric evidence. The length of cold exposure and the temperature can have significant effects on tissue swelling. (Some animal laboratory studies will be discussed in this section, while clinical reports will be presented subsequently under Clinical Indications for Cryotherapy.)

In most of the animal experiments, trauma was induced through some type of crushing force, resulting in soft-tissue damage or fracture. Cold was then applied for varying lengths of time. Masten[22] used ice bags following tibial fractures in rabbits. Animals treated with ice, at temperatures ranging from 5°C to 15°C for 24 hours and at 10°C for 6 hours, had more swelling than control animals. The swelling in a group cooled at 20°C to 25°C did not differ from that of the control group.

Jezdinsky and associates[23] also gave prolonged cold for 2, 5, 7, or 10 hours, with a constantly maintained temperature of 11.5°C to 12.5°C for postcrush edema in the rat. They reported a slight tendency for increased edema in the cold-treated animals. In a later group of experiments from the same laboratory,[24] the degree of cooling was less. Cold compresses at an initial temperature of 15°C to 18°C were applied to traumatized rat paws and were changed at 30-minute intervals. Tissue cooling was probably not as great as with the first set of experiments,[23] because the compresses increased in temperature during each 30-minute period. There was no apparent reactive hyperemia after the compresses, as was reported after constant cold of 11.5°C to 12.5°C. Also, there was less tendency for edema formation if cold was applied at 2 hours post-trauma rather than immediately postinjury.

Four different protocols were given by McMaster and Liddle[25] to treat crush injuries to rabbit forelimbs. The protocols included limb immersion in: (1) 20°C water bath for 1 hour; (2) 30°C water bath for 1 hour; (3) 20°C water bath for 1 hour in, 1 hour out, 1 hour in; and (4) 30°C water bath for 1 hour in, 1 hour out, 1 hour in. Results are detailed in Figure 4–4. It is interesting to note that both groups treated at 20°C had greater residual edema at 24 hours postinjury than did the control group. It would have been interesting to see the results if compression wraps had been applied to all groups after immersion in the baths.

No attempt was made by the investigators described so far to correlate changes in tissue swelling with inflammatory exudates. Farry and Prentice[26] applied crushed-ice packs to treat experimentally induced radiocarpal ligament sprains in pigs. Cold was given for 20 minutes, followed by a 1-hour rest period, followed by another 20 minutes of cold. This protocol was probably similar to actual clinical practice. Even though the cold produced an increased swelling in subcutaneous tissues, there was histologic evidence of decreased inflammation. Only 1 out of the 20 treated limbs had signs of a pronounced inflammatory response (that is, numerous polymorphonuclear leukocytes, plasma cells, lymphocytes, and fibrinous exudate). All the others had either no inflammatory cells or occasional to moderate amounts of polymorphs and lymphocytes.

The increases in edema that were observed in the animal experiments described could have been due to cold-induced vasodilation or thermal damage secondary to prolonged cold exposures. The animal studies reviewed do not seem to support the

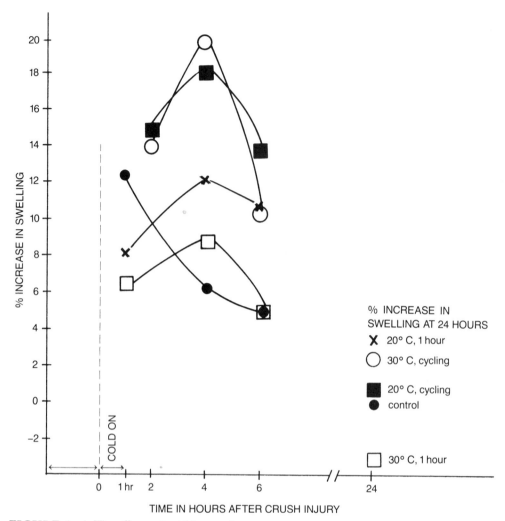

FIGURE 4–4. The effects of cold immersion on post-crush injury swelling in rabbits. Animals treated by "cycling" had three consecutive cycles of 1 hour immersion, 1 hour no immersion. (Adapted from McMaster and Liddle.[25])

notion that cold prevents or reduces edema. Certainly, more animal studies using shorter duration cold followed by compression or elevation are warranted. These would more closely simulate clinical conditions and perhaps further add to our understanding of the effects of cold on edema.

Effects on Peripheral Nerves

Cold can alter the conduction velocity and synaptic activity of peripheral nerves. If the temperature of the nerve is decreased, there will be a corresponding decrease in sensory and motor-conduction velocities, or even a failure of the nerve to conduct impulses. Synaptic transmission can be impeded or blocked. The quantity of the change elicited depends upon the duration and the degree of the temperature alteration.

Nerve fibers of different diameters and degrees of myelination appear to have different thresholds, or sensitivities, to the effects of cold.[27] The most sensitive fibers (for instance, those that exhibit changes in nerve-conduction velocity first) are small-diameter myelinated fibers. The fibers least responsive to decreasing temperature are unmyelinated, small-diameter fibers. A fibers were blocked before C fibers in the saphenous nerve (afferent). Of the A fibers, the fibers with the smallest diameters—the deltas—were blocked first; the largest fibers—the alphas—were blocked last. In motor fibers of the sciatic nerve, the gammas were blocked before the alphas.

Cold can decrease nerve-conduction velocity. Motor-conduction velocity of the ulnar nerve after cold application has been investigated by two groups of researchers.[28,29] Following his study of 5 minutes of cold to the elbow, Zankel[28] recorded an average of a six-percent decrease in motor-conduction velocity in 8 out of 10 subjects. In those 8, conduction velocity returned to precooled values within 15 minutes. Zankel[28] postulated that cold can alter the rate of transmembrane ionic flow.

With longer durations of cold, a greater decrease in temperature and conduction velocity is predicted. Ice packs over the ulnar nerve for 20 minutes resulted in an average decrease in motor-conduction velocity of 29.4 percent from precooling values.[29] Thirty minutes after the ice packs were removed, the conduction velocity was still 8.3 percent lower than before ice application, suggesting a long-lasting effect when ice is given for a longer duration than in the experiments of Zankel. One group of investigators could find no direct correlation between percentage of body fat and velocity or temperature changes.[29]

Li[30] demonstrated in the rat that neuromuscular synaptic transmission was impeded when temperatures dropped as low as 15°C, and that it was blocked at 5°C. The peripheral nerve stopped conducting impulses at 4°C.

Cryotherapy resulted in four cases of neurapraxia and one of axonotmesis, in young athletes.[31] The ice packs were applied either over a major nerve branch that was superficially located (for example, over the peroneal nerve at the lateral border of the knee) or around the thigh for up to 2 hours (as in the case of axonotmesis). One hour of cryotherapy (on two occasions) around the knee of a male patient with a post-hamstring strain was reported as causing an axonotmesis of the peroneal nerve.[32]

Muscle Strength

When designing and implementing exercise programs, the clinician should be aware of the effect of a thermal agent on the ability of a muscle to generate tension. If cold is applied before exercise, could this be expected to alter muscle strength? And if it is applied after fatiguing exercise, will this have an effect on the course of postexercise recovery? Both questions have been examined in part. Most investigators to date have addressed only isometric strength.

McGown[33] measured isometric strength of the quadriceps before and after 5 minutes of ice massage to the entire anterior thigh of normal subjects. After icing, there was an increase in strength compared with pretest values and with changes among a control group. There was no further follow-up reported to see whether strength changed over time. Because muscle temperature was not expected to be lowered by such a short period of ice massage to this large muscle mass, the author felt the increase in strength may have been due to increased muscle blood flow via sympathetic changes. In addition, those who received ice could have been psychologically motivated to perform better post-test.

Perhaps the short-duration cold had a facilitatory effect on the alpha motoneuron pool.[34] This notion is also supported by the finding that the facilitation of single motor unit activity is seen after 1 to 2 minutes of icing over the biceps brachii muscle in healthy subjects.[35]

When the duration of cold exposure is lengthened, muscle temperature can be expected to decrease. Following cold immersion of normal legs for 30 minutes at 10°C to 12°C, Oliver and associates[9] found that muscle temperature and plantarflexion strength decreased. This decrease could have been the result of reduced muscle blood flow at these lowered temperatures or an increase in the viscous properties of the muscle. At 45 minutes postimmersion, plantarflexion strength began to increase over pretreatment values and continued to do so for the next 3 hours (Fig. 4–5).

The findings of Johnson and associates[36] were similar to those of Oliver.[9] Following 30 minutes of immersion of the hand and forearm in a bath of 10°C to 15°C, grip strength was decreased for up to 1 hour, then increased over the pretest values for the next 2 hours.

Neither Johnson and colleagues[36] nor Oliver[9] carried out post-test measurements past 3 hours. Therefore, time to recovery of the pretest values is not known. Also, both groups only tested one repetition of isometric strength at each interval. This paradigm is

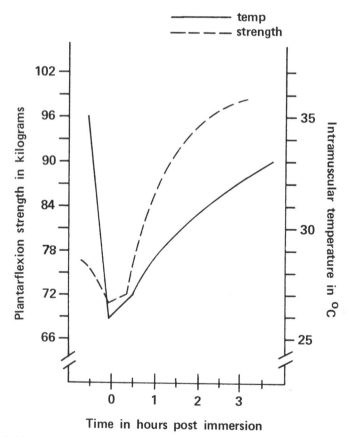

FIGURE 4–5. Plantarflexion strength and intramuscular temperature measurements post-cold immersion at 10°C. (Adapted from Oliver, et al.[9])

not representative of a therapy setting in which a patient often is expected to perform multiple repetitions within a few minutes. On the other hand, Clarke[37] reported that cold baths at 10°C following fatiguing isometric exercise did not alter the period of recovery.

The fact that cold can change muscle strength can have important implications when evaluating patients and carrying out treatment plans. Short-duration cold could perhaps be used to enhance muscle performance during a therapy program, thus maximizing muscle performance. Because cold can change muscle strength, caution should be taken when performing initial and follow-up evaluations on patients during a therapy program. Strength evaluation should be done before cold application to that muscle and not for at least a few hours after cooling.

Neuromuscular Effects

Spasticity limits a person's ability to carry out purposeful movements at the varying speeds required to perform activities of daily living. Spasticity is associated with an increased resistance to passive stretch, increased deep-tendon reflexes, and clonus. Many therapeutic agents and regimens are used to reduce spasticity. Cryotherapy can temporarily reduce spasticity. Although the mechanisms responsible for the changes seen have not been fully elucidated, many animal and human studies have been designed to clarify and provide a rationale for these observed responses.

Eldred and associates[38] directly cooled the gastrocnemius muscle in cats and recorded the discharge of muscle spindle primary (Ia) and secondary (II) sensory endings and Golgi-tendon organs (GTOs). The muscle spindles were de-efferented in these experiments. As the muscle temperature dropped from 38°C to 28°C, there was a linear decrease in the frequency of discharge of Ia and II afferents. GTO discharge decreased by approximately 50 percent. Between temperatures of 25°C and 20°C, firing became irregular and, in some instances, ceased altogether.

Newton and Lehmkuhl[39] also directly cooled cat gastrocnemius muscles. Recordings from dorsal-root filaments revealed a decrease in action-potential firing when muscle was cooled to 25°C. This finding indicates a decrease in muscle-spindle-afferent discharge secondary to cooling. When isolated muscle is cooled, the axonal discharge in cutaneous sensory afferents may be different than when cold is applied transcutaneously.

Twenty minutes of cold packs were applied to the calves of normal humans by Knuttsson and Mattsson.[34] Skin temperature dropped abruptly (by as much as 25°C) within the first few minutes, and the H response increased in amplitude. This increase in H amplitude would suggest facilitation of alpha motoneuron activity by short-duration cold. The amplitude of the Achilles tendon reflex (ATR) decreased shortly after the cold was started and continued to do so during the 20-minute period. Because ATR amplitude decreased before intramuscular temperature fell, activation of cutaneous afferents could cause reflex changes in muscle activity. The ATR continued to decrease as muscle temperature dropped. Therefore, changes in muscle-spindle sensitivity secondary to cooling could also have contributed to the total response. The changes seen probably involve a series of complex mechanisms.

A decrease in monosynaptic reflexes following gastrocnemius cooling in the decerebrate cat was reported by Eldred.[38] Wolf and Letbetter[40] also examined the effects of short-duration cold stimulus on spontaneous electromyogram (EMG) activity of decerebrate cats. Cold was applied to the skin overlying the gastrocnemius muscle. EMG activity and subcutaneous and muscle temperatures were recorded. Rigidity, as measured by integrated EMG activity, decreased within 1 to 5 seconds after the skin was cooled. The decrease in muscle temperature was not as great as that predicted to change muscle-spindle-afferent activity. Therefore, Wolf and Letbetter[40] concluded that a change in cutaneous afferent firing through reflex mechanisms produced a decrease in skeletal muscle activity.

Ten patients with spasticity were studied by Hartvikksen.[11] Twenty minutes of iced towels over the calf resulted in abolition of ATR and clonus. Decreasing ATR activity was seen before intramuscular temperature dropped; therefore, a reflex decrease in gamma-motoneuron activity activated through skin receptors was proposed. These findings were in general agreement with those by Mecomber and Herman,[41] who recorded a decreased tendon-jerk response before intramuscular temperature drop.

After 10 minutes of cooling muscle temperature, decreases in ATR were recorded by Hartvikksen.[11] This observation may be due to a decrease in muscle-spindle firing. The ATR remained depressed for 30 minutes following removal of cold; clonus disappeared for 1½ to 2 hours.

Fifteen minutes of cold whirlpool to the leg also at 18.3°C was successful in decreasing the frequency of clonus or totally abolishing it for 4 to 5 hours.[42] Miglietta[43] studied clonus and muscle-contraction time on a large series of patients with spasticity. Cold baths were given for 10, 20, and 30 minutes at 7°C. Muscle-twitch time was prolonged before intramuscular temperature decreased, but clonus was not abolished in the majority of the patients until intramuscular temperature dropped. Even though contraction time increased and clonus decreased, the author thought they were not directly related to each other.

Knuttsson[44] used 15 minutes of cold packs to the upper extremity, or 20 minutes to the lower extremity, of patients with spasticity. Ten out of 15 patients had a decrease in resistance to passive motion, two had no change, and three had an increase. Clonus decreased in frequency, duration, and threshold in all patients who had displayed it initially. Voluntary range of motion improved in two thirds of those who had reduced range of motion.

Urbscheit and associates[45] reported inconsistent findings following cooling of the calf of hemiplegics for 12 to 20 minutes. H responses and ATRs were measured. In addition to having no consistent changes among the patients in H response and ATR, the patients' uninvolved side often responded differently than the involved side.

This finding points out that the change in spasticity following cold cannot always be accurately predicted. The underlying pathophysiology of the spasticity must be considered in predicting the responses to cold.

In many patients with spasticity, cold application can temporarily decrease the amplitude of deep-tendon reflexes and the frequency of clonus and can improve the patient's ability to participate in therapy programs. Cold facilitates alpha-motoneuron activity and decreases gamma-motoneuron firing. In order for spasticity to be reduced, the reduction in gamma activity should be proportionally greater than the increase in alpha activity. In summary, spasticity reduction with cold may occur through at least two mechanisms: (1) a reflex decrease in gamma-motoneuron activity through stimulation of cutaneous afferents and, (2) a decrease in afferent-spindle discharge by direct cooling of the muscle.

CLINICAL INDICATIONS FOR CRYOTHERAPY

Most clinicians will agree that in the acute stages (24 to 48 hours) following trauma, cold should be the thermal agent of choice. Even though cold may be uncomfortable for the patient during the first few minutes, pain will ultimately be reduced, and edema, inflammation, and muscle spasm will most likely be lessened. Beyond the acute phase of injury, heat may be the first agent for treatment. But in many cases, cold has been a successful part of a therapeutic regimen to reduce spasticity, facilitate muscle contraction, reduce arthritic joint pain, and lessen muscle spasm.

Musculoskeletal Trauma

One of the most common applications of cryotherapy is for musculoskeletal trauma or postorthopedic surgical swelling and pain. One of the earliest clinical reports supporting cold therapy for edema control and pain management appeared in 1946.[46] A comparison was made between two groups of patients who had undergone a variety of orthopedic procedures. One group (n = 479) had no ice packs, while the other (n = 345) had ice bags over their soft casts for a 48-hour period. Even though the cooling period was prolonged, the decrease in tissue temperature was probably minimal, owing to the cast interference between the ice pack and the skin.

The group treated with ice packs required less splitting of casts (5.31 percent) compared with that of the noniced group (41.3 percent). In addition to the benefit of less swelling, the ice-treated group had less inflammation, as evidenced by a lower white blood cell count, and fewer elevated temperatures. None of the experimental group had apparent hematomas or hemarthrosis, compared with 16 of those in the group receiving no ice. Fewer narcotics were taken by those who were ice treated, indicating that their pain was less. Reduction of analgesic intake following cold also has been reported by others.[47]

In most acute-trauma situations, cold is used in conjunction with compression and elevation. The cold can reduce pain and fluid infiltration into the area, but the compression wraps usually are necessary to maintain the decreased tissue swelling. In the animal studies discussed earlier under the heading of Biophysical Effects, it was noted that the cold regimens did not incorporate compression as part of the study design. Basur and associates[48] looked at the more common clinical practice of cold and compression compared with compression only in patients following ankle sprain. One group of patients received cold packs once every 4 hours, followed by a compression wrap using a crepe bandage. The patients treated with cold had a mean period of disability of 9.7 days, compared with 14.8 days for patients receiving only crepe bandaging. Swelling was better controlled in the group treated with ice. The use of ice in combination with intermittent compression pumps is discussed in Chapter 11.

The duration of cold and the extent of temperature drop are important to the final outcome. To lessen the risk of thermal damage and an increase in limb volume during the acute post-trauma or postoperative phases, cold given for 20 to 30 minutes a few times a day, in combination with compression and elevation, would seem to be a logical treatment.

If cold is applied for edema or pain control over casts or bandages, the application time is usually longer than when cold is applied on the bare extremity. Kaempffe[49] recorded a reduction of 3.5 °C when cold gel packs were applied for 60 minutes to upper extremities casted with plaster and with fiberglass. Maximal temperature reduction occurred by 12 minutes over the plaster cast and by 40 minutes over the fiberglass. It should be noted, however, that in Kaempffe's work the casts were allowed to dry for 72 hours before the study. Temperature changes may be different during the initial hours after cast application, particularly over plaster, when an exothermic reaction of the plaster may occur.

Although intuition might lead us to believe that cold rather than heat, during the early phases postinjury, would lead to a faster recovery, this comparison was not reported until 1982 by Hocutt and associates.[50] One group of patients with ankle sprains was treated with superficial heating agents 1 to 3 times a day for 15 minutes and wore Ace wraps within the first 36 hours postinjury. Other ankle-sprain patients had cold whirlpools of 7°C to 10°C or ice packs for the same duration and frequency as the heat-treated group. A third group of patients was seen after 36 hours and treated with cold. Treatment was continued for a minimum of 3 days among all patients. The patients treated with early cold (within the first 36 hours) returned to full activity (running and jumping without pain) an average of 8 days before the other two groups. Therefore, the time at which thermotherapy is initiated following trauma can be expected to influence the time course for functional outcome.

As sequelae to trauma, skeletal-muscle spasm and pain limit mobility and function. Many therapeutic techniques, including thermal agents, electrical stimulation, and massage are given with the common goals of reducing pain and muscle spasm, thus facilitating a more expedient recovery to normal function. In addition, many of these agents could be given in lieu of pain medication. Patients easily can be instructed in the use of cold packs or ice massage for control of pain and muscle spasm at home.

Cooling the skin can elevate pain threshold[51] and reduce pain by acting as a counterirritant,[52] thus making motion more comfortable. During an acute episode of tendinitis or bursitis, severe pain can limit motion and could ultimately lead to joint stiffness. To avoid this, a therapeutic regimen should be aimed at reducing pain and inflammation and maintaining range of motion. Lane[53] reported a patient with bicipital tendinitis who regained full, pain-free range of motion after four treatments with ice massage.

Cryokinetics (cold and exercise) was a technique popularized in the 1960s by Hayden[54] and Grant.[55] Hayden wrote about a group of 1000 military patients who sustained sprains, strains, and contusions during training. Ice massage or ice-water immersion was used to provide analgesia before range-of-motion exercises. All but three of the patients returned to active duty within 2 days; most of them required only one physical therapy treatment. Of the 7000 patients reported by Grant[55] 80 percent had no more than three formal treatments with ice massage. Both Grant[55] and Hayden[54] cite that ice massage and exercise have the additional advantage of allowing patients to be more easily instructed in self-treatment.

Cold in combination with static stretch or contract–relax techniques has been recommended for reducing muscle spasm or decreasing exercise-induced muscle soreness, thus increasing range of motion. Cold is applied over the painful muscle using ice massage, ice packs, or iced towels. Either during or immediately following the cold application, the exercise is carried out with the idea of returning the muscle to its normal resting length. Knight[21] suggests that, when cold is used in conjunction with exercise, the area is first cooled, followed by exercise (active or passive stretch). This cycle is then repeated.

Prentice[56] induced muscle soreness in normal subjects through fatiguing concentric and eccentric contraction of the hamstrings. The following day, EMG activity of the exercised muscle was increased from the pre-exercise measurement. EMG activity was measured as an indicator of muscle pain and spasm.[57] Following 20 minutes of cold packs and static stretch to the hamstrings, EMG activity was reduced, suggesting a decrease in muscle soreness and spasm. Cold application, followed by a proprioceptive neuromuscular facilitation (PNF) technique, slow–reversal–hold, was done with another group. This technique was also successful in reducing EMG activity. These techniques were compared with an untreated control group and two groups who were given hot packs and static stretch or PNF. Those who received cold had less measured EMG activity.

With 15 minutes of ice massage only, pain and range of motion did not improve in subjects with exercise-induced soreness in the biceps.[58] No stretching or other form of exercise was given. The combination of ice and exercise may successfully decrease muscle soreness. The cold may be used to reduce the pain, thus permitting stretching to be carried out. In addition, cooling of 10 or more minutes may reduce muscle temperature and decrease the sensitivity of the muscle spindle to stretch.

Vapocoolant sprays also can be used as a counterirritant to decrease pain, thus allowing an increase of range of motion. In a study on normal subjects, Fluori-Methane was sprayed along the length of the hamstrings as a static passive stretch was applied. In one report, passive hip-flexion measurements were increased more significantly in the group receiving stretch and spray versus a control group who received only passive stretch.[59] A later study, although designed as the first, did not report changes in passive hip flexion.[60] Perhaps different results would be obtained on a patient population with muscle spasm and pain.

A series of patients with low back pain was studied by Landen.[61] Patients with chronic pain (an onset of greater than 2 weeks pretreatment) received ice massage or hot packs followed by flexion exercises. Those patients who were treated with ice had a significantly shorter hospitalization period than did those treated with heat—an average of 6.27 days compared with 9.29 days, respectively. Interestingly enough, however, those patients classified as acute had a shorter hospitalization when given hot packs instead of ice massage, an average of 4.08 days compared with 5.53 days, respectively.

Myofascial Pain Syndrome

Myofascial pain syndrome is defined as "pain and/or autonomic phenomena referred from active myofascial trigger points with associated dysfunction."[13] The dysfunction can be manifested as decreased range of motion in the area of the myofascial trigger point or area of referred pain. A trigger point in muscle may result from muscular strain and may be associated with sensitized nerves, increased metabolism, and decreased circulation. Trigger points also are thought to be present in skin, ligaments, and nonmuscular fascia.

The pioneering work in trigger-point localization and therapy was done by Dr. Janet Travell. She has designated active and latent trigger points. Active points are associated with a decrease in motion and moderate to severe pain. With latent trigger points, the person may have restricted range of motion, but pain is present only on palpation. Trigger points can be located by digital pressure, electronic point locators such as the Neuroprobe (Physio Technology, Inc., Topeka, KS), and thermography.

Trigger points can be treated using a variety of techniques, including stretch and spray, ice massage, deep pressure, ultrasound, electrical stimulation, and low-power laser. The choice of treatment seems to be based upon empiricism.

Stretch and spray is a method taught by Travell that involves putting the affected muscle on passive stretch, then spraying over the area with a vapocoolant while maintaining the stretch (Figs. 4–6 and 4–7). The skin is then rewarmed by the therapist's hand or moist hot pack, and the stretch and spray is repeated if necessary. Spraying over the trigger point and area of referred pain is thought to stimulate cutaneous afferents, producing a reflex decrease in gamma-motoneuron firing and, thus, permitting more passive stretch of the muscle.

Common areas of trigger points can be around the cervical spine, shoulder girdle, and low back. Poor body mechanics and faulty posture are probably contributing factors. Therefore, in addition to stretch-and-spray techniques, a complete therapeutic program should include postural exercises and instruction in proper body mechanics.

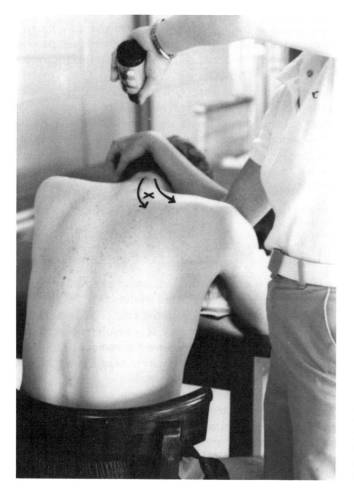

FIGURE 4–6. Stretch and spray with Fluori-Methane. A trigger point has been identified in the levator scapula muscle (noted by the X). The muscle is put on passive stretch and then sprayed.

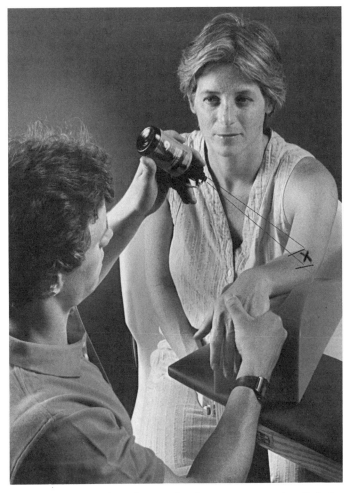

FIGURE 4–7. Stretch and spray for the extensor carpi radialis brevis.

Reduction of Spasticity

Spasticity associated with upper motoneuron lesions often interferes with the performance of activities of daily living and gait. Cryotherapy can be used as an adjunct in the total treatment plan of the patient with spasticity to reduce temporarily the hypertonicity, thus permitting instruction in purposeful movements and activities.

Levine and associates[62] suggested cryotherapy as part of the treatment regimen. Cold is applied over the hypertonic muscle for 10 to 30 minutes. The method of application (for example, iced towels and cold packs) depends on accessibility, size, and contour of the body area to be treated. Once the area has been cooled and the spasticity reduced, an exercise program is carried out. The effects of the cold can be expected to last about 1 to 1½ hours.

As discussed earlier in the chapter, many researchers have documented decreases in ATR and clonus following cold. These measures, though, do not directly relate to an ability to perform skillful and purposeful activities. Hedenberg[63] reported on a series of hemiplegic patients with onset of their disability from 3 months to 10 years. All patients had hypertonia and hyperreflexia in the involved arm. The study was designed to measure upper extremity function, using a standardized test to evaluate if cryotherapy contributed to improvement of function. The hemiplegic upper extremities of the patients were immersed in a 12°C water bath for 15 minutes. Following immersion, all patients improved test scores. Seventeen of the 24 had significant improvements. The greatest improvements in skill were with precision movements involving the thumb and the index and middle fingers.

Certainly more clinical documentation and information sharing on the use of cryotherapy for patients with spasticity should be encouraged. In fact, this technique could be appropriate for patients, caretakers, and family members to apply in the home before exercise and selected activities of daily living.

GENERAL GUIDELINES FOR METHODS OF CRYOTHERAPY

Cold is administered by a variety of means. The methods discussed include cold packs, ice massage, iced towels, cold baths, vapocoolant sprays, and controlled cold-compression units. The choice of which agent to use depends on accessibility, body part to be treated, and size of the area to be cooled. The foot may be best covered by a cold immersion bath, for example, and the knee by a cold pack wrapped circumferentially. Treating the ankle and leg can be done more efficiently with cold packs than with ice massage.

When considering cryotherapy, the therapist must be familiar with the patient's medical status. (Precautions for cryotherapy are discussed in a later section.) Before actual treatment, particularly before ice massage or cold immersion bath, a small area of skin should be tested for hypersensitivity.[64] If hypersensitivity is apparent, this should be documented and the cold discontinued. Generally speaking, conductive cooling is administered for 10 to 30 minutes, with the longer time periods recommended for obese patients.[6]

Often, the skin underlying the cooling agent will redden. This may occur for one of two reasons. First, oxygen does not dissociate as freely from hemoglobin at lowered temperatures; therefore, the blood passing through the venous system is highly oxygenated, giving a red color to the skin. Second, after a 10- to 15-minute period of chilling, or upon removal of the cold stimulus, a reactive hyperemia may occur, bringing a greater amount of blood to the area.

For an hour or two after cryotherapy, patients should avoid stresses that could potentially reinjure or aggravate the pathologies for which they were treated. The analgesia produced by the cold could mask exercise-induced pain, thus giving patients false senses of security. Lowering of joint temperature can increase stiffness,[65] thereby decreasing reaction time and velocity of motion.[66] This fact, in combination with analgesia, predisposes patients to further injury.

Cold Packs

Cold packs can be inexpensively purchased or easily made. The commercial brands usually contain a silica gel or sand-slurry mixture encased in vinyl and are available in a variety of sizes and shapes to contour the area to be treated. The packs can be stored in a special refrigeration unit or in a household freezer. Storage temperature should be approximately $-5°C$ for at least 2 hours before use. For hygienic reasons, a layer of towel should be placed between the pack and the skin surface. Air is a poor thermal conductor; therefore, a moist towel will facilitate energy transfer by eliminating as much air interference as possible. If the towel is wet with room temperature or lukewarm water, the initial contact will be more comfortable for the patient. The packs can be secured by a strap, with the patient positioned so that the area is well supported.

There are some cold packs chemically activated by squeezing or hitting them against a hard surface. These packs are usually marketed for first aid and designed for one-time use only. The chemical reaction inside some of the packs is at an alkaline pH and can cause skin burns if the package splits open and the contents spill out.

Commercial gel packs are suitable for home use. Cold packs remain at a sufficiently low temperature for 15 to 20 minutes. If longer treatment time is desired, the pack should be replaced.

Ice Massage

Ice massage is usually done over a small area—over a muscle belly, tendon, or bursa, for instance, or over trigger points—before deep-pressure massage. The technique is simple and can be taught to reliable patients for home use.

Water is frozen in paper cups to make handling of the ice by the therapist easier. The cup is pealed back as the ice melts. As an alternative, ice "lollipops" can be made by putting a wooden tongue depressor in the cup with the water. The ice pop can be taken out of the cup and held by the tongue depressor for application. An area 10 cm by 15 cm can be covered in 5 to 10 minutes.[67] The ice is rubbed over the skin using small overlapping circles.

During ice massage, the patient will most likely experience four distinct sensations, including intense cold, burning, aching, then analgesia. The stages of burning and aching should pass rapidly within about 1 to 2 minutes. A prolonged phase of aching or burning may result if the area covered is too large, or if a hypersensitive response is imminent (see Precautions for Cryotherapy). Skin temperature will usually not drop below $15°C$ when this technique is employed; therefore, the risk of damaging tissue is minimal.

Ice Towels

If a terrycloth towel is put in a bucket of crushed ice and then removed and lightly shaken, ice particles will adhere to the towel. Alternatively, towels can be soaked in a slush mixture, then wrung out. The towel can be wrapped around a joint or over a muscle from origin to insertion, providing good contact. The towels can be held on by the therapist or strapped on while exercises are performed. This approach allows the clinician easily to do contract–relax procedures for increasing range of motion. The towel must be changed after 4 to 5 minutes, because it will warm fairly rapidly. This method of cold application probably is the most impractical.

Cold Baths

When cooling the distal extremities, immersion of those parts in a cold bath is most practical (unless simultaneous elevation is desired). This approach ensures circumferential contact of the cooling agent. Water temperatures for immersion vary from $13°C$ to

18°C. The lower the temperature range, the shorter the duration of immersion. In fact, immersion at 13°C often will be very uncomfortable. A basin of water or a small whirlpool filled with water and crushed ice can be used. The patient can also be instructed to use this technique at home.

Vapocoolant Sprays

Fluori-Methane spray is a nonflammable and nontoxic vapocoolant spray. This combination of 15% dichlorodifluoromethane and 85% trichloromonofluoromethane is bottled under pressure and emitted as a fine spray when the bottle is inverted. Ethyl-chloride spray, a topical anesthetic, was originally used for trigger-point treatment, but it is no longer recommended because it is volatile, flammable, and can freeze the skin.

After locating the treatment area, the patient is comfortably positioned and the muscle is maintained on passive stretch. The bottle of vapocoolant spray is inverted and held at an acute angle (30°) approximately 45 cm from the skin. Further stretch is applied as tolerated.

When treating trigger points, spraying is done in unidirectional parallel sweeps along the muscle over the trigger area, then over the area of referred pain. If muscle is sprayed to increase range of motion when no specific trigger areas have been identified, then the entire length of muscle from proximal attachment to distal attachment should be covered (Fig. 4–8). The skin should be covered 2 to 3 times, at a rate of about 10 cm per second. Further treatment, whenever necessary, should be undertaken after re-warming, to avoid frosting of the skin. If spraying is done around the face, the eyes should be covered and precautions should be taken to avoid inhalation of the vapors.

Controlled Cold-Compression Units

Controlled cold-compression units like the Cryotemp (Jobst Corporation, Toledo, OH) can be adjusted to selected temperatures (ranging from approximately 10°C to 25°C) and can be maintained during the time the unit is turned on. Cooled water is circulated through a sleeve that is applied over an extremity. The sleeve is inflated intermittently to pump edema fluid from the extremity.

These units are probably most commonly seen in centers that treat a multitude of acute musculoskeletal injuries.

SELECTING A COOLING AGENT

When selecting a cooling agent, the clinician should consider which body area, and how much of the body surface, is to be cooled. For small areas (such as over a tendon, bursa, or small muscle belly), ice massage may effectively produce the cooling desired. If a distal extremity is to be cooled, as mentioned previously, a cool bath will most efficiently cover all surfaces.

When cooling around a joint such as the knee, elbow, or shoulder, or a larger muscle mass, such as lumbar or cervical paravertebral muscles, a cold pack or chipped ice wrapped in a terrycloth towel may be the best choice. Belitsky and colleagues[68] compared the abilities of three cooling agents—wet ice, dry ice, and a commercial gel

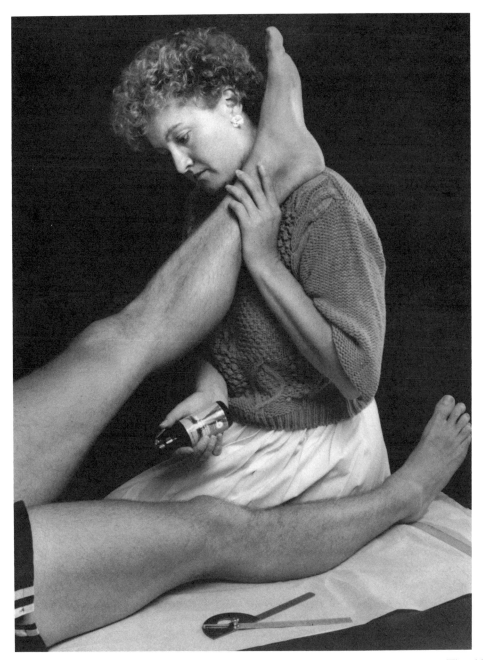

FIGURE 4–8. Stretch and spray with Fluori-Methane spray for hamstring tightness. The skin over the hamstrings is sprayed from proximal muscle attachment toward distal muscle attachment, while the therapist holds the leg with the muscle in a stretched position.

pack—in reducing skin temperature over the gastrocnemius muscle. Average skin temperature before cooling was 29.5°C to 30°C. The greatest temperature reduction, 12°C, was recorded after wet ice (chipped ice in a terrycloth towel) was applied for 15 minutes, while cold gel packs applied for the same amount of time reduced skin temperature by 7.3°C. These authors emphasize the importance of accurate placement of a cold agent over, and completely covering, the area to be treated. Skin temperatures proximal and distal to the ice or other cooling agent were not significantly lowered.

DOCUMENTATION OF TREATMENT

The use of cold in a therapy program, as that of any therapeutic technique, should be based on the goals of the treatment. These goals are determined after a thorough evaluation of the patient, including history of present problem, subjective measures, and objective measures. In order to assist in determining treatment outcome and to be able to reproduce or modify the treatment as appropriate, accurate recording of the technique used and the patient response to that treatment should be documented. Specific to cold application, the type of cold agent (i.e., cold pack, cold bath, etc.) and duration and site of application should be recorded on the patient's chart. Appropriate outcome measures should also be periodically recorded. For example, if cold is used as part of a program to control edema, then this should be noted and quantified. Either volume-displacement techniques or girth measures are used to quantify swelling (see Chapters 1 and 10). If pain reduction is desired, pain assessment should include localization by body diagrams, quantification by numerical or visual analogue scales, and qualification with word descriptors (see Chapters 2 and 10).

PRECAUTIONS FOR CRYOTHERAPY

Cryotherapy should be avoided in patients with cold-sensitivity symptoms. These symptoms include, but are not limited to, cold urticaria, cryoglobinemia, cold intolerance, Raynaud's phenomenon, and paroxysmal cold hemoglobinurias.[69]

Cold urticaria, or hypersensitivity, can include both local and systemic reactions. In patients experiencing local reactions, wheals occur, having erythematous, raised borders with blanched centers.[70,71] Mast cell degranulation causes histamine release into the area, thus markedly increasing capillary permeability.[72] This phenomenon can lead to local redness and swelling, in addition to the wheals. Systemic reactions can include flushing of the face, a sharp drop in blood pressure, increased pulse rate, and syncope.[73]

Cryoglobinemia is a disorder characterized by an abnormal blood protein that forms a precipitate or gel at low temperatures. Precipitate or gel formation can lead to ischemia or gangrene. This condition can be found in association with multiple myeloma, leukemia, systemic lupus erythematosus, rheumatoid arthritis, and some other disorders.[69]

Cold intolerance can occur in some types of rheumatic diseases, following crush injuries, and following digital or partial extremity-replantation surgery. It can manifest itself by severe pain, numbness, and color changes including redness, cyanosis, and mottling.

Raynaud's phenomenon, a vasospastic disorder, can be idiopathic or associated with some rheumatic diseases, particularly scleroderma and systemic lupus erythematosus. In addition, about 50 percent of patients with thromboangiitis obliterans (Buerger's disease) have cold sensitivity of Raynaud's type.[74] Attacks of cyanosis, blanching, or rubor, as well as numbness of distal parts of extremities, can be precipitated by cold exposure or emotional stress.[70]

Paroxysmal cold hemoglobinuria can occur following local or general exposure to cold. Hemoglobin, which is normally found within red blood cells (RBCs), is released from lysed RBC and appears in the urine.

Cold should not be applied over circulatory-compromised areas. In particular, in patients with peripheral vascular disease affecting the arterial system, the vasoconstrictive effects of cold could further compromise an already nutritionally deprived area.

Because cold can cause a transient increase in systolic and diastolic blood pressure,[75,76] care should be taken when considering cryotherapy for the hypertensive patient. If the decision is made to use cold, the patient's blood pressure should be monitored throughout treatment. Treatment should be discontinued if an elevation of blood pressure is noted.

Wound healing may be impaired by cold temperatures. Lundgren and associates[77] demonstrated a 20-percent reduction in wound tensile strength in rabbits kept at environmental temperatures of 12°C, compared with those kept at 20°C. The decreased healing might be caused by a decreased blood supply to the area. Only innervated animals showed this impaired healing response, suggesting a reflex cutaneous vasoconstriction. Until demonstrated otherwise, it is probably a prudent decision to avoid vigorous cold application directly over a wound during the initial 2- to 3-week period of healing.

As mentioned earlier, prolonged cold application, from 1 to more than 2 hours, over an area containing a superficial peripheral nerve (for example, around the medial epicondyle of the elbow or fibular head) can lead to neuropraxia or axonotmesis.[31,32]

In addition to certain physiologic reasons contraindicating use of cryotherapy, the psychologic response of the patient to this form of treatment should be taken into account. Some people have an aversion cold and, thus, would not tolerate this thermal agent. This consideration is particularly important if cold is being used to decrease pain and promote skeletal-muscle relaxation.

SUMMARY

The use of cryotherapy is based on the physiologic responses to a decrease in tissue temperature. Cold decreases blood flow and tissue metabolism, thus decreasing bleeding and acute inflammation. Spasticity and muscle-guarding spasms can be diminished, allowing for a greater ease of motion. Pain threshold is elevated, allowing exercises to be carried out with increased comfort.

Cold can be easily applied through a variety of means, including cold packs, ice massage, ice-soaked towels, cool baths, vapocoolant sprays, or controlled cold/compression devices. Caution should be taken, though, to avoid undue exposure to cold in persons with cold-hypersensitivity syndromes, impaired circulation, and hypertension.

REFERENCES

1. Nave, CR and Nave, BC: Physics for the Health Sciences, ed 2. WB Saunders, Philadelphia, 1980, p 178.
2. Clarke, RSJ, Hellon, RF, and Lind, AR: Vascular reactions of the human forearm to cold. Clin Sci 17:165, 1958.

3. Abramson, DI: Physiologic basis for the use of physical agents in peripheral vascular disorders. Arch Phys Med Rehabil 46:216, 1965.
4. Wolf, SL and Basmajian, JV: Intramuscular temperature changes deep to localized cutaneous cold stimulation. Phys Ther 53:1284, 1973.
5. Bierman, W and Friedlander, M: The penetrative effect of cold. Arch Phys Ther 21:585, 1940.
6. Lehmann, JF and DeLateur, BJ: Cryotherapy. In Lehmann, JF (ed): Therapeutic Heat and Cold, ed 4. Williams and Wilkins, Baltimore, 1990, pp 590–632.
7. Lowdon, BJ and Moore, RJ: Determinants and nature of intramuscular temperature changes during cold therapy. Am J Phys Med 54:223, 1975.
8. Wakim, KG, Porter, AN, and Krusen, KH: Influence of physical agents and of certain drugs on intra-articular temperature. Arch Phys Med 32:714, 1951.
9. Oliver, RA, et al: Isometric muscle contraction response during recovery from reduced intramuscular temperature. Arch Phys Med Rehabil 60:126, 1979.
10. Johnson, DJ, et al: Effect of cold submersion on intramuscular temperature of the gastrocnemius muscle. Phys Ther 59:1238, 1979.
11. Hartvikksen, K: Ice therapy in spasticity. Acta Neurol Scand 38:79, 1962.
12. McMaster, WC, Liddle, S, and Waugh, TR: Laboratory evaluation of various cold therapy modalities. Am J Sports Med 6:291, 1978.
13. Travell, JG and Simons, DG: Myofascial Pain and Dysfunction. The Trigger Point Manual. Williams & Wilkins, Baltimore, 1983.
14. Perkins, J, et al: Cooling and contraction of smooth muscle. Am J Physiol 163:14, 1950.
15. Guyton, AC: Textbook of Medical Physiology, ed 7. WB Saunders Co, Philadelphia, 1986, pp 344–345.
16. Folkow, B, et al: Studies on the reactions of the cutaneous vessels to cold exposure. Acta Physiol Scand 58:342, 1963.
17. Cobbold, AF and Lewis, OJ: Blood flow to the knee joint of the dog: Effect of heating, cooling and adrenaline. J Physiol 132:379, 1956.
18. Lewis, T: Observations upon the reactions of the vessels of the human skin to cold. Heart 15:177, 1930.
19. Fox, RH and Wyatt, HT: Cold-induced vasodilatation in various areas of the body surface in man. J Physiol 162:289, 1962.
20. Major, TC, Schwinghamer, JM, and Winston, S: Cutaneous and skeletal muscle vascular responses to hypothermia. Am J Physiol 240 (Heart Circ Physiol 9):H868, 1981.
21. Knight, KL: Cryotherapy: Theory, Technique, Physiology. Chattanooga Corp., Chattanooga, TN, 1985, p 154.
22. Matsen, FA, Questad, K, and Matsen, AL: The effect of local cooling on post fracture swelling. Clin Orthop 109:201, 1975.
23. Jezdinsky, J, Marek, J, and Ochonsky, P: Effects of local cold and heat therapy on traumatic oedema of the rat hind paw. I: Effects of cooling on the course of traumatic oedema. Acta Universitatis Palackianae Olomucensis Facultatis Medicae 66:185, 1973.
24. Marek, J, Jezdinsky, J, and Ochonsky, P: Effects of local cold and heat therapy on traumatic oedema of the rat hind paw. II: Effects of various kinds of compresses on the course of traumatic oedema. Acta Universitatis Palackinanae Olomucensis Facultatis Medicae 66:203, 1973.
25. McMaster, WC and Liddle, S: Cryotherapy influence on post traumatic limb edema. Clin Orthop 150:283, 1980.
26. Farry, PJ and Prentice, NG: Ice treatment of injured ligaments: An experimental model. NZ Med J 9:12, 1980.
27. Douglas, WW and Malcolm, JL: The effect of localized cooling on conduction in cat nerves. J Physiol 130:53, 1955.
28. Zankel, HT: Effect of physical agents on motor conduction velocity of the ulnar nerve. Arch Phys Med Rehabil 47:787, 1966.
29. Lee, JM, Warren, MP, and Mason, SM: Effects of ice on nerve conduction velocity. Physiotherapy 64:2, 1978.
30. Li, C-L: Effect of cooling on neuromuscular transmission in the rat. Am J Physiol 194:200, 1958.
31. Drez, D, Faust, DC, and Evans, JP: Cryotherapy and nerve palsy. Am J Sports Med 9:256, 1981.
32. Collins, K, Storey, M, and Peterson, K: Peroneal nerve palsy after cryotherapy. The Physician and Sports Medicine 14:105, 1986.
33. McGown, HL: Effects of cold application on maximal isometric contraction. Phys Ther 47:185, 1967.
34. Knuttsson, E and Mattsson, E: Effects of local cooling on monosynaptic reflexes in man. Scand J Rehabil Med 1:126, 1969.
35. Clendenin, MA and Szumski, AJ: Influence of cutaneous ice application on single motor units in human. Phys Ther 51:166, 1971.
36. Johnson, J and Leider, FE: Influence of cold bath on maximum handgrip strength. Percept Mot Skills 44:323, 1977.
37. Clarke, DH: Effect of immersion in hot and cold water upon recovery of muscular strength following fatiguing isometric exercise. Arch Phys Med Rehabil 44:565, 1963.
38. Eldred, E, Lindsley, DF, and Buchwald, JS: The effect of cooling on mammalian muscle spindles. Exp Neurol 2:144, 1960.

39. Newton, M and Lehmkuhl, D: Muscle spindle response to body heating and localized muscle cooling: Implications for relief of spasticity. J Am Phys Ther Assoc 45:91, 1965.
40. Wolf, SL and Letbetter, WD: Effect of skin cooling on spontaneous EMG activity in triceps surae of the decerebrate cat. Brain Res 91:151, 1975.
41. Mecomber, SA and Herman, RM: Effects of local hypothermia on reflex and voluntary activity. Phys Ther 51:271, 1971.
42. Miglietta, O: Electromyographic characteristics of clonus and influence of cold. Arch Phys Med Rehabil 45:508, 1964.
43. Miglietta, O: Action of cold on spasticity. Am J Phys Med 52:198, 1973.
44. Knuttsson, E: Topical cryotherapy in spasticity. Scand J Rehabil Med 2:159, 1970.
45. Urbscheit, N, Johnston, R, and Bishop, B: Effects of cooling on the ankle jerk and H-response in hemiplegic patients. Phys Ther 51:983, 1971.
46. Schaubel, HH: Local use of ice after orthopedic procedures. Am J Surg 72:711, 1946.
47. Conolly, WB, Paltos, N, and Tooth, RM: Cold therapy—an improved method. Med J Aust 2:424, 1972.
48. Basur, R, Shephard, E, and Mouzos, G: A cooling method in the treatment of ankle sprains. Practitioner 216:708, 1976.
49. Kaempffe, FA: Skin surface temperature reduction after cryotherapy to a casted extremity. Journal of Orthopaedic and Sports Physical Therapy 10:448, 1989.
50. Hocutt, JE, et al: Cryotherapy in ankle sprains. Am J Sports Med 10:316, 1982.
51. Benson, TB and Copp, EP: The effects of therapeutic forms of heat and ice on the pain threshold of normal shoulder. Rheumatol Rehabil 13:101, 1974.
52. Gammon, GD and Starr, I: Studies on the relief of pain by counterirritation. J Clin Invest 20:13, 1941.
53. Lane, LE: Localized hypothermia for the relief of pain in musculoskeletal injuries. Phys Ther 51:182, 1971.
54. Hayden, CA: Cryokinetics in an early treatment program. J Am Phys Ther Assoc 44:990, 1964.
55. Grant, AE: Massage with ice (cryokinetics) in the treatment of painful conditions of the musculoskeletal system. Arch Phys Med Rehabil 45:233, 1964.
56. Prentice, WE: An electromyographic analysis of the effectiveness of heat or cold and stretching for inducing relaxation in injured muscle. Journal of Orthopaedic and Sports Physical Therapy 3:133, 1982.
57. Cobb, CR, et al: Electrical activity in muscle pain. Am J Phys Med 54:80, 1975.
58. Yackzan, L, Adams, C, and Francis, KT: The effects of ice massage on delayed muscle soreness. Am J Sports Med 12:159, 1984.
59. Halkovich, LR, et al: Effect of Fluori-Methane® spray on passive hip flexion. Phys Ther 61:185, 1981.
60. Newton, RA: Effects of vapocoolants on passive hip flexion in healthy subjects. Phys Ther 65:1034, 1985.
61. Landen, BR: Heat or cold for the relief of low back pain? Phys Ther 47:1126, 1967.
62. Levine, MG, et al: Relaxation of spasticity by physiological techniques. Arch Phys Med Rehabil 35:214, 1954.
63. Hedenberg, L: Functional improvement of the spastic hemiplegic arm after cooling. Scand J Rehabil Med 2:154, 1970.
64. Olson, JE and Stravino, VD: A review of cryotherapy. Phys Ther 52:840, 1972.
65. Wright, V and Johns, RJ: Physical factors concerned with the stiffness of normal and diseased joints. Bull Johns Hopkins Hosp 106:215, 1960.
66. Fox, RH: Local cooling in man. Br Med Bull 17:14, 1961.
67. Waylonis, GW: The physiologic effect of ice massage. Arch Phys Med Rehabil 48:37, 1967.
68. Belitsky, RB, Odam, SJ, and Hubley-Kozey, C: Evaluation of the effectiveness of wet ice, dry ice, and Cryogen packs in reducing skin temperature. Phys Ther 67:1080, 1987.
69. Ritzmann, SE and Levin, WC: Cryopathies: A review. Arch Intern Med 107:186, 1961.
70. Austin, KD: Diseases of immediate type hypersensitivity. In Isselbacher, KJ, et al (eds): Harrison's Principles of Internal Medicine, ed 9. McGraw-Hill, New York, 1980.
71. Day, MJ: Hypersensitive response to ice massage: Report of a case. Phys Ther 54:592, 1974.
72. Shelley, WB and Caro, WA: Cold erythema: A new hypersensitivity syndrome. JAMA 180:639, 1962.
73. Horton, BT, Brown, GE, and Roth, GM: Hypersensitiveness to cold with local and systemic manifestations of a histamine-like character: Its amenability to treatment. JAMA 107:1263, 1936.
74. Strandness, DE: Vascular diseases of the extremities. In Isselbacher, KJ et al (eds): Harrison's Principles of Internal Medicine, ed 9. McGraw-Hill, New York, 1980.
75. Boyer, JT, Fraser, JRE, and Doyle, AE: The haemodynamic effects of cold immersion. Clin Sci 19:539, 1980.
76. Claus-Walker, J, et al: Physiological responses to cold stress in healthy subjects and in subjects with cervical cord injuries. Arch Phys Med Rehabil 55:485, 1974.
77. Lundgren, C, Muren, A, and Zederfeldt, B: Effect of cold vasoconstriction on wound healing in the rabbit. Acta Chir Scand 118:1, 1959.

CHAPTER 5

Biophysical Principles of Heating and Superficial Heat Agents

Susan L. Michlovitz, M.S., P.T.

Warmth is associated with tranquility and relaxation. Heating injured tissue has been used for centuries for pain relief and reduction of muscle spasm. In physical rehabilitation, locally applied heat agents are used, not only to promote relaxation and pain relief, but also to increase blood flow, to facilitate tissue healing, and to prepare stiff joints and tight muscles for exercise.[1] The physiologic effects that occur as a result of temperature elevation are the rationales for including these agents as part of a therapy protocol. Elevation of collagen tissue temperature, for example, can alter viscoelastic properties, thus enhancing the effects of passive stretch for increasing range of motion.[2]

There are numerous thermal agents available for tissue heating. These generally fall within one of two broad categories: superficial and deep-heating agents. The former are agents that primarily increase skin temperature with little change in the temperature of underlying structures. Superficial, or surface, heat agents, such as hot packs or paraffin, are used (1) to heat joints, such as those of the hand, that have relatively little soft-tissue covering or, (2) to cause an effect in deeper structures, such as muscle, through reflex mechanisms. When the goal of treatment is to elevate tissue temperature at a deeper-seated pathology level (for example, the knee joint or the muscle belly of cervical muscles), then a deep-heating agent is logically chosen. Deep-heating agents, including the diathermies and continuous-wave ultrasound, can increase tissue temperature at depths ranging from 3 to 5 cm without overheating skin and subcutaneous tissue. These deep-heating agents will be discussed in Chapters 7 and 8.

The objectives of this chapter are to 1) discuss biophysical responses to local heating; 2) describe the biophysical principles underlying application of superficial heating agents; 3) discuss clinical techniques and rationales for the use of superficial heating agents; 4) discuss safety and precautions to be taken with these agents; and 5) discuss clinical decision-making principles for logical and effective application of thermal agents.

BIOPHYSICAL EFFECTS OF TEMPERATURE ELEVATION

Many sequelae can occur as a result of an increase in temperature of body tissues. The occurrence and magnitude of these physiologic changes will be dependent upon a number of factors, including: (1) the extent of the temperature rise, (2) the rate at which energy is being added to the tissue, and (3) the volume of tissue exposed. In order to meet therapeutic levels of vigorous heating, Lehmann and deLateur[1] state that temperature must be elevated to between 40°C and 45°C. Within these temperatures, hyperemia, which is indicative of increased blood flow, will occur. Above this range, there is potential for tissue damage. Below 40°C, heating is considered to be only mild.[1,2]

The rate of rise in temperature in response to the addition of thermal energy can influence physiologic responses. Temperature elevation increases local blood flow;[3-9] thus, cooler blood comes into the area and acts to remove some of the heat produced. If the rate of temperature increase is very slow, the amount of heat added could be balanced out by the convective effect of cooler blood so that therapeutically effective levels may not be obtained. On the other hand, if temperature rises faster than excess heat can be dissipated, heat may build up to a point that stimulates pain receptors. The goal of heating is to achieve a therapeutic level of temperature elevation without causing adverse responses.

Physiologic alterations can occur at the site of local temperature rise and in areas remote from the area of heat absorption. Usually, the larger the tissue volume affected by the addition of thermal energy, the greater the likelihood for reflex, or consensual, changes in other areas and for systemic alterations. An increase in forearm temperature as a result of hot pack application could be expected to cause an increase in local blood flow, with no or minimal alterations in overall peripheral-vascular resistance. On the other hand, immersion of a person in a water bath of 40°C could result in systemic changes, such as a decrease in mean blood pressure, an increase in heart rate, and an increase in pulmonary minute ventilation.[1]

A number of physiologic responses to temperature elevation are important to understand when considering a heat agent for therapeutic intervention. The most relevant changes to address include alterations in metabolic activity, hemodynamic function, neural response, skeletal-muscle activity, and collagen-tissue physical properties. These changes, in part, serve as a foundation for the use of heat as an effective therapeutic agent. An understanding of adverse reactions to the addition of thermal energy is imperative for the execution of a safe treatment.

Metabolic Reactions

Chemical reactions in cells of the body are influenced by temperature. Generally speaking, chemical activity in cells and metabolic rate will increase twofold to threefold for each 10°C rise in temperature.[6,10] Therefore, energy expenditure will increase with increasing temperature. As temperature rises past a certain point, usually 45°C to 50°C, human tissues will burn because the metabolic activity required to repair tissue is not capable of keeping up with thermally induced protein denaturation.

An increase in chemical reaction rate can also have positive effects on human function. Oxygen uptake by tissues will increase.[3] Theoretically, therefore, more nutrients will be available to promote tissue healing.

Vascular Effects

Increasing tissue temperature is usually associated with vasodilation and, thus, with an increase in blood flow to the area.[3-9] This blanket statement, however, can be misleading. It is important to know which regions have an increased blood flow. The control mechanisms for flow to different structures—for example, skin versus skeletal muscle—are different. Therefore, responses to temperature change will not always be the same; or if a response is in the same direction, it may not be of the same magnitude.

Skin blood flow has an important role in the maintenance of constant body core temperature of 37°C and is primarily under the control of sympathetic adrenergic nerves.[11] Vasodilation of resistance vessels of the skin will occur as a means of losing heat through local or reflex mechanisms. The skin is unique in that it has specialized vessels, arteriovenous (A–V) anastomoses, which have an important role in heat loss.[11] These shunt vessels go from arterioles to venules and venous plexuses, thus bypassing the capillary bed. The blood flow through these anastomoses is under neural control. Activation occurs in response to reflex activation of temperature receptors or stimulation of heat-loss mechanisms triggered in part by the circulation of warmed blood through the preoptic region of the anterior hypothalamus. These A–V shunt vessels are found in the hands (palms and fingertips), feet (toes and soles), and face (ears, nose, and lips).

Blood flow changes in the skin, as mentioned earlier, can be due to local[5,12] or reflex mechanisms. Vasodilation of the heat-exposed skin can be proposed to occur owing to three factors: (1) an axon reflex; (2) release of chemical mediators secondary to temperature elevation; and, (3) local spinal cord reflexes. Heat applied to the skin stimulates cutaneous thermoreceptors. These sensory afferents carry impulses to the spinal cord. Some of these afferent impulses are carried through branches antidromically toward skin blood vessels, and a vasoactive mediator is released. This results in vasodilation through an axon reflex (Fig. 5–1).

Heat produces a mild inflammatory reaction. Chemical mediators of inflammation, including histamine and prostaglandin, are released in the area and act on resistance vessels to cause vasodilation. In addition, temperature elevation causes sweat secretion;

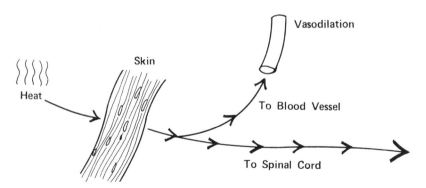

FIGURE 5–1. Schematic diagram of an axon reflex.

the enzyme kallikrein is released from sweat glands. This enzyme acts on a globulin, kininogen, to release bradykinin.[13] Vasodilation of resistance vessels and an increase in capillary and postcapillary venule permeability occur due to the action of these chemical mediators on smooth muscle tone and endothelial cell contractility, respectively. Because of an increase in capillary hydrostatic pressure and permeability, outward fluid filtration from vascular to extravascular space is favored. Therefore, heat within the therapeutic range can potentially increase interstitial fluid and cause a mild edema.

A local spinal-cord reflex is elicited through heat-activated cutaneous afferent stimulation. This reflex results in a decrease in postganglionic sympathetic adrenergic nerve activity to the smooth muscles of blood vessels.[14] A schematic of the reflex is diagrammed in Figure 5–2.

Vasodilatory effects of this reflex response are not only limited to the area heated, but there will be a consensual response in areas remote from the site of application. When one area of the body (for instance, the hand or low back) is heated, increases in skin blood flow occur in distal extremities at areas of the body that are not directly heated.[15–17] This principle of reflex vasodilation is felt to be safe to use with patients with peripheral vascular disease.[15] For example, cutaneous blood flow to the feet could be increased by heat application to the low back.

Skeletal-muscle blood flow is primarily under metabolic regulation and demonstrates the greatest response to increases or decreases in levels of exercise. When surface heat agents are given, minimal to no change in skeletal-muscle blood flow is expected. This notion is supported by two reports on infrared application. Crockford and Hellon[4] measured venous oxygen content following 20- to 30-minute exposures of the forearm. Superficial venous oxygen content increased, but there was no change in muscle blood flow. Wyper and McNiven[18] reported no change in muscle blood flow following infrared treatment.

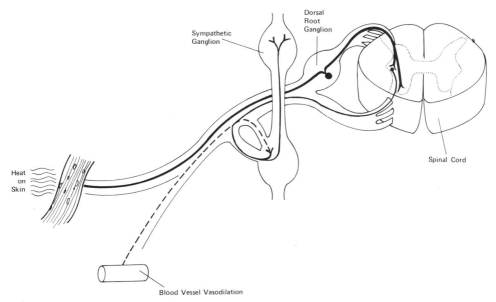

FIGURE 5–2. Heat applied to the skin leads to vasodilation. The change in activity of postganglionic sympathetic adrenergies secondary to local heating is diagrammed.

Cobbold and Lewis[19] measured blood flow to the knee joint of the dog following exposure to radiant heat. The magnitude of temperature change was not as great, though, as when ice packs were applied to the animals. Their work does not support the earlier suggestion of Horvath and Hollander[20] that heat will cause a reflex decrease in joint temperature and blood flow, and cold will cause the opposite response.

Heat is often used before exercise. Both modalities will increase local blood flow. Hot packs alone, exercise alone, and hot packs plus exercise were compared by Greenberg.[7] Heat application was for 20 minutes; exercise consisted of squeezing a rubber ball once per second for 1 minute. The increase in blood flow from exercise was greater than that with heat; but the effects of hot packs and exercise in combination were additive and greater than either modality used alone.

Neuromuscular Effects

Heat is used therapeutically to provide analgesia and assist in the resolution of muscle-guarding spasms. Although the mechanisms of action are not totally understood, the underlying basis for use may relate to the ability of heat to elevate pain threshold,[21] alter nerve-conduction velocity,[22-24] and change muscle-spindle firing rates.[25] In addition, temperature elevation of skeletal muscle can temporarily change the ability to build tension and sustain prolonged activity.[26,27]

Raising subcutaneous tissue temperature by $1.2\,°C$[24] to $23\,°C$[23] using infrared radiation has been reported to increase sensory nerve conduction velocity. The most pronounced changes appear to occur during the first $1.5\,°C$ to $2.0\,°C$ temperature increase.[23] The relevance of these findings, however, to the therapeutic use of heat is not readily apparent.

Heating over the area of a peripheral nerve can elevate pain threshold. Fifteen minutes of high-intensity infrared radiation was administered over the medial aspect of the elbow — that is, over the ulnar nerve. Pain threshold measurements distal to the site of application, over the tip of the little finger, revealed analgesia.[21] Direct heating over the area where pain was measured also produced analgesia. Therefore, heat can be a useful adjunct to reduce pain before stretching exercises, joint mobilization techniques, or active exercise.

Muscle spasms can result from overuse of a muscle during exercise or from activation of a protective mechanism to guard against movement of painful joints. Pain can be the event triggering a reflex, tonic muscle contraction, thus beginning the pain–spasm–pain cycle.[28] The muscle-spindle afferents that alter their rate of firing primarily in response to tonic or static stretch are the II afferents. Elevation of muscle temperature to about $42\,°C$ will decrease firing rate of the II afferents and increase firing of the Ib fibers from Golgi tendon organs (GTOs).[25] Therefore, with decreased firing of II afferents and increased GTO activity, we could predict a decreased firing of the alpha motoneuron, thus reducing tonic extrafusal fiber activity.

Surface-heating agents most likely will not elevate muscle temperature to the degree necessary to alter II or Ib afferent activity. Therefore, another mechanism must be postulated to account for the reduction in muscle spasm when the skin overlying the muscle is heated. Heating the skin has been demonstrated to produce a decrease in gamma (γ) efferent activity.[6] With a decrease in gamma activity, the stretch on the muscle spindle would be less, thus reducing afferent firing from the spindle. This indirect method ultimately results in decreased alpha motoneuron firing.

Elevating muscle temperature can also alter strength and endurance. In a study of normal volunteers, Chastain[26] used a deep-heating agent, shortwave diathermy, over the quadriceps. During the first 30 minutes following discontinuance of the heat, isometric strength was decreased, followed by an increase for the next 2 hours of measurement. Strength and endurance decreases following heating also have been reported in other studies on humans.[27,29] Immediately after immersion in whirlpools ranging from 40°C to 43°C, quadricep strength and endurance were reduced. Edwards and associates[27] found similar results following immersion of the lower extremity in a water bath of 44°C for 45 minutes. The muscle temperature following the 45-minute immersion had reached a value of 38.6°C from a normal mean of 35.1°C.

The physical therapist should be aware of the changes in muscle performance following heat application, particularly when planning strengthening programs or doing valid assessments of performance.

Connective Tissue Effects

Temperature elevation in combination with a stretch can alter the viscoelastic properties of connective tissues.[30] The viscous properties of connective tissue permit a residual elongation of connective tissue after stretch is applied, then released. This is referred to as "plastic" deformation, or elongation. An elastic structure will stretch under tension, but will return to its original length when the load is removed. The elastic properties of connective tissue result in recoverable deformation.[31]

Connective tissue will progressively shorten, and joint contractures will develop following injury, if full range-of-motion exercises are not performed.[32] Adhesions, or the loss of ability for tissue layers to glide past one another, also will develop. Lacerations and crush and burn injuries will result in scar tissue, further limiting mobility.

Heat and stretch of connective tissue will result in plastic elongation. Two factors must be considered in determining effective treatment strategies, including: (1) temperature elevation—site, time, and amount; and, (2) stretch—duration, amount, and velocity.

Greater residual length changes with less damage will occur when a stretch is applied during the time tissue temperature is elevated at therapeutic levels; that is, between 40°C and 45°C.[2] For in vivo experiments on rat-tail tendon, temperature was elevated in a water bath of 45°C for 10 minutes, then elongation was performed and maintained until cooling to resting values occurred.[33] This was compared with stretch in a water bath of 25°C. Length increases were greater in the 45°C bath, with less evidence of tissue damage.[34]

There are three techniques for proposed permanent elongation of collagen tissue: (1) constant load of enough magnitude to overcome tissue elasticity; (2) rapid stretch followed by a period of holding in that position; and, (3) constant rate of stretch using a slow, low, steady stretch.[2] Lower loads of longer duration result in less tissue damage[34] and greater increases in range of motion.[32,34,35]

Joint stiffness is a common complaint among patients with rheumatoid arthritis and osteoarthritis. Joint stiffness has the physical components of elasticity, viscosity, inertia, plasticity, and friction. Joint stiffness in normal subjects and in patients with rheumatoid arthritis is mainly attributable to the elastic properties of joint capsular structures.[36] Following immersion of the hands into a water bath of 43°C for 10 minutes, in one study, there was a slight decrease in finger joint stiffness.[37] Surface heating of the hand to 45°C with infrared resulted in a 20 percent reduction in metacarpophalangeal stiff-ness, when compared with heating to a temperature of 33°C.[36] Clearly, heating can result in decreased joint stiffness and increased tissue extensibility, thus facilitating ease of motion and gains in motion.

PRINCIPLES AND TECHNIQUES OF SUPERFICIAL HEATING

Changes in surface tissue temperatures from superficial heat agents depend on the intensity of the heat applied, the time of heat exposure, and the thermal medium (product of thermal conductivity, density, and specific heat) for surface heat.[38] Superfi-cial heating agents elevate skin temperature and tissues within 0.5 cm from the surface to the greatest degree. In areas of adequate blood supply, temperature will increase to a maximum within 6 to 8 minutes of exposure.[3,7,39] Muscle temperature at depths of 1 to 2 cm will increase to a lesser degree and will require longer durations of exposure (15 to 30 minutes) to reach peak values.[3,39] At a depth of 3 cm, using clinically tolerable intensi-ties, muscle temperature elevation can be expected to be 1°C or less.[3,40] Fat provides an insulation against heat; it has a low thermal conductivity (see Table 4–1). Therefore, tissues below adipose may be minimally affected by surface-heating agents. In order to elevate deep temperatures to therapeutically desirable levels without burning skin and subcutaneous tissue, a deep-heat agent, such as continuous wave ultrasound or dia-thermy, should be chosen.

In joints of the hand and wrist or foot and ankle, with relatively little soft-tissue covering, superficial heat agents can raise intra-articular temperatures.[41–43] In fact, a 20-minute exposure of the foot to dry heat at 47.8°C was shown to increase joint capsule temperature in the foot by as much as 9°C.[41] Even though there can be a reflex vasodilatory response on the unheated opposite extremity, no reflex temperature changes would be expected to occur.[43]

After the peak temperature is obtained, there is a plateauing effect, or slight decrease in skin temperature, over the remainder of the heat exposure.[3,7,39] Typical temperature responses of areas with intact circulation are diagrammed in Figure 5–3.

Conductive Heat Agents: Hot Packs and Paraffin

Commonly used superficial heat agents are hot packs and paraffin. These both transfer their heat energy to the body by conduction. The hot pack or paraffin is at a much higher temperature than the skin surface to which it is applied. Thermal energy is lost from the agent and gained by the tissues. The quantity of heat gained and the subsequent physiologic responses to that heat gain are dependent on several factors, including but not limited to: (1) thermal conductivity of tissues; (2) body volume exposed; and, (3) time of exposure (see previous discussion of conduction in Chapter 4).

HOT PACKS

Hot packs provide a superficial, moist heat. Commercial packs consist of canvas cases, usually filled with bentonite, a hydrophilic silicate, or some other hydrophilic substance. The packs are stored in a thermostatically controlled cabinet in water at a temperature of approximately 71.1°C (160°F).[1]

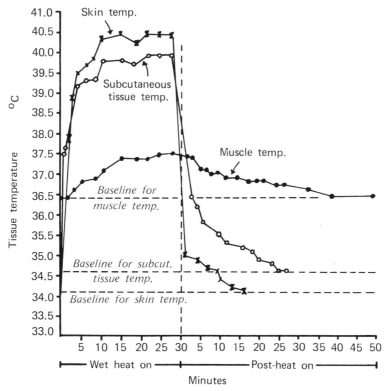

FIGURE 5–3. Curves representing changes in skin, subcutaneous tissue, and muscle temperatures, obtained during and after 30 minutes of wet heat topically applied to the forearm. (From Abramson, et al,[3] with permission.)

The packs are wrapped in toweling before application. Typically, towel layers range from six to eight, depending on individual towel thickness, storage temperature of the pack, and patient tolerance. Commercially available hot-pack covers can also be used. These require additional towel layers, however, to assure safety in application. (As with all the superficial heats, the patient should only experience a mild to moderate sensation of heat during application; following the old adage, "the hotter the better," could result in skin burns). Between treatments, the packs should be completely immersed in water in the heating unit. Reheating usually takes about 30 minutes. Old, worn packs will leak bentonite; they should be discarded when this occurs. For home use, electrically controlled, moist heating packs such as the Thermophore (Battle Creek Equipment Company, Battle Creek, MI) are practical. There are also gel packs available, which can be heated in a microwave oven.

Hot packs come in a number of sizes and shapes and should be chosen on the basis of the size and contour of the surface to be covered. The packs should totally cover the intended area and then should be secured in place (Fig. 5–4). Five minutes after initiating heating, the therapist should remove the pack and check the patient's skin for any blotching—mottled erythema. An uneven, blotchy red and white areas in whites, or darker and lighter areas in blacks, could be a sign of overheating. If the heat is too intense, more toweling can be added.

Patients should not lie on top of the hot packs, particularly when the intended area of treatment is on the trunk. Body weight will squeeze water from the pack and

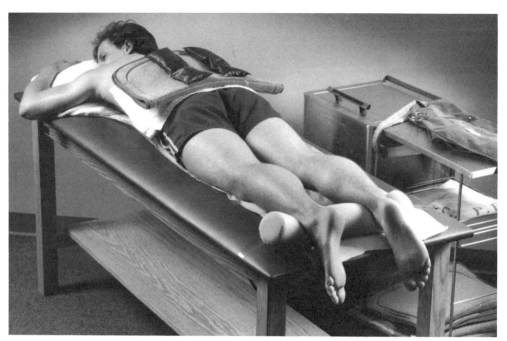

FIGURE 5–4. Application of hot packs for low back pain. Note: the patient is in the prone position. If indicated for patient comfort, a pillow may be added under the abdomen.

accelerate the rate of heat transfer. In addition, local circulation could be reduced, thus reducing convective cooling. Both of these factors could cause overheating of the skin. If packs are recommended for home use by the reliable patient, adequate instruction should be provided.

PARAFFIN

Paraffin wax, with a melting point of 54.5°C, will stay liquid at temperatures greater than 47.8°C when mixed with mineral oil. The mineral oil acts to lower the paraffin melting point; this combination has low specific heat. Therefore, the ability for someone to tolerate paraffin at these temperatures, ranging from 47.0°C to 54.4°C (118°F–130°F), is better than it would be to water within the same temperature range.[44] The lower end of the temperature range is used for newly healed skin, such as skin after a burn.[45,46] The paraffin mixture comes commercially available and is melted and stored until use in a thermostatically controlled, stainless steel or plastic container. There are a number of paraffin units available for home use.

Paraffin is most commonly used for heat application to the distal extremities. (Application of paraffin to the foot is depicted in Fig. 5–5.) There are two principle techniques of application — dip and wrap and dip and reimmerse. For both methods, the hands or feet to be treated should have jewelry removed, then should be washed and dried. If treating the hand, the fingers are spread apart gently; then the hand and wrist are quickly dipped into and out of the tank. This dipping is repeated for a total of 8 to 10 times, until a solid glove is formed. The hand should be wrapped in a plastic bag, then a towel, to help retain heat. If there is a potential for edema to increase secondary to the heat, the part should be elevated above heart level until treatment time is over.

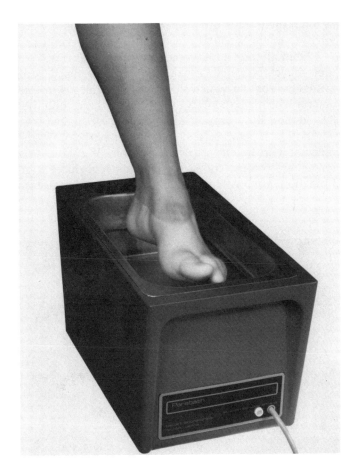

FIGURE 5–5. Application of paraffin to the foot. (Courtesy of Talcott Laboratories, Houston, PA.)

With the dip-and-reimmerse technique, after the glove is formed, the area covered by the glove is put back into the wax bath and kept there for the duration of the heat treatment. The most vigorous responses with respect to temperature elevation and blood-flow changes will occur with the dip-and-reimmerse technique.[47] This technique will not be well suited for most patients, particularly if they are predisposed to edema, or if they cannot sit comfortably in the position required for treatment.

When using paraffin to improve skin pliability over healed burn areas, temperatures of 47°C have been suggested. If wax is applied over a skin grafted area, the graft should be stable, nonfragile, and at least 10 days postgraft.[45] Treatment is daily for 2 to 3 weeks. If areas are treated that are not easily amenable to the dip-and-wrap technique, then the paraffin wax can be painted on the skin surface, using up to ten coatings.

Paraffin should not be applied over open wounds, owing to the risk of burning of the area, nor should it be applied over infected skin lesions, since it could exacerbate these lesions.

Convective Heating: Fluidotherapy

Fluidotherapy (Henley International, Sugar Land, TX) is a dry heat agent that transfers energy by forced convection. Warm air is circulated through a container holding fine cellulose particles. The solid particles become suspended when air is forced through them, thus the properties of Fluidotherapy are similar to those of liquids. The viscosity of the air-fluidized system is low, permitting exercise with relative ease.[48]

Fluidotherapy units come in varying sizes (Fig. 5–6 and 5–7). Whereas the smaller units have the capability of treating only distal extremities, two larger models are available—one in which the lower extremity is inserted to above the knee level, and one on which a patient can lie. With the latter unit, netting covers the area the patient lies on, and the warm air and particles hit against the netting.

Both temperature and amount of particle agitation can be varied. Temperature ranges for treatment are typically from 38.8°C to 47.8°C (102°F–118°F). The lower ranges are recommended for patients who have a greater predisposition for edema formation or who are in beginning programs for desensitization, when they may not be

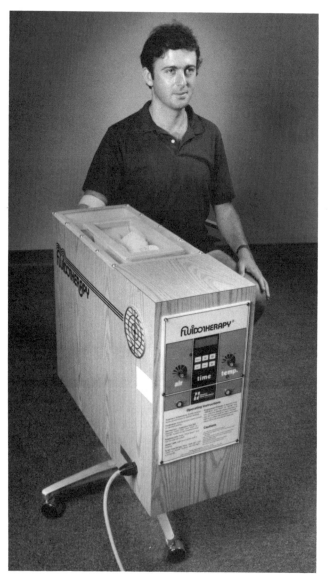

FIGURE 5–6. Fluidotherapy to the hand and wrist.

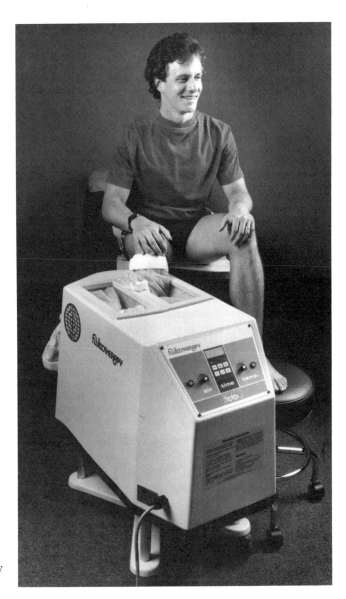

FIGURE 5–7. Fluidotherapy to the foot and ankle.

able to tolerate higher temperatures. Agitation can be controlled for patient comfort. In addition, varying degrees of agitation can be used in a program of desensitization for hypersensitive areas.

Patients can carry out exercises while their hand and wrist or foot and ankle are within the cabinet. If heat and stretch are desired, dynamic splinting can be used during the time of heat treatment to provide a gentle stretch, or stretching techniques can be used immediately following immersion in Fluidotherapy.

If areas with open wounds are placed in the cabinet, the wounds can be protected by a plastic bag to prevent particles from becoming embedded in the wound land to minimize the risk of cross-contamination.

Radiant Heating: Infrared Lamps

Radiant energy is emitted from a substance with a temperature greater than absolute zero. Unlike conductive heating, which requires an intervening medium, this form of energy can flow without a medium for support at an approximate velocity of 3×10^8 m per second. Radiant energy can be absorbed 100 percent by "black bodies," but can also be reflected off reflecting surfaces. The net transfer of heat by thermal radiation is the difference between the radiation emitted by a surface and that which it receives.[10] Human skin acts as a black body — as a nonreflecting surface for the infrared spectrum. Infrared lamps provide a superficial, dry heat.

The energy for clinical use falls within both the near and far infrared spectrum (see Fig. 3–1) on the electromagnetic spectrum. Near infrared lamps, also called "luminous," because they have some visible light in their design, are within the wavelength range of 770 to 1500 nanometers. The generators usually consist of a tungsten or carbon filament that heats up very rapidly when a current is introduced across the element. Because of the visible light emitted, some of the energy is reflected at the skin surface.

Far infrared, also called "nonluminous," is within the 1500 to 12,500 nanometer range on the electromagnetic spectrum. The depth of penetration is slightly less (2 mm compared with 5–10 mm) than with near infrared; therefore, the skin may feel warmer during treatment. With infrared heating, only one body surface at a time can be heated, unlike hot packs, which can easily heat all sides of an extremity. But there is no discomfort from the weight of an object when infrared is used, compared with that of hot packs.

The output of infrared lamps is determined by the wattage. Intensity is controlled by varying the wattage and the distance of the lamp from the surface to be heated. Distance is typically 45 to 60 cm. Using an inverse square relationship, we could predict that the intensity would increase fourfold if the distance is halved. This relationship cannot be taken as an exact measure of intensity, because the metal reflectors surrounding the infrared source must be taken into account. The angle at which the light beam is incident to the skin will also change the intensity. A larger area of skin will be covered by an infrared beam of perpendicular incidence. If the beam is at an acute angle to the skin, it will reduce the intensity by the cosine of the angle (cosine law).[1]

There are low wattage, hand-held infrared devices available for "spot" heating, but the advantage of using this type of device is not readily apparent. Because tissue temperature rises and physiologic responses are very similar with either far or near infrared, the choice of lamp should really depend on accessibility of equipment and staff preference. (It should be noted, however, that infrared is not commonly used in clinical practice today.)

CLINICAL APPLICATION: PRINCIPLES AND INDICATIONS

Surface-heat agents are used in therapeutic programs to assist in reduction of pain and stiffness, to alleviate muscle spasm, to increase range of motion, and to improve tissue healing by increasing blood flow and nutrients to an area. When superficial heat is applied to the trunk, shoulders, hips, or knees, it is usually considered a mild heat. The site of dysfunction often is well below the surface and the heat will produce desired responses through reflex mechanisms by stimulation of cutaneous afferents. Mild heat-

TABLE 5-1. A Comparison of Mild and Vigorous Heating[1]

	Mild	Vigorous
Temperature elevation at site of pathology	Low	High
Degree of temperature increase	Comfortable sensation of warmth — up to 40°C	Near tolerance levels up to 45°C
Rate of rise of temperature	Slowly	Rapid
Duration of peak temperature elevation	Relatively short period	Relatively long period
Clinical examples	Hot packs to cervical area for reducing muscle spasm in upper trapezius	Fluidotherapy at 45°C to the hand for increasing tissue extensibility

ing usually elevates temperature at the site of pathology to less than 40°C and may be thought of as having a soothing counterirritant effect.[2]

When a higher temperature, between 40°C and 45°C, is desired at the involved structure, then the appropriate agent for the job must be chosen. Paraffin, for example, may be a vigorous heater of the finger joints, but only a mild heater of the shoulder. The principles of mild versus vigorous heating are summarized in Table 5-1.

Treatment time with all superficial heating agents varies from 20 to 30 minutes. After this time, no further significant increases in blood flow occur.[3] This duration will allow time for maximal tolerable increases in tissue temperatures and blood flow.

Despite the widespread clinical use of surface-heat agents, there is a dearth of well-designed clinical studies that address the efficacy of these modalities in a therapeutic regimen. In the remainder of this chapter, some of those studies will be discussed, but most of the text will serve as treatment suggestions based on suspected physiologic rationales and on the author's clinical experience.

Reduction of Pain and Muscle Spasm

Symptomatic resolution of pain or elevation of pain threshold can be justification for giving a superficial heat agent before exercise, posture training, or gait training. Muscle spasm can perpetuate pain and limit motion. Alleviation of the spasm can be accomplished by using a heat agent.

Heat may be used before stretching exercises to reduce pain. A comparison was made among normal subjects of the effects of heat alone, stretch alone, and heat plus stretch.[49] In one group, an electric heating pad, at a temperature of 43°C, was used for 20 minutes over the back and sides of each subject's thigh. Then range-of-motion measurements were taken and compared to pretest values. The second group had exercise only, including contract-relax, followed by passive stretch of the hamstrings. The third group had heat and exercise as described for the first two groups. No changes in range of motion were measured with the heat-only group. This greatest change was measured in hip flexion in the heat-and-stretch group, compared with the stretch-only group. This technique of heat application would not be expected to alter the viscous properties of underlying muscle due to minimal or no temperature elevation of those structures. Therefore, range-of-motion increases could probably be attributed to the analgesic effect of heat, which allowed the person to tolerate the stretch better.

A comparison between hot packs and shortwave diathermy (SWD) was made for trigger-point therapy.[50] Hot packs or shortwave diathermy were administered for 20 minutes over trigger points in the thoracic, lumbar, or gluteal region. Heat was adjusted to patient tolerance. Pain was measured at the trigger points by tolerable grams of pressure from a pressure algometer. Both hot packs and SWD were effective in reducing pain at the most sensitive trigger points. SWD was more effective in treating less-sensitive trigger points. (An interesting comparison would be between cold versus heat for trigger-point therapy.)

Cervical pain of varying origins (injury, arthritis, or tension) was treated with hot packs, deep massage, and exercise.[51] About one half of all patients were reported to have "good improvement," but the criteria for improvement were not defined by the investigators.

Hot packs reduced muscle spasms in patients with cervical osteoarthritis and neck or hamstring spasms secondary to poliomyelitis.[52] A decrease in spasm was correlated with a decrease in resistance to passive stretch. A static force balance, which measures the force required to initiate movement about a joint, was the measurement tool used. No comparisons were made to nonheat-treated patients.

Alcorn and associates[53] reported a decreased length of hospitalization in children with pain and loss of motion secondary to sickle cell anemia crises, when Fluidotherapy and exercise were used in combination. The authors also reported decreased dosage of analgesics, increased range of motion, and improved gait. This was compared to the same population of children who were previously hospitalized with sickle cell crises. Fluidotherapy at 45.6°C (114°F), with the unit on which the patient lies, was used 2 times per day for 30 minutes. This was usually followed by 10 to 30 minutes of exercise. It would be interesting to compare this treatment regimen with one using whirlpools or hot packs.

When treating a patient with pain, muscle spasms, or both, the patient's position for treatment must be carefully selected and should be the most comfortable position possible. If muscle spasm is present, the muscle should not be in a position of "undue stretch" until some analgesia has occurred. If the patient has joint pain, the joint should be positioned in an open-packed position,[54] with the ligaments and joint capsule in a slackened position. In this position, intra-articular pressure[55] and stress on joint structures will be lessened.

Improving Range of Motion

In addition to heat decreasing the pain associated with stretching, if the temperature of tightened structures is elevated to high but tolerable levels, then tissue is stretched so that range of motion can improve. The stretch should begin after temperature levels reach their maximum, and a slow, prolonged stretch should be held throughout the period necessary for the tissues to cool back to preheat values. This increased tissue "length" should be maintained over a long duration, that is, up to hours. Devices such as dynamic splints and continuous passive-motion machines can be used to further facilitate increases in range of motion.[56]

Range of motion during one treatment session could be expected to increase up to 5 to 10 degrees.[2] If increases are more dramatic, one could predict that either tissue was overzealously stretched (thus, damaged) or that the cause of limited motion was not due to alterations in connective tissue.

Even though heat and stretch has been well tested in the laboratory on normal tissue, little clinical evidence on contracted tissue has appeared in the literature. There was, however, a clinical report on techniques for stretching burn contractures. Paraffin and sustained stretch reduced contractures in freshly healed burns.[46] Owing to the decreased viability of newly healed skin, more mineral oil than usual was added to the paraffin mixture to lower temperature to 38°C. Certainly more studies or reports on the efficacy of heat and stretch would be a welcome addition to our current body of knowledge.

CONTRAINDICATIONS AND PRECAUTIONS IN SUPERFICIAL HEATING

Before the decision to use heat in a therapeutic regimen, sensitivity to temperature and to pain, as well as the status of the patient's circulation, should be made known to the therapist. An area of skin overlying the intended treatment surface can be tested for sensation using warm and cool objects and a pinprick for pain. This information is necessary, because determining the safe level of heat requires that the patient be able to perceive when pain threshold has been reached.

Patients with circulatory impairment, particularly arterial disease, should be treated by heating with caution, or not at all, over areas of arterial insufficiency.[57] Dangerous levels of heat could accumulate in the area. Metabolic demands will increase and not be satisfied owing to impaired arterial inflow. Therefore, there is a high risk of tissue burns.

A mottled erythema may be an indication of overheating, but is not always a reliable sign. Persons who have had prolonged, repeated use of superficial heat may have a mild erythema ab igne, which mimics a mottled erythema.

Areas that are prone to increased bleeding or hemorrhage should not be treated with heat because of the ability of heat to increase blood flow. Conditions included in this category are hemophilia, postacute trauma (when bleeding may not be controlled), and patients on long-term steroid therapy who have capillary fragility.

Elevating tissue temperature at the site of malignancy may increase the rate of growth of a cancer.

CLINICAL DECISION MAKING

The decision to use a thermal agent as *part* of a total treatment program should be based on a combination of factors, including the patient's diagnosis and medical status, and the objective findings on physical therapy assessment. It is not until this information is gathered that treatment goals are established. The plan of treatment to obtain these goals can include a thermal agent, when indicated. It should be noted that, in most situations, it is only appropriate to apply one type of surface heat modality. To include two, such as paraffin and whirlpool, to the hand in one treatment session would most likely be redundant. Treatment is executed and follow-up done. The procedures for clinical decision making and carrying out the treatment are outlined in Table 5–2.

TABLE 5–2. Procedure for Clinical Decision Making and Execution of
Treatment with a Thermal Agent

1. Assess patient
2. Establish treatment goals based on results of patient assessment.
3. Select treatment plan including thermal agent when applicable to meet these goals.
4. Choose thermal agent.
5. Select position for treatment.
6. Apply thermal agent (followed by exercise or other appropriate techniques).
7. Reassess and determine if treatment will continue or be modified or discontinued.
8. Establish home program (which can include a thermal agent).

Heat Versus Cold

There are clinical situations when either heat or cold may be selected to meet treatment objectives, or when one is clearly preferred over the other. Often the choice between heat and cold is empirical, but before the decision is made, certain factors should be considered: (1) stage of injury or disease; (2) area of body treated; (3) medical status; (4) patient preference, which may be determined by cold or heat hypersensitivity; and (5) decision to use thermal agents as part of a home program. Cold is the preferred agent during the acute stages of inflammation; heat at this stage may further aggravate inflammation. In patients who can tolerate cryotherapy, this may be chosen for reduction of muscle spasm (see discussion, Chapter 4). Cold also can reduce pain around joints before range-of-motion exercises and may be easier for the patient to apply at home. On the other hand, heat may be better psychologically tolerated by persons with pain or muscle spasm, thus increasing patient compliance with treatment programs. Temperature elevation will decrease joint stiffness and increase connective tissue extensibility; so, clearly, if the treatment goal is either of these, heat is the agent of choice. In addition, heat to distal extremities seems to be tolerated better than cold.

A sample clinical case is described in Figure 5–8, in which either heat or cold can be considered as part of the therapeutic program. The advantages and disadvantages of the thermal agents are listed and the outcome determined from the process.

Superficial Versus Deep Heat

The decision to use superficial versus deep heat primarily depends on the location of the involved structure and the degree of temperature elevation desired. Generally speaking, though, deep heat is usually selected during the phases after an injury or a disease when tissue contracture persists.

Wet Versus Dry Heat

Many patients say they have heard that moist heat is more penetrating, and thus more effective, than dry heat. Clinical studies that examine the efficacy of one versus the other in obtaining treatment goals are not available. It has been determined, however, that dry heat can elevate surface temperatures to a greater degree, but that moist heat can elevate temperature to a slightly deeper tissue level.[58]

PATIENT CASE

A 25-year old female is seen in physical therapy 8 weeks following reduction and casting of a right Colles' fracture. The cast was removed yesterday. There is mild swelling on the dorsum of the hand. Range of motion of the wrist is limited in all planes. Metacarpophalangeal (MCP) flexion is reduced in all digits. Pain is present on active and passive motion but not at rest.

Assessment Techniques

  1. Volumetrics of hand and wrist
  2. Pain quantity, quality, and location
  3. Range of motion measurement

Goals

  1. Reduce and maintain reduction of edema.
  2. Reduce pain.
  3. Increase range of motion of wrist and MCPs.

TREATMENT CHOICE: HEAT VS COLD

Heat		Cold	
Advantages: ↓ pain ↑ tissue extensibility ↓ stiffness	*Disadvantages:* May cause ↑ swelling	*Advantages:* May prevent further swelling ↓ pain	*Disadvantages:* ↑ stiffness ↓ tissue extensibility

DECISION

Heat agent—paraffin

RATIONALE

Owing to the period of immobilization, one would expect that decreased range of motion is due to capsular shortening and adhesions. Heat followed by exercise can increase tissue extensibility. Paraffin application can be expected to increase temperature of the involved structures. With paraffin on, the hand can be elevated during treatment to help prevent further edema. Passive and active exercises can be performed in elevation following the removal of the paraffin glove.

FIGURE 5–8. Clinical decision making: heat versus cold. A patient case is presented, goals are defined, and advantages and disadvantages of heat and cold for this case are then outlined. The treatment decision and rationale for the choice is given. (Note: The reader should first cover over the decision and rationale, then uncover them after having had time to formulate a decision.)

Until otherwise proven, it is probably safe to say that the choice between moist and dry heat depends on patient preference and availability or accessibility of the thermal agent in the clinical setting or for home use.

Home Application of Superficial Heat Agents

In most cases, it is desirable to provide a patient with a means for pain control and reduction of stiffness before exercise, when they are not within the confines of a supervised clinical situation. Electric moist-heat pads or gel packs, which can be heated in a microwave oven, are available; so are both paraffin and Fluidotherapy units for the hand and wrist. Adequate instructions should be written down, to include treatment time, method, and frequency of application and special precautions.

DOCUMENTATION OF TREATMENT

The astute clinician realizes the importance of documenting the specifics of treatment techniques and patient response to therapeutic intervention. Information included in the treatment record should include the thermal agent used, duration of application, body area treated, and patient position for treatment. If the technique is modified, this also should be noted in the patient record. Without such information, it is often difficult to replicate techniques and to adjust the plan of care as needed. A copy of home instructions should be kept with the patient's file.

SUMMARY

The use of heat in a therapeutic program is predicated on the biophysical effects of temperature elevation, including elevation of pain threshold, decrease in muscle spasm, decrease in joint stiffness, increase in blood flow, and increase in collagen tissue extensibility.

Superficial heat agents include hot packs, infrared, Fluidotherapy, and paraffin. Guidelines for their clinical and home uses and safety precautions have been presented.

REFERENCES

1. Lehmann, JF and deLateur, BJ: Therapeutic heat. In Lehmann, JF (ed): Therapeutic Heat and Cold, ed 4. Williams & Wilkins, Baltimore, 1990.
2. Warren, CG: The use of heat and cold in the treatment of common musculoskeletal disorders. In Kessler, RM and Hertling, D: Management of Common Musculoskeletal Disorders. Harper & Row, Philadelphia, 1983.
3. Abramson, DI, et al: Changes in blood flow, oxygen uptake and tissue temperatures produced by the topical application of wet heat. Arch Phys Med Rehabil 42:305, 1961.
4. Crockford, GW and Hellon, RF: Vascular responses of human skin to infra-red radiation. J Physiol 149:424, 1959.
5. Crockford, GW, Hellon, RF, and Parkhouse, J: Thermal vasomotor response in human skin mediated by local mechanism. J Physiol 161:10, 1962.
6. Fischer, E and Solomon, S: Physiological responses to heat and cold. In Licht, S (ed): Therapeutic Heat and Cold, ed 2. Waverly Press, Baltimore, 1965.
7. Greenberg, RS: The effects of hot packs and exercise on local blood flow. Phys Ther 52:273, 1972.
8. Krusen, EM, et al: Effects of hot packs on peripheral circulation. Arch Phys Med 31:145, 1950.

9. Randall, BF, Imig, CJ, and Hines, HM: Effects of some physical therapies on blood flow. Arch Phys Med 33:73, 1952.
10. Hardy, JD and Bard, P: Body temperature regulation. In Mountcastle, VB (ed): Medical Physiology, Vol 2, ed 13. CV Mosby, St. Louis, 1974.
11. Berne, R and Levy, MN: Cardiovascular Physiology, ed 4. CV Mosby, St. Louis, 1981.
12. Fox, HH and Hilton, SM: Bradykinin formation in human skin as a factor in heat vasodilation. J Physiol 142:219, 1958.
13. Milnor, WR: Autonomic and peripheral control mechanisms. In Mountcastle, VB (ed): Medical Physiology, Vol 2, ed 13. CV Mosby, St. Louis, 1974.
14. Guyton, AC: Textbook of Medical Physiology, ed 7. WB Saunders, Philadelphia, 1986.
15. Abramson, DI, et al: Changes in blood flow, O_2 uptake and tissue temperatures produced by therapeutic physical agents. III. Effect of indirect or reflex vasodilation. Am J Phys Med 404:5, 1961.
16. Abramson, DI, et al: Indirect vasodilation in thermotherapy. Arch Phys Med Rehabil 46:412, 1965.
17. Wessman, MS and Kottke, FJ: The effect of indirect heating on peripheral blood flow, pulse rate, blood pressure and temperature. Arch Phys Med Rehabil 48:567, 1967.
18. Wyper, DJ and McNiven, DR: Effects of some physiotherapeutic agents on skeletal muscle blood flow. Physiotherapy 62:83, 1976.
19. Cobbold, AF and Lewis, OJ: Blood flow to the knee joint of the dog: Effect of heating, cooling and adrenaline. J Physiol 132:379, 1956.
20. Horvath, SM and Hollander, JL: Intra-articular temperature as a measure of joint reaction. J Clin Invest 28:469, 1949.
21. Lehmann, JD, Brunner, GD, and Stow, RW: Pain threshold measurements after therapeutic application of ultrasound, microwaves and infrared. Arch Phys Med Rehabil 39:560, 1958.
22. Abramson, DL, et al: Effect of tissue temperatures and blood flow on motor nerve conduction velocity. JAMA 198:1082, 1966.
23. Currier, DP and Kramer, JF: Sensory nerve conduction: Heating effects of ultrasound and infrared. Physiother Can 34:241, 1982.
24. Halle, JS, Scoville, CR, and Greathouse, DG: Ultrasound's effect on the conduction latency of the superficial radial nerve in man. Phys Ther 61:345, 1981.
25. Mense, S: Effects of temperature on the discharges of muscle spindles and tendon organs. Pflugers Arch 374:159, 1978.
26. Chastain, PB: The effect of deep heat on isometric strength. Phys Ther 58:543, 1978.
27. Edwards, HT, et al: Effect of temperature on muscle energy metabolism and endurance during successive isometric contractions, sustained to fatigue, of the quadriceps muscle in man. J Physiol 220:335, 1972.
28. DeVries, H: Quantitative electromyographic investigation of the spasms theory of muscle pain. Am J Phys Med 45:119, 1966.
29. Wickstrom, R and Polk, C: Effect of whirlpool on the strength endurance of the quadriceps muscle in trained male adolescents. Am J Phys Med 40:91, 1961.
30. LeBan, MM: Collagen tissue: Implications of its response to stress in vitro. Arch Phys Med Rehabil 43:461, 1962.
31. Sapega, AA, et al: Biophysical factors in range-of-motion exercise. Phys Sports Med 9:57, 1981.
32. Kottke, FJ, Pauley, DL, and Ptak, RA: The rationale for prolonged stretching for correction of shortening of connective tissue. Arch Phys Med Rehabil 47:345, 1966.
33. Lehmann, JF: Effect of therapeutic temperatures on tendon extensibility. Arch Phys Med Rehabil 51:481, 1970.
34. Warren, GC, Lehmann, JF, and Koblanski, JN: Heat and stretch procedures: An evaluation using rat tail tendon. Arch Phys Med Rehabil 57:122, 1976.
35. Light, KE, et al: Low-load prolonged stretch vs. high-load brief stretch in treating knee contractures. Phys Ther 64:330, 1984.
36. Wright, V and Johns, RJ: Physical factors concerned with the stiffness of normal and diseased joints. Bull Johns Hopkins Hosp 106:215, 1960.
37. Backlund, L and Tiselius, P: Objective measurement of joint stiffness in rheumatoid arthritis. Acta Rheum Scand 13:275, 1967.
38. Hendler, E, Crosbie, R, and Hardy, JD: Measurement of heating of the skin during exposure to infrared radiation. J Appl Physiol 12:177, 1958.
39. Lehmann, JF, et al: Temperature distributions in the human thigh produced by infrared, hot pack and microwave applications. Arch Phys Med Rehabil 47:291, 1966.
40. Whyte, HM and Reader, SR: Effectiveness of different forms of heating. Ann Rheum Dis 10:449, 1951.
41. Borrell, RM, et al: Comparison of in vivo temperatures produced by hydrotherapy, paraffin wax treatment and Fluidotherapy. Phys Ther 60:1273, 1980.
42. Mainardi, CL, et al: Rheumatoid arthritis: Failure of daily heat therapy to affect its progression. Arch Phys Med Rehabil 60:390, 1979.
43. Wakim, KG, Porter, AN, and Krusen, KH: Influence of physical agents and of certain drugs on intra-articular temperature. Arch Phys Med Rehabil 32:714, 1951.
44. Zeiter, WJ: Clinical application of the paraffin bath. Arch Phys Ther 20:469, 1939.

45. Burns, SP and Conin, TA: The use of paraffin wax in the treatment of burns. Physiother Can 39:258, 1987.
46. Head, MD and Helms, PA: Paraffin and sustained stretching in the treatment of burn contractures. Burns 4:136, 1977.
47. Abramson, DI, et al: Effect of paraffin bath and hot fomentation on local tissue temperature. Arch Phys Med Rehabil 45:87, 1965.
48. Borrell, RM, et al: Fluidotherapy: Evaluation of a new heat modality. Arch Phys Med Rehabil 58:69, 1977.
49. Harrison, AS, et al: The effect of heat and stretching on the range of hip motion. Journal of Orthopaedics and Sports Physical Therapy 6:110, 1984.
50. McGray, RE and Patton, NJ: Pain relief at trigger points: A comparison of moist heat and shortwave diathermy. Journal of Orthopaedics and Sports Physical Therapy 5:175, 1984.
51. Cordray, YM and Krusen, EM: Use of hydrocollator packs in the treatment of neck and shoulder pains. Arch Phys Med Rehabil 39:105, 1959.
52. Fountain, FP, Gersten, JW, and Senger, O: Decrease in muscle spasm produced by ultrasound, hot packs and IR. Arch Phys Med Rehabil 41:293, 1960.
53. Alcorn, R, et al: Fluidotherapy® and exercise in the management of sickle cell anemia. Phys Ther 10:1520, 1984.
54. Kessler, RM and Hertling, D: Management of Common Musculoskeletal Disorders. Harper & Row, Philadelphia, 1983.
55. Eyring, EJ and Murray, WR: The effect of joint position on the pressure of intra-articular effusion. J Bone Joint Surg 46-A(6):1235, 1964.
56. Flowers, K and Michlovitz, SL: Assessment and management of loss of motion in orthopaedic dysfunction. Postgraduate Advances in Physical Therapy, APTA, 1988.
57. Abramson, DI: Physiologic basis for the use of physical agents in peripheral vascular disorders. Arch Phys Med Rehabil 46:216, 1965.
58. Abramson, DI: Comparison of wet and dry heat in raising temperature of tissue. Arch Phys Med Rehabil 48:654, 1967.

CHAPTER 6

Hydrotherapy: The Use of Water as a Therapeutic Agent

Mark T. Walsh, M.S., P.T.

Hydrotherapy is one of the oldest therapeutic methods for managing physical dysfunctions.[1] It has been advocated for the treatment of joint stiffness, painful scars, adhesions, and arthritis, and as a warm-up to assist with exercise.[2] Water therapy is used for the effects on body tissues of heating,[3] cooling, debridement,[4,5] pain relief, and relaxation of muscles. When treatment is not well planned or well executed, it can have adverse side effects, primarily on the cardiovascular system.

Hydrotherapy achieves its desired effects through the physical properties of water, temperature, and agitation. A basic understanding of these physical principles, normal physiology, and the pathology involved serves as a foundation for the decision to use hydrotherapy in the treatment of a specific dysfunction. The objectives of this chapter are to (1) provide the reader with a knowledge of the physical principles underlying hydrotherapy, (2) discuss the biophysical effects of water immersion, (3) describe equipment preparation and maintenance, (4) discuss specific clinical techniques and pathologies, and (5) discuss safety in hydrotherapy.

PHYSICAL PRINCIPLES

Forces Existing in Water

Water has the inherent forces of buoyancy, pressure, cohesion, and viscosity, which play a role in the effects produced on the body from hydrotherapy. The most important of these is Archimedes' principle of buoyancy. This principle states that a body immersed in a liquid experiences an upward force equal to the weight of the displaced liquid.[6] Thus, the body appears to weigh less in water than it does in air. Buoyancy may be affected by (1) postural alignment; (2) the surface area immersed; (3) the weight of the bones in relationship to muscle and fat; and, (4) vital capacity. The buoyancy of water can be used to assist with exercise in the extremities and to minimize stress of joints and muscles. Work can be done in the opposite direction, against the assist of buoyancy, so that resistance to motion can be exerted. In addition, by varying the speed of exercise in water, the difficulty of the exercise can be changed or graded. These concepts will be discussed in more detail.

Specific gravity is the ratio of the weight of a volume of substance to the weight of an equal volume of water. The specific gravity of the body is approximately 0.974. Objects with a specific gravity less than 1.0 will float in water. The specific gravity of the body, therefore, can be advantageous to exercise in water.

Water exerts a perpendicular pressure against the surface of the body. This hydrostatic pressure is the ratio of the magnitude of the force exerted by the fluid per body surface area. This pressure is dependent on the depth of the submerged part and the density of the liquid. Hydrostatic pressure increases as depth and density of the liquid increase. Therefore, motion is performed more easily near the surface of the water than at greater depths.

Water molecules are cohesive; they have a tendency to attract each other. This results in an increase in viscosity of the medium, as compared with that of air, and an increase in resistance to motion. Viscosity is internal friction, the property of liquids that resists relative motion within it. The greater the speed of the liquid, the higher the viscosity. Resistance to motion is also dependent on the shape of the body. The more streamlined the body or object, the less force is required to move it through the water. The larger and more spread out the object moving through the water, the greater the resistance to motion.

Methods of Heat Transfer

Hydrotherapy is performed in water tanks of varying sizes and shapes. Tanks used for partial body immersion (that is, immersion of one or two extremities) are termed whirlpools. (Often the terms hydrotherapy and whirlpool are used interchangeably.) Tanks used for full-body immersion are referred to as Hubbard tanks, or walking tanks. Thermal energy is exchanged by water in the tank when the body is immersed by two methods: conduction and convection.

CONDUCTION

Conduction is an exchange of thermal energy in which there is physical contact between two surfaces. If water temperature is higher than skin temperature, heat will be conducted to the skin and temperature will rise. Since fat acts more as an insulator than as a conductor, it has a tendency to hold heat in or to keep it out. This point is important for two reasons: (1) The effect of superficial heating by conduction will be lessened as the body fat composition increases and (2) the higher the body fat content, the less able the body is to dissipate heat, which may cause an increase in body-core temperatures to dangerous levels. With the obese person, therefore, superficial heating with the whirlpool may not achieve the intended effects. Caution must be taken when a large body surface area is immersed; the person may not be able to dissipate internal heat and maintain proper core temperature. This may present a dangerous situation, requiring other methods of heat loss, such as evaporation and convection, to work overtime causing dehydration and increased cardiac output. A particular patient's medical condition may not tolerate this situation, such as a patient with cardiac or peripheral vascular diseases.

CONVECTION

Convection, which occurs when a portion of the fluid moves from one place to another, is a more rapid process of thermal energy exchange than conduction. Energy transfer by convection occurs when the patient is moving in the water or when the water swirls across the skin surface. Convection plays an important role in heating or cooling tissues, as well as in dissipating or retaining body heat.

Convection occurs between the core and the shell of the body. Surface body heat can be carried by the venous blood toward the core, thus potentially increasing core temperature. Conversely, convection will help with heat dissipation by carrying heat away from areas of the body that are being heated. This method of heat transfer is compromised when the patient has cardiovascular or peripheral vascular disease. In this case, heating an entire extremity or full body may create dangerous overheating, because the extremity or body is unable to dissipate heat from the treated area to maintain tissue temperature at safe levels.

Thus far, the methods of heat transfer discussed were used to transport heat in either direction in the body. Two other methods of heat transfer, of dissipating heat from the body during or following therapy, will be discussed.

RADIATION

Radiation is the exchange of electromagnetic energy that occurs when there is a difference in temperature between the skin and the surrounding environment. As convection and conduction bring the heat from within the body to the level of the skin, radiation assists in the transfer of this heat from the skin to the air. This ability to eliminate heat through radiation will be lost in the areas immersed in the whirlpool.

EVAPORATION

The other heat transfer mechanism used to dissipate heat is *evaporation*. No temperature gradient is necessary. Evaporation occurs through the loss of fluid from sweating and by the pulmonary system during exhaling. Any disturbance with the autonomic nervous or pulmonary systems' functions may interfere with loss of heat by evaporation. Therefore, when administering hydrotherapy, sufficient body surface must be exposed to the air to allow heat loss; otherwise, water temperatures must be kept below a body temperature between 33.3° and 36.6°C.

Heat loss is affected not only by the medical condition of the patient and his or her ability to cope with heat, but also by the environmental factors of humidity and temperature. If either humidity or ambient temperature, or both, are too high, the body will have great difficulty with heat loss. On the other hand, should the ambient temperature be too low and the area dry, heat loss may occur to a greater extent than needed, thereby causing a chill. Therefore, muscle and joint stiffness secondary to the reduction in peripheral circulation could occur. Strong consideration, therefore, should be given to the design and environment of the hydrotherapy area.

BIOPHYSICAL EFFECTS

Thermal Effects

One of the principal reasons for using hydrotherapy is to gain the therapeutic value of heat or cold. The same physiologic effects of heat and cold apply to hydrotherapy as to other thermal agents, except that a larger body surface area usually is immersed in water than that covered by a hot or cold pack. Therefore, exposure of the body to varying temperatures will have, not only a local effect (see Chapter 5), but systemic effects on the cardiovascular and other organ systems as well. The greater the difference in temperature between the water and skin, the more intense the reaction. Cold application to the whole body decreases heart rate and lengthens diastole. The tone of the cardiac muscle is enhanced, and blood pressure is raised, as a result of peripheral vasoconstriction. The increase in peripheral resistance requires the heart to work harder to maintain adequate blood flow to the periphery. Other effects of cold immersion can be reviewed in Chapter 4.

The application of heat to the entire body will cause an initial increase in blood pressure, followed by a decrease in blood pressure as a result of vasodilation. The initial rise in blood pressure may be quite marked and prolonged if the temperature of the bath is very high, above 40°C. Respiratory rate will increase owing to application of heat *or* cold, although the increase may be less marked with the application of heat. Dawson and associates[7] studied the effects of hydrotherapy on cardiac output, oxygen consumption, heart rate, and blood pressure, while study subjects were in the resting state (positioned supine and sitting) and while exercising (the step test). The subjects were immersed in the whirlpool to hip level for 20 minutes in 40°C water. The mean cardiac output and oxygen consumption increased, but not significantly. Pulse rate increased 1.3 to 1.5 times over the sitting or supine resting level, and the mean blood pressure increased 1.1 times over the supine resting values.

In addition, sweating will increase; the amount is dependent on the temperature, size of body surface exposed, and the length of treatment. Whether the use of hydrotherapy bath increases diuresis remains controversial,[8,9] but diuresis seems to be affected by the hydrostatic pressure, which increases with depth of immersion. This influence of hydrostatic pressure may have more of an effect on urinary output than does water temperature itself.

Increasing tissue temperature and blood flow are physiologic effects of heat that can have therapeutic value. The depth to which this vasodilation occurs, and its relationship to tissue temperature, are important. If whirlpool does not increase circulation and temperature to sufficient levels to meet therapeutic goals, it may not be the agent of choice. When one arm was immersed in a water bath 45°C for 20 minutes, there was a 4.17°C rise in subcutaneous-tissue temperature, a 1.4°C rise in muscle temperature of the forearm, and an increase in blood flow.[10,11] There is a direct relationship between the increase in superficial blood flow and temperature with the arm immersed in a water bath from 37°C to 42°C. Borrell and coworkers[13] confirmed the penetrating ability of whirlpool in their study in which the thumb-joint capsule temperature rose 4°C in a whirlpool bath of 38.9°C when given for a 20-minute period.

Mechanical Effects

WHIRLPOOL AGITATION

Whenever the effects of both cold or superficial heat and water are indicated for a rehabilitation program, the use of whirlpool has been advocated. Physiologically, the whirlpool acts as an analgesic agent, relaxes muscle spasm, relieves joint pain and stiffness, improves mechanical debridement,[14] and facilitates exercise.[15] Based on these facts, its use has been suggested for debriding necrotic tissue and dirt[3,5,8,14,15] before exercising,[3] and for various musculoskeletal problems.[2] The agitation created by the whirlpool serves as a source of mechanical stimulation to skin receptors, which may explain its sedative and analgesic effects. The agitation may act as a counterirritant, or it may act as a stimulus to large sensory afferents, thus blocking pain input.

Cohen and associates[16] studied the effects of agitation on blood flow by comparing agitation and nonagitation on diseased and normal extremities. There was no significant affect on blood flow in limbs immersed in whirlpool baths of 38.6°C without agitation and 37.7°C with agitation.[16]

Determining what affects agitation has on body tissues requires some understanding of the pressure and turbulence created in the whirlpool. This has been studied in several types of whirlpools. In general, pressure was significantly increased by greater amounts of air allowed to enter into the agitation, and there was more turbulence toward the surface than deeper in the water.[17] The importance of these concepts will be clarified further on in this chapter, especially regarding exercise and open-wound care.

GENERAL DESCRIPTION AND UNIT OPERATION

Whirlpool Types

There are basically two types of whirlpools, portable and fixed. In most cases, with the exception of full-body therapeutic tubs, such as the Hubbard tank or walk tank, any size or style of whirlpool can be either fixed or portable. There are basically three styles of whirlpool baths. They are depicted in Figure 6–1, along with their usual dimensions.[18] The "extremity" tank is used for the treatment of arms and legs. The "lowboy" and "highboy" (hip or leg tank) can be used for lower extremity or trunk immersion. Each of these tank styles has specific applications that will be discussed later.[18]

All tanks require an ample supply of hot and cold water and some means of blending them for the desired temperature. The water may be mixed by a thermostatic control valve or manually. Both means of introducing water should include a vacuum breaker on the faucets to prevent the suctioning of water from the whirlpool into the water system. These tanks are routinely drained and cleaned between patient treatments. The larger walk tanks or therapeutic tanks are used for exercising and conditioning. These are not routinely drained between patients and should be equipped with a filtration system and a means by which to add chemicals.

Hydrotherapy Area

The room temperature in the hydrotherapy area should be higher than in other treatment areas in the physical therapy department. The area should be adequately ventilated (1) to prevent the condensation of moisture on the walls, floors, and equip-

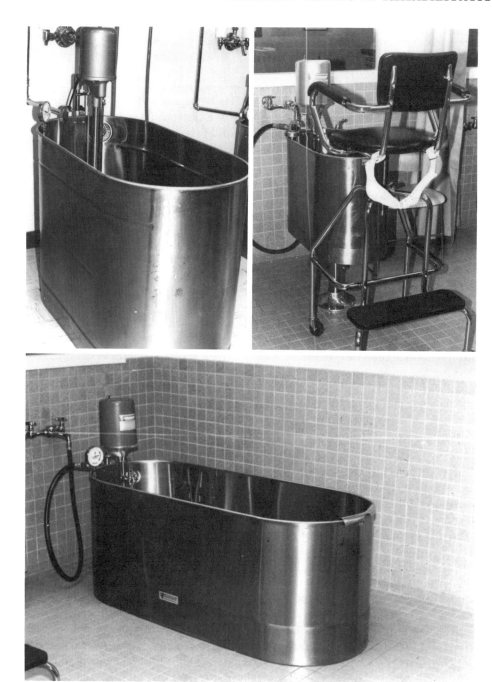

FIGURE 6–1. Styles of whirlpool baths. (*Top left*) extremity tank width 15#, length 28–32″, depth 18–25″; (*top right*) leg or hip tank (high boy) width 20–24″, length 36–48″, depth 28″; bottom, lowboy width 24″, length 52–66″, depth 18″.

ment and (2) to remove aerosols of water and additives induced into the air by water turbulence in the whirlpool.[5] The hydrotherapy area is best designed and used when it is kept separate from other treatment areas and when it contains adequate storage for bandages and other supplies. It should also contain a sink for hand and equipment washing and an area for dressing wounds. The room should be of adequate size to allow for maneuvering of wheelchairs and stretchers.

Turbine

The movement of water and air is regulated by the water pump, or turbine. The whirlpool operates by mixing water and air to control turbulence. Turbulence is created and controlled by combining aeration (the amount of air mixed with the water) and agitation (the movement of the water). In general, the more aeration, the greater the turbulence. Agitational patterns are not uniform from one piece of equipment to another. In any piece of equipment, though, the turbulence is greater toward the surface of the water.[17]

The turbine is mounted on a tubular column, which is often a springloaded circular vice attached to the whirlpool. The circular vice functions to help with raising and lowering the turbine, as well as rotating it horizontally. The turbine assembly consists of an electrical motor pump located above the water to which two tubular shafts are connected. The first tube is the drive shaft, which contains an impeller, housed in a casing at the bottom of the tube. A control valve located near the whirlpool motor regulates the opening at the end of the tube, to control the amount of water introduced into the whirlpool system. At the top of the second tube, which is called the breather tube, is a variable-pressure-control valve to control the amount of aeration; a water jet is attached at the bottom of this tube. Therefore, by regulating the water and air intake by these valves, the turbulence or pressure can be controlled. The various parts of the whirlpool are shown in Figure 6–2.

The agitational pattern may be controlled by rotating the turbine assembly to direct the air or water jet stream to the right or left, creating a circular pattern, or to direct it at various points toward the center of the tub, which decreases the circular motion but

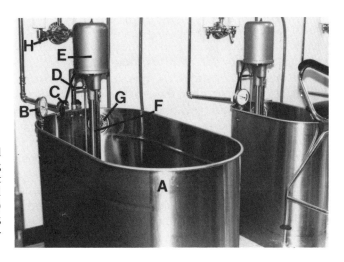

FIGURE 6–2. Whirlpool parts. (*A*) Stainless Steel Tank; (*B*) Thermometer; (*C*) Inlet Spout; (*D*) Water Control Valve; (*E*) Turbine Motor; (*F*) Impellor and Breather Tubes; (*G*) Overflow Drain; (*H*) Mixing Valve.

increases central turbulence. The agitation can be further controlled by raising or lowering the assembly.

Whirlpool Care and Safety Precautions

Care of the whirlpool entails cleansing the tank and turbines after each use. The external surface of the tank can be polished with a commercial stainless steel polish. Cleansing the inside can be a problem, especially when patients with contagious or infected open lesions are treated in the tank. Proper cleansing can be performed in two steps depending on the whirlpool additive and disinfectant system chosen. The inside of the tank, after emptying, should be scrubbed with a commercial disinfectant that will not cause corrosion, rinsed thoroughly with clean water, and dried. Scrubbing alone, however, is not effective in eradicating possible contaminants[19] on the bottom, edges, drains, overflow pipe, thermometers, and agitators, the most frequently contaminated sites. Disinfecting these hard-to-reach places can be achieved through several methods. Chlorine at 200 ppm (parts per million) has been found to be effective in eradicating the common forms of bacteria—clostridium and Pseudomonas. However, only glutaralde-hydes, formatin alcohol, ethylene oxide, and beta propriolactone have been found to be effective against spore-forming bacteria.[20] A hydrotherapy sterilizing system is probably the most practical system.[21] The exact disinfecting protocol is available from the various manufacturers. The use of povidone–iodine surgical scrub (0.75% available iodine) has also been found to be effective in significantly reducing colony counts.[22] Finally, the use of a commercial additive, Chloramine-T (chlorazene), in concentrations of 100 to 200 ppm has proven to be effective at reducing gram-negative organisms and Pseudo-monas.[23] The benefit of this system is, it is also used at the same time as a whirlpool additive for disinfecting the wound, thus diminishing the amount of time required for sterilization, and it is not corrosive.[23] Routine culturing of the tanks should be performed. Guidelines for culturing can be obtained through an appropriate clinical laboratory or hospital infection-control department.

Recent concern over the transmission of the HIV (AIDS) virus deserves special attention, especially for protection of the health-care worker. The Centers for Disease Control recommends "blood and body fluid precautions be consistently used for *all* patients regardless of the blood-borne infection status."[24,25] (Note: For the most current update on AIDS precautions, contact the Centers for Disease Control, Atlanta, GA) This would include blood, body fluids containing visible blood, tissues, cerebrospinal fluid, synovial fluid, pleural fluid, peritoneal fluid, pericardial fluid, and amniotic fluid. When treating open wounds with hydrotherapy, protective barriers such as gloves, masks, gowns, and goggles should be used, particularly when dealing with large wounds, an infectious patient, or when there is the possibility of splashing. While cleansing the tank, general-purpose utility gloves should be used at all times, whether or not an open wound was treated in the tank. A solution of sodium hypochlorite, in concentrations ranging from 500 ppm (1:100 dilution) to 5000 ppm (1:10 dilution) can inactivate the HIV rapidly.[25] Sterilization of the tank and its components can be performed in the same manner as previously discussed.

Electrical safety is an important matter to consider when using hydrotherapy equipment. The turbines must be grounded. A ground-fault circuit interrupter should be installed either at the receptacle or with the circuit breaker for the receptacle. A GFCI eliminates the hazard of ground-fault circuits (see Chapter 3). Also included would be any electrical motors that may be used to help with patient transfers, such as with the Hubbard tank or walk or therapeutic tanks. Finally, if the motor support, which is springloaded and controlled by the vice grip, is released with the counterbalance of the weight of the whirlpool turbine, the assembly spring may catapult the support, creating a hazardous situation.[26] If the support becomes stuck, there should be no attempt to correct this situation while water or a patient is in the tank.

CLINICAL TECHNIQUES

Preparatory Considerations

Before initiating a whirlpool treatment, objectives of treatment should be determined and may include (1) stimulation of circulation for wound care; (2) promotion of muscle relaxation and pain relief; (3) removal of exudates and necrotic tissue; and (4) facilitation of exercise, either as assistance or resistance.

Next, the proper temperature should be selected, based on the patient's medical condition and treatment objectives. Commonly used temperatures and their corresponding generic names are located in Table 6–1. In general, temperatures from 36.5°C to 40.5°C are accepted temperatures when using heat,[2] except in the presence of peripheral vascular disease, sensory loss, or full-body immersion. With peripheral vascular disease, the skin temperature of the extremity to be immersed can be a guideline to help determine water temperature and should not be greater than 1°C above skin temperature to a maximum of body temperature. In the presence of cardiovascular or pulmonary disease, the temperature should not exceed 38°C.

The part to be treated should be inspected for its temperature, presence of edema, open lesions, color, muscle spasm, sensation, and conditions previously noted. The treatment procedure and unit operation should be explained to the patient to reduce anxiety and promote safety. The patient should be positioned comfortably. The whirlpool may then be activated and the agitation force adjusted initially at a minimal level and increased as desired. Be sure not to direct the agitation specifically toward any body area that could suffer further damage or not withstand the force of the agitation. The patient should not be left unattended during the treatment session. Whenever immersed in a lift chair or stretcher, the patient should be strapped in place. The patient should be strapped into the elevated chair, if used, when employing the extremity tank for treatment of the lower extremities.

TABLE 6–1. Whirlpool Water Temperatures and Frequent
Descriptive Terminology

Descriptive Terminology	F°	C°
Very Cold	35–55	1–13
Cold	55–65	13–18
Cool	65–80	18–27
Tepid	80–92	17–33.5
Neutral	92–96	33.5–35.5
Warm	96–98	35.5–36.5
Hot	98–104	36.5–40
Very Hot	104–115	40–60

Whirlpool Duration

The decision on the length of time for treatment in a whirlpool must be based on sound physiologic judgment and on the treatment objectives the therapist is attempting to achieve through use of the whirlpool. The duration of treatment will change, depending on the specific pathologies involved. When used strictly as a heating modality and the patient's medical condition permits, the usual duration is 20 minutes. Borrell and colleagues[13] demonstrated that 20 minutes was a long enough time to increase skin, muscle, and joint capsule temperature in the hand and foot. Abramson and associates[11] demonstrated that a 20-minute application of moist heat increased blood flow, and that further exposure of up to 2 hours had no real affect on increasing the peak response obtained at the 20-minute mark. When using the whirlpool for debridement, the duration is 5 to 20 minutes, depending on the amount of necrotic tissue; for exercising, a duration of 10 to 20 minutes is recommended, depending on the patient's medical status. When the treatment is concluded, the agitator should be turned off and the patient should be helped out of the tub. At no time should the patient operate the agitator controls. Occasionally, when full-body immersion has been performed, the patient may experience some lightheadedness. This may be avoided by having the patient sit for 5 to 10 minutes before standing.

Documentation of Treatment

After removal from the tank or hydrotherapy pool, the patient should be checked for any evidence of adverse reaction, and the effects of the treatment should be documented. This would include inspection of the patient's skin for marked temperature change, any evidence of dermatologic eruption, erythema, and blanching time. When treating an open wound, re-evaluation of the wound's appearance and surrounding margins, evidence of exudate and its description, and the amount and type of necrotic tissue present should be noted. If the whirlpool were used for exercising, any change in range of motion, strength, joint appearance, and edema should be noted. Keep in mind that warmer temperatures and full-body immersion may have a tendency to cause transient weakness. If the patient has a medical history of cardiac or pulmonary disease, including hypertension, the patient's respirations, pulse, and blood pressure should be monitored and recorded to determine tolerance to the treatment. Finally, of equal importance are the patient's subjective comments regarding an increase or decrease in pain, joint stiffness, and fatigue. The duration of the treatment, water temperature, and additives used also should be documented.

Treatment Techniques

LOWER EXTREMITY TECHNIQUES

Lower-extremity immersion, or immersion to the midthoracic level, can be achieved with two of the basic whirlpool types. The highboy tank requires the patient to be able to flex the hip and knee. The length of this tub does not allow for full extension of the average adult lower extremity and limits the amount of range-of-motion exercise or activity a person can perform while in this whirlpool. However, its depth allows a greater body-surface area to be submerged safely and comfortably, to as high as the midthoracic region.

The lowboy tank is not as deep, but has greater length, than the highboy, and it affords the patient the ability to fully extend the lower extremities and perform full-motion exercises for the knees. When only the distal portion of the lower extremity has to be immersed, the extremity tank, with the use of the whirlpool chair, is the appropriate choice.

In summary, the highboy and lowboy afford greater body-surface immersion than the extremity tank does, while the lowboy may allow for greater lower extremity extension than the highboy does. In the event that the patient is unable to negotiate transfer into any of the tubs, the highboy and lowboy each can be fitted with a hydraulic-chair lift, or "hoyer lift," to assist the patient in and out of the tub.

UPPER EXTREMITY TECHNIQUES

When treating the upper extremity, the patient should be seated comfortably next to the extremity tank, with a towel or other form of padding on the tank edge to avoid constriction of the circulatory and lymphatic system of the upper extremity (Fig. 6–3). The use of the whirlpool for the upper extremity deserves special consideration, because edema can form. It is well accepted that edema of the hand is one of the adverse effects of whirlpool, and the reduction of edema is the primary concern of the treating therapist.[27] Magness and coworkers[28] studied the affect of whirlpool on volume in the upper extremity. They measured upper-extremity volume in 20 normal male and female volunteers before and after the immersion of this same extremity in a whirlpool bath at temperatures ranging from 33.5°C to 44.4°C for 20 minutes. In addition, 20 patients with various upper-extremity disorders were also treated by whirlpool in the same

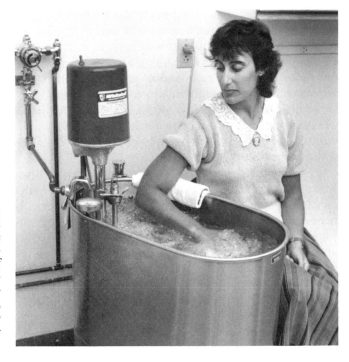

FIGURE 6–3. Whirlpool treatment to the hand and forearm. Caution should be used to avoid a totally dependent position of the hand. If possible, active range-of-motion exercises should be performed during the treatment, to encourage venous and lymphatic return, thus minimizing edema formation.

manner, at temperatures from 37.8°C to 40°C for 20 minutes. The results revealed a significant increase in volume for the normal subjects, which was directly related to the increase in water temperature. There was also a significant increase in volume of the patient's extremity, and the rise in volume was greater than in the normal subjects at the specific temperatures treated.

Several attempts have been made to determine the causes of this edema and how it can be controlled. Schultz[29] used 20 normal subjects and 20 upper-extremity-injured patients to determine the effect of active exercise on edema formation during whirlpool treatment at 37°C. She found no significant difference in edema formation, when comparing active exercise during whirlpool treatment with no exercise during whirlpool treatment, for both normal subjects and upper-extremity-injured patients. Walsh[30] studied the effect of elevation versus nonelevation of the upper extremity during whirlpool on 30 healthy volunteers, at temperatures of 37.6°C and 40°C. He also found a significant increase in extremity volume in the 40°C whirlpool group. Although not statistically significant, the data supported the theory of nondependency toward the reduction of edema. Recently Hoyrup and Kjorrel[31] studied the effect of whirlpool and paraffin dips on the hand volume, range of motion, and pain of traumatic-hand-injured patients. The patients received whirlpool at 43°C and paraffin dips at 50°C. One half of each group performed exercises, the other half did not. A significant reduction in pain and increase in motion were found. There was no significant change in hand volume during a 3-week period. Daily increases in volume, however, were significant, and the changes were significantly greater in the whirlpool group. Therefore, these studies suggest exercising discrimination when choosing whirlpool for the treatment of upper-extremity disorders in patients for whom edema is a primary concern.

FULL-BODY IMMERSION

A tank available for full body-immersion is the Hubbard tank, as shown in Figure 6–4. The tank is usually used in conjunction with an overhead lift or stretcher to place the patient into the water. Examples of uses for the Hubbard tank can include treatment of (1) an arthritic patient who is at present in an exacerbation phase and is unable to negotiate transfer into the smaller tank, but who requires the use of heat and water to help with exercising, maintaining range of motion, and providing pain relief; (2) a patient with neurologically involved paralysis who is actively able to move his or her extremities in the buoyancy of water, but unable to do so in air; (3) a burn patient; or, (4) an elderly or debilitated patient with an open wound. The major advantage of the Hubbard tank is that its design allows for motion of all the extremities and accessibility of the patient by the therapist.

The Hubbard tank (Fig. 6–4) is shaped with 15-inch insets, which permit the therapist access to the patient. Its dimensions are a length of 7 feet 2 inches; upper width 6 feet, middle width 35 inches, and lower width 4 feet 2 inches; and a usual depth of 22 inches. It has approximately a 425-gallon capacity, unless the tank has a walking trough, which requires approximately 700 gallons of water. It is equipped with two whirlpool turbines that can be moved around the perimeter of the tank to direct and control the agitation pattern. Other accessories include an optional walking trough with parallel bars for gait training. For treating open wounds, the Hubbard tank should be drained and cleaned, as previously discussed, and the same preparatory techniques should be observed.

The walking tank, or larger therapeutic exercise units, because of the greater

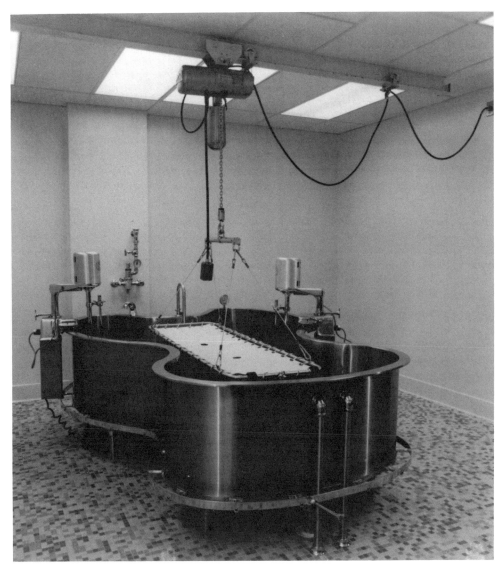

FIGURE 6–4. Hubbard tank with overhead lift (Courtesy of Whitehall Electro Medical Co., Inc., Hackensack, NJ 07602.)

gallonage, frequently is hooked to its own filtration system. One of the many available therapeutic hydrotherapy units is pictured in Figure 6–5. The primary purpose of these tanks is for exercising or conditioning, while using the inherent forces of water. The patient may be placed into the tank either with or without a flotation device to assist them. Full-body immersion systems require some special considerations. They should be housed in a separate area, with the temperature controlled ideally at 25.5°C, with 50 percent humidity.[32] An area for showering and cool-down should be available to the patient.

The therapist should be aware of the increased demand placed on the patient's cardiovascular and pulmonary systems. Core temperature can be increased by the water

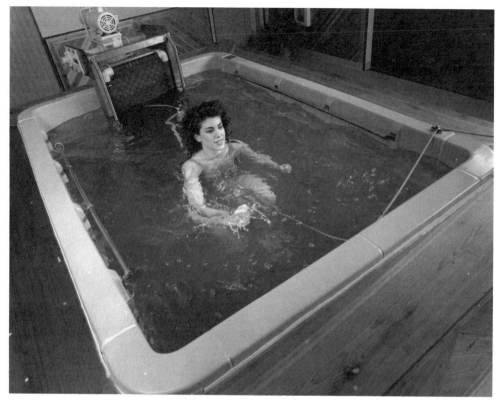

FIGURE 6–5. Therapeutic hydrotherapy unit. Note patient hydraulic lift and flotation device and tethering system. (Courtesy of Aqua Ark Therapeutic Systems, Inc., Doylestown, PA 18901.)

temperature, and muscular contraction places a greater demand on heat dissipation, the respiratory system, and the exposed integument. General considerations should include a maximum immersion time of 20 minutes for noncompromised cardiopulmonary patients, and less time for the elderly, hypertensive, and cardiopulmonary patients. It may be advisable to initiate treatment for 10 minutes and increase as tolerated. Contraindications are patients who are incontinent of bowel or bladder, presence of skin infection, unstable blood pressure, uncontrolled epilepsy, acute febrile episode, and tuberculosis. Caution should be exhibited with those patients whose vital capacity is less than 1000 cc or in the presence of pulmonary disease.

CONTRAST BATH

One special technique in the treatment of distal extremities for which the whirlpool can be used is the contrast bath. This requires the use of whirlpool at a temperature from 38°C to 44°C, and an additional basin containing water kept at a temperature from 10°C to 18°C. The basin should be large enough to enable immersion of the extremity to cover at least the level of the injury. The extremity to be treated is placed into the warm whirlpool for 10 minutes, then immersed in the cold water in the basin for 1 minute, and returned to the warm whirlpool for 4 minutes. The cycle continues for 30 minutes, with the last immersion in the warm whirlpool. Although these specific times do not have to be followed, the generally accepted hot:cold ratio is 3:1 or 4:1. The theory, although not well researched, involves the vasodilation (hot water) and vasoconstriction (cold water) caused by the contrast bath. The net result is hypothesized to stimulate local circulation in the treated extremity and, to a lesser extent, to increase circulation in the contralateral untreated extremity. This last point is important and can be of assistance to the therapist when treating a patient with peripheral vascular disease. If the use of heat or cold is contraindicated for a specific extremity, the contralateral extremity may be treated using the contrast bath, causing an increase in circulation in the affected extremity by this crossover phenomenon.

Contraindications for the use of the contrast bath would be small-vessel disease secondary to diabetes or arteriosclerotic endarteritis and Buerger's disease. Caution should be exercised in patients with any peripheral vascular disease if the water temperature is higher than 40°C. Contrast baths have been advocated for arthritis of peripheral joints, joint sprains, muscular tenderness strains, some peripheral vascular diseases (in selected cases), and to toughen amputation stumps. No well-controlled studies, however, discussing the efficacy of contrast baths are available in the literature.

INDICATIONS FOR HYDROTHERAPY

Wound Care

The whirlpool is commonly used in the care of open wounds. The whirlpool provides an effective method of debriding a wound to remove necrotic material and of cleansing, through the addition of a bactericidal agent. In addition, the mechanical effects of the whirlpool help to stimulate formation of granulation tissue and, in conjunction with the appropriate water temperature, can help to soften tissues and stimulate circulation of the affected area. The increase in local circulation raises the levels of oxygen, antibodies, leukocytes, and nutrition supplied to the tissues, and enhances the removal of metabolites. In addition, the amount of systemic medications, such as antibiotics, available to the wound area is increased by the improved circulation, which helps to diminish or to prevent infection. The whirlpool also creates sedation and analgesia, which may aid in reducing pain caused by the open wound or surrounding tissues.

Whirlpool Additives

The first consideration in the treatment of wounds with whirlpool is deciding which whirlpool additive to use. An antibacterial agent added to the whirlpool water helps prevent or reduce infection. Common additives are a povidone–iodine solution (4 ppm),[22] especially prepared for whirlpools, and sodium hypochlorite 5.25 percent, household bleach, and Chloramine-T.[21] Sodium hypochlorite has been found to be effective at reducing colony counts in dilution up to 1:160.[33] The Centers for Disease Control recommend sodium hypochlorite in concentrations of 70 percent per 100 gallons, which produces 15 mg pure chlorine per liter.[34] The 1:60 dilution is sometimes painful, however, and may cause irritation to the surrounding tissues. The aerosols formed from the turbulence also may cause irritation to the eyes with prolonged exposure. Zigenfuls and associates[35] found that concentrations of povidone–iodine solution in a minimum concentration of 3 ppm, rounded by 1.2 cc per 1 gallon H_2O, to

TABLE 6–2. Betadine and Chlorine Bleach Concentrations in
Standard Whirlpools at Therapeutic Levels

Whirlpool Type	Average Capacity	Povidine Iodine (Oz)	Chlorine Bleach (Oz)	Chloramine-T (Chlorazene)
Foot/Hand	22–36 gls	4	26	20–36 gms
Leg/Hip	100–110 gls	13.5	102	88 gms
Low boy	93–137 gls	10	96	50–88 gms

be effective in reducing wound and water colony counts after 18 minutes of exposure. McGuckin and associates[36] studied the cross contamination of 10 Hubbard-tank wound patients with pseudomonas aeruginosas. The outbreak began after discontinuing sodium hypochlorite additive. The outbreak ceased after reinstituting the sodium hypochlorite additive and disinfecting the tank between treatments for 30 minutes with 12 ppm iodine and 1000 ppm sodium hypochlorite.

The use of Chloramine-T (chlorazene) in concentrations of 100 ppm virtually eliminated positive cultures of all micro-organisms on the equipment. Concentrations of 150 to 200 ppm also reduce colonization of a gram-negative organism of the patient's wound. Due to its chemical configuration and stability, Chloramine-T is effective in releasing free chlorine, throughout a 20-minute treatment, at effective levels and in reducing the irritating qualities of chlorine. This same solution, with continued agitation of 5 minutes after patient removal, is all that is necessary to sterilize the tank. This is followed by scrubbing with a disinfectant and rinsing. The use of this substance can greatly diminish the amount of sterilization time necessary between treatments. The exact amount of povidone–iodine and Chloramine-T to be added for each tank type can be obtained from the manufacturers. The proper dilutions of povidone–iodine, chlorine bleach, Chloramine-T for common tanks can be found in Table 6–2.

Therapists should be aware that addition of an antibacterial agent in the stronger concentrations, or simultaneous use of more than one whirlpool with additives, can produce vapors that have the potential to cause lightheadedness, dizziness, and even syncope. Continuous monitoring of the patient during treatment and adequate ventilation of the hydrotherapy area therefore are essential.

WOUND TYPE AND CONDITION

The second consideration in determining the proper use of whirlpool for wound care is the wound itself. The therapist must consider what affects water temperature, agitation, and duration will have on the wound and surrounding tissues. Evaluation and recognition of the various components of a wound are essential. Tables 6–3 and 6–4 will help the reader to organize wound evaluation and to identify wound characteristics and exudates.

Wounds can be classified, based on a time frame for closure, as: (1) primary; (2) delayed primary; and (3) healing by secondary intention. Primary wounds are surgically closed or closed within 5 days. Delayed primary closures are wounds that are surgically closed after 5 days. Secondary-intention wounds are allowed to close by granulation, marginal or budding epithelization, and wound-margin contracture. To treat the latter two wound classifications, the clinician would most appropriately use the whirlpool for

TABLE 6-3. Components of Wound Evaluation

A. History
   1. Injury—etiology, date onset, injury components
   2. Social/Occupational—age, dominance, vocational/avocational, alcohol, nicotine, caffeine, family support
   3. Medical—system review, previous injury, medications, allergies
B. Subjective Report
   1. Pain, sensory changes
   2. Functional problems
C. Objective Evaluation
   1. General observation
      a. Wound, surrounding tissue, extremity
      b. Location
   2. Wound
      a. Size, shape, depth measurement
      b. Classification
         1.) Primary/delayed primary
         2.) Secondary
      c. Exudate characteristics
      d. Wound bed
         1.) Necrotic, granulative, epithelial budding
         2.) Vital structure involvement
      e. Wound margins
         1.) Extent
         2.) Change
      f. Grafts/flaps
         1.) Adherence
         2.) Drainage
         3.) Vascularity

cleansing, debridement, antibacterial action, and circulation enhancement. An example of a delayed primary wound would be a dog bite. Primary closure is not advocated because of the risk of infection and abscess formation. Daily whirlpool could be used until delayed closure is carried out, or until the wound heals by secondary intention. An example of secondary intention would be a stasis ulcer. The whirlpool could be carried out until the wound closes or is surgically closed with skin graft or a tissue flap.

TABLE 6-4. Wound Exudate Characteristics and Relationship to Wound Type

	Serous	Sanguineous	Fibrous/ Proteinious	Purulent
Color	Yellow	Yellow red to red	White to white–yellow	Green Brown White
Odor	No	No	No	Yes
Adherency	No	No	Yes	No
Consistency (Viscosity)	Thin Transparent to wound base	Thin–thick Transparent	Gel-like Nontransparent	Viscous Nontransparent
Wound type	Primary Secondary	Primary Secondary	Secondary	Secondary Primary

SKIN GRAFT AND TISSUE FLAP

Skin-graft viability is still delicate 3 to 5 days postgrafting. The graft may not adhere well to the granular bed, or there may not be sufficient capillary infiltration to provide nutritional support to the graft. A graft will not tolerate the high shearing forces and turbulence that can be created in the whirlpool; therefore, whirlpool aeration is adjusted to minimal levels or it is absent and is only administered for 5 minutes. This would allow for softening of the tissues and cleansing with the antibacterial agent, in preparation for mechanical debridement. The whirlpool also would help with the removal of superficial wound exudates. As a graft ages, and stability improves, the duration and aeration may be increased.

Whirlpool also can be used in the care of tissue flaps, whether they are cutaneous, muscular, or myocutaneous (free or pedicle type). Again, consideration must be given to the viability and circulation of the flap. Is the flap free, where arteries have had to be anastomosed? Or is the flap a pedicle type, where the major circulatory supply to the flap has not been interfered with? If the whirlpool is too cold, or should the patient suffer a chill while in the whirlpool, this may cause vasoconstriction of the small infiltrating vessels. The vasoconstriction may result in ischemia of a portion, or all, of the flap, leading to partial or full loss of the skin flap. Therefore, temperature of the whirlpool and hydrotherapy area, as well as agitation, are important considerations. In general, the younger the flap (in postoperative days), the less turbulence and shear force it will be able to tolerate. The common characteristics of skin grafts and tissue flaps are highlighted in Table 6–5.

TABLE 6–5. Skin Graft and Flap Characteristics

	Tissue Layers	Vascularity/Take	Common Drainage	Donor Site Closure
Split Thickness	Epidermis and supperficial dermis	3 days	Serous Sanguineous	Secondary Intention
Full Thickness	Epidermis and protein dermal layer	5–7 days	Serous Sanguineous	Primary
Pedicle Flap Random Axial	Dermis and subcutaneous fat	Approximately 3 weeks	Serosanguineous	Primary or skin graft
Free Flap		Immediate	Serosanguineous	Primary or skin graft
Cutaneous	Dermis and subcutaneous fat			
Myocutaneous	Dermis and subcutaneous fat Muscle			
Myo	Muscle only			
Osteo	Bone alone or in combination			
Joint	Joint and bone			

PAINFUL OPEN LESIONS

When the open wound is painful, as in the case of an ischemic ulcer or a burn, agitation should be gentle to avoid stimulating the neural tissue, thereby increasing pain. If used properly, with the correct temperature and agitation, the whirlpool may actually help to relieve the discomfort created by the wound and provide a gentle method of debridement. Agitation should be kept at a minimal level and should not be directed at the wound. In the case of a pressure sore, stasis ulcer, or traumatic open wound, debridement may be the main objective, and the maximal agitation level may be used. A final consideration is prevention of edema, which whirlpool may create. The edema could cause compromise by compressing the venous and lymphatic systems, possibly delaying healing or preventing systemic medication from reaching the wound, retarding the development of capillary formation, and removing wound-healing byproducts.

SURROUNDING TISSUE CONDITION

A third and final consideration for the treatment of open wounds with whirlpool is the condition of the surrounding tissues, or of the extremity, being treated. The circulation, both arterial and venous, must be able to tolerate the increased temperature and turbulence created by the whirlpool. The surrounding soft tissue's neurologic status must also be considered. The sensation in the area must not be compromised to a level that would prevent the patient from being able to protect himself or herself from further injury (caused by the agitation or rise in tissue temperature). Traumatized tissues may not be able to tolerate whirlpool because of underlying fractures, joint injuries, or soft-tissue damage.

In summary, the same indications and contraindications discussed for superficial heating must be considered with whirlpool, in addition to (1) the objectives of the whirlpool treatment, (2) the desired physiologic effect; (3) the condition and type of wound; and, (4) the condition of the surrounding tissues or extremities.[1]

Pool Therapy and Use of Hydrotherapy for Exercise

Pool therapy combines the physical forces of water (buoyancy, pressure, and viscosity) with therapeutic exercise.[11] Buoyancy can be used to help with exercises, as a means of resistance to improve strength, or to reduce undue stress on joints by providing support.[38] The general aims of pool therapy are to promote patient relaxation, improve circulation, restore mobility, strengthen muscles, provide gait training with less stress on the weight-bearing joints, and improve psychologic and emotional outlook (patients are often able to move or ambulate in water in ways they could not achieve without the aid of buoyancy).[39,40]

PRINCIPLES OF EXERCISE IN WATER

Hydrostatic pressure, the pressure exerted equally on all body surfaces of an immersed body, increases proportionally to the depth of immersion. Hydrostatic pressure decreases the tendency for blood to pool in the lower portion of the body. Viscosity is the property of friction in fluids. Since the viscosity of water is low, there is little friction with body movement at low speeds. As speed increases, however, this friction increases, making the movement more difficult and requiring greater muscle strength to perform the exercise. In addition, as speed increases so does turbulence (positive pressure), in the direction of the movement and drag (negative pressure), behind the moving part. One way of varying resistance, therefore, is by regulating the speed at which the body part moves; the greater the speed, the greater the resistance.

The principle of relative density is used to provide support of the body or its limb in water. When the specific gravity of an object is less than one, it will float. The average specific gravity of the body is 0.974.[37] The body or limb is supported, therefore, and the stresses placed on weight-bearing joints, as when a patient is ambulating in a pool, is decreased.

The final principle is buoyancy. Based on Archimedes' principle, a body when immersed in fluid will experience an upward force or thrust equal to the weight of the fluid displaced. Buoyancy can be used to provide either assistance or resistance with exercise. Buoyancy will assist with any exercise when the movement is performed in a direction toward the water surface, such as when abducting the shoulder in the standing position. Buoyancy produces resistance when the motion occurs in a direction away from the surface of the water, such as when adducting the shoulder in the standing position. The effect of buoyancy can also be varied by (1) changing the length of the lever arm, (2) by adding flotation devices to the extremity, or (3) by performing all extremity exercises in the horizontal position, or when the patient is floating on his or her back. In this position, resistance can be adjusted by altering the speed of the movement.

In summary, hydrostatic pressure helps circulation, depending on the depth of immersion. Specific gravity provides support of the body and limbs. Viscosity and the turbulence and drag created by body-parts movement can be used to vary the resistance. The faster the motion, the greater the resistance. Buoyancy can be used to support the body or the limb and provide assistive or resistive exercises.

PATIENT SELECTION

Proper patient selection for the use of pool therapy is very important. The patient should not be incontinent (feces or urine), unless catheterized. No patient for whom exposure to warm water or exercising is contraindicated (including those with open or discharging wounds, upper respiratory infection, uncontrolled blood pressure, febrile conditions, severe mental disorders, uncontrolled epilepsy, or cardiac or pulmonary conditions [especially with vital capacity less than 1500 ml]),[41] and no patient who fears water, should be allowed to participate in pool therapy. When pool therapy is chosen for cardiac- or pulmonary-compromised patients, the intensity of the exercise should be kept at low levels. It has been shown that there is an increase in oxygen consumption as the exercise level intensifies in young, healthy subjects.[42] Debilitated patients not usually suited to this treatment may be considered when the treatment, for some reason, seems desirable and is given for short periods of time. Pool therapy has been recommended for treatment of patients with rheumatoid arthritis,[39] orthopedic patients with joint injuries or replacements,[40] patients with neurologic disorders (such as paraplegia), or those with poliomyelitis, polyneuritis, multiple sclerosis, and (in certain cases) cerebral palsy.[43]

TREATMENT CONSIDERATIONS, EQUIPMENT, AND ENVIRONMENT

Treatment should last from 10 to 20 minutes, with the therapist monitoring vital signs, and neither the therapist nor the patient should remain in the pool for too long. In general, the more debilitated or medically compromised the patient, the shorter the duration should be initially. High temperatures of 36°C to 37°C are most suitable for patients with arthritis. Lower temperatures of 30°C to 34.5°C are recommended for patients with spasticity and for any patient whose immersion may last for 20 to 45 minutes. The lower temperatures are chosen to reduce fatigue.[40]

The pool should be at least 12 feet by 16 feet in area, with a built-in filtration and chlorination system; and 3 to 4 feet in depth, with easy accessibility to either a ramp, a ladder or stairs, and a mechanical overhead lift. Adequate room ventilation, which does not allow condensation to accumulate on the walls or windows, is important.[30] There should be a regular maintenance schedule for cleaning at least weekly and tests for water chlorine and pH levels should be performed twice a day.[40,44] Floats (such as rings for the trunk and extremities), paddle boards, slippers, parallel bars or hand rails, as well as weighted stools and chairs, are necessary equipment. There also must be established safety rules and regulations, as well as established procedures for emergencies, including at least one member of the staff present at all times being certified in cardiopulmonary resuscitation (CPR).

The environment should be established as previously discussed for the full-body immersion systems. There should be shower facilities for cleansing before therapy (36°C) and for cooling down after therapy (30–32°C).[32] In addition, adequate space for patients to rest after therapy for 20 minutes and fluid replenishment should be available. Adequate staffing in the pool depends on the condition of the patient population being treated, and there should always be one person present to help the patient outside the pool.

Hot Tubs and Jacuzzis

With the increase in public awareness for physical fitness, health clubs have been increasing in number and have been including hot tubs or whirlpools as part of their facilities. In addition, Jacuzzis and hot tubs are becoming more popular in the home. One of the rising problems is infection with *Pseudomonas aeroginosa*, causing folliculitis.[45] Organic contaminates reduce the effectiveness of the chlorine as a bactericidal agent. Heavy use of whirlpool increases the total organic carbon as well as ammonia and organic nitrogen. Since these events are accelerated by high temperatures and turbulence, there is an increased potential for pathogens to be present.

In order to prevent infection, the following steps should be taken. The pool should have a good filtration and chlorination system. Chlorine and pH levels should be monitored as often as hourly during periods of heavy use, and calcium hardness should be checked weekly. Superchlorination should be performed after each cleaning; and the water should be drained, cleaned, and refilled once every 3 months. Finally, the water temperature should not exceed 38.9°C to 40.5°C. Maintaining the appropriate temperature is also important because of the physiologic effects of total-body heating and heat dissipation. High temperatures will put a greater demand on the cardiovascular and pulmonary systems. The same precautions and contraindications should be observed for any whirlpool.

TABLE 6–6. Clinical Decision Making for Various Forms of Heating/Cooling Modalities

Healing Phase	Characteristics	Desired Effects	Mild Heating	Vigorous Vigorous Heating	Cooling	Whirlpool
Active/exudative phase (0–5 days)	Inflammation Vasoactive agents (histamine) Pain at rest Pain before limitation of motion	Vasoconstriction Dec vasoactive agents Pain relief Dec edema Dec muscle guarding	Contraindicated	Contraindicated	Whirlpool 13–18°C Mild–moderate agitation (extremity) Cold packs	For debridement only 34.4°C (open wounds)
Subacute/ fibroblastic phase (5–21 days)	Inflammation Fibroblastic proliferation Stiffness, pain Pain at resistance of motion	Vasodilation Dec edema Dec muscle guarding Dec pain	Paraffin Moist heat	Fluidotherapy Circumferential moist heat (latter portion of phase)	Whirlpool 13–18°C Conductive Cooling methods (post-treatment)	Extremity Debridement Only 34.4°C 36.7–38.8°C with caution (open wounds)
Chronic/ maturation phase (21 days)	Collagen remodeling Stiffness Pain Pain beyond motion restriction	Vasodilation Tissue Extensibility Sedation, analgesia for exercise	Paraffin Moist Heat (inc superficial) temperature	Fluidotherapy Circumferential Moist heat (greater penetration depth)	Whirlpool 13–18°C Conductive cooling methods (post treatment)	Extremity Debridement 34.4°C Heating extremity 36.7–38.8°C w/caution

TABLE 6–7. Clinical Decision Making in Hydrotherapy (Clinical Problems Given with Supporting Rationale and Treatment Guidelines)*

Case	Rationale for Treatment with Hydrotherapy	Water Temperature and Tank Chosen	Additional Considerations
65-year-old diabetic woman with draining ulcer on left heel	Mechanical debridement of ulcer	At extremity skin temperature to avoid increase in metabolic needs of tissue; foot/ankle tank	Carefully dry and dress ulcer after treatment. Proper whirlpool sterilization, through evaluation of soft tissues, circulation, and neurologic status.
45-year-old man with post-shotgun wound to dorsum of left wrist, with soft tissue loss; wound open, draining; motion of wrist, particularly in flexion, painful and limited	Mechanical debridement of wound Pain reduction to facilitate ease of exercise (buoyancy-assisted exercise)	34.4°C, neutral, comfortable; do not want to cause swelling; hand/arm tank	Carefully dry and dress wound after treatment; encourage patient to keep hand elevated and to do active exercise after whirlpool.
40-year-old woman with flareup of rheumatoid arthritis; ROM of all extremities limited, owing to pain; requires maximal assistance to transfer from supine to sit	Pain reduction; buoyancy-assisted exercise	37–38°C, Hubbard tank	Physical therapist present during session to supervise ROM exercises; overhead lift available; related medical problems of the pulmonary, cardiovascular, and peripheral vascular systems.

*The rationale should be covered when the reader reviews problem, then uncovered to compare choices with those of the author.

SUMMARY

Only with a thorough knowledge and understanding of normal physiology and pathology; the biophysical, thermal, and mechanical effects of whirlpool; and the various physical properties of water and methods of heat transfer can the therapist decide on the proper use of whirlpool treatment for the patient. This knowledge plays an important part in the decision-making process and helps with the recognition of contraindications and precautions to be observed in the use of hydrotherapy. Table 6–6 summarizes the clinical decision-making process. Knowledge of the contraindications and precautions (such as those to be considered with patients with medically compromising cardiovascular or pulmonary pathology, peripheral vascular disease—including acute phlebitis—extremely debilitating or disorienting illness, severe infection or febrile process, renal failure, or gangrene), combined with general knowledge, will help the therapist in problem solving in the borderline case. Safe and effective operation of the whirlpool involves a combination of common sense values and an understanding of the whirlpool's operation and components. Another aspect of the decision-making process is recognition of the special consideration that must be taken when using whirlpool for various anatomic parts, such as upper and lower extremities, or for full-body immersion.

Wound management, especially, requires that we not only understand the aspects of hydrotherapy, but also have a thorough knowledge of the nature of the wound, its physiology, and the condition of the surrounding tissues.

As we have seen in the example of pool therapy, hydrotherapy does not require agitation to be valuable. The inherent properties of water can be combined with therapeutic exercise to effectively treat a portion of the patient population. Finally, we have seen that the use of whirlpool outside the therapist's domain can create potential problems and dangerous situations. Our knowledge, however, can help in properly educating those individuals involved in preventing such situations. The real challenge in hydrotherapy is not necessarily its technical use, but the decision-making process that must occur before its use to achieve the end result of safe, effective treatment for the patient. Examples of clinical decision making in hydrotherapy are briefly outlined in Table 6–7.

REFERENCES

1. Holmes, G: Hydrotherapy as a means of rehabilitation. Br J Phys Med 5:93, 1942.
2. Zislis, J: Hydrotherapy. In Krusen, F (ed): Handbook of Physical Medicine and Rehabilitation, ed 2. WB Saunders, Philadelphia, 1971.
3. Beasley, R and Kester, N: Principles of medical-surgical rehabilitation of the hand. Med Clin North Am 53:645, 1969.
4. Abraham, E: Whirlpool therapy for treatment of soft tissue wounds complicated by extremity fractures. J Trauma 4:222, 1974.
5. Koepke, G: The role of physical medicine in the treatment of burns. Surg Clin North Am 50:1385, 1970.
6. Nave, CR and Nave, BC: Physics for the Health Sciences, ed 2. WB Saunders, Philadelphia, 1980.
7. Dawson, WJ, et al: Evaluation of cardiac output, cardiac work, and metabolic rate during hydrotherapy exercise in normal subjects. Arch Phys Med Rehabil 46:605, 1965.
8. Epstein, M: Water immersion: Modern researchers discover the secrets of an old folk remedy. The Sciences, November: 12, 1979.
9. Boyle, RW, Balisteri, F, and Osborne, F: The value of the Hubbard tank as a diuretic agent. Arch Phys Med Rehabil 45:505, 1964.
10. Abramson, D: Physiologic basis for the use of physical agents in peripheral vascular disorders. Arch Phys Med Rehabil 46:216, 1965.

11. Abramson, D, et al: The effects of altering limb position on blood flow, O_2 uptake and skin temperature. J Appl Physiol 17:191, 1962.
12. Abramson, D, et al: Changes in blood flow, oxygen, uptake and tissue temperatures produced by a topical application of wet heat. Arch Phys Med Rehabil 42:306, 1961.
13. Borrell, R, et al: Comparison of in vivo temperatures produced by hydrotherapy, paraffin wax treatment, and Fluidotherapy. Phys Ther 60:1273, 1980.
14. Nylin, J: The use of water in therapeutics. Arch Phys Med Rehabil 13:261, 1932.
15. Pope, C: Physiologic action and therapeutic value of general and local whirlpool baths. Arch Phys Med Rehabil 10:498, 1929.
16. Cohen, A, Martin, G, and Wakim, K: The effect of whirlpool bath with and without agitation on the circulation in normal and diseased extremities. Arch Phys Med Rehabil 130:212, 1949.
17. Hellerbrand, T, Holutz, S, and Eubank, I: Measurement of whirlpool temperature, pressure and turbulence. Arch Phys Med Rehabil 32:17, 1950.
18. Whitehall Hydrotherapy Equipment, Catalog No. 680, Hackensack, NJ.
19. Turner, AG, Higgins, MM, and Craddock, JG: Disinfection of immersion tanks (Hubbard) in the hospital burn unit. Arch Environ Health 28:101, 1974.
20. Miller, JK, et al: Surveillance and control of Hubbard tank bacterial contaminants. Phys Ther 50:1482, 1970.
21. Ascenzi, J: The need for decontamination and disinfection of hydrotherapy equipment, Vol 1. Asepsis Monograph, Surgikos, Inc, 1989.
22. Simonetti, A, Miller, R, and Gristin, J: Efficacy of povidone-iodine in the disinfection of whirlpool baths and Hubbard tanks. Phys Ther 52:450, 1972.
23. Steve, L, Goodhart, P, and Alexander, J: Hydrotherapy burn treatment: Use of chloramine-T against resistant micro-organisms. Arch Phys Med Rehabil 60:301, 1979.
24. Update: Universal precaution for prevention of transmission of human immunodeficiency virus, hepatitis B virus, and other bloodborne pathogens in health care settings. CDC, MMWR 37:377, 1988.
25. Supplement: Recommendations for prevention of HIV transmission in health-care settings. CDC, MMWR 36:15, 1987.
26. Gieck, J: Precautions for hydrotherapeutic devices. Clinical Management 3:44, 1983.
27. Hunter, JM and Mackin, EJ: Management of edema. In Hunter, JM, et al (eds): Rehabilitation of the Hand: Surgery and Therapy, ed 3. CV Mosby, St. Louis, 1990, pp 187–194.
28. Magness, J, Garrett, T, and Erickson, D: Swelling of the upper extremity during whirlpool baths. Arch Phys Med Rehabil 51:297, 1970.
29. Schultz, K: The effect of active exercise during whirlpool on the hand. Unpublished thesis. San Jose State University, San Jose, CA, 1982.
30. Walsh, M: Relationship of hand edema to upper extremity position and water temperature during whirlpool treatments in normals. Unpublished thesis. Temple University, Philadelphia, 1983.
31. Hoyrup, G and Kjorvel, L: Comparison of whirlpool and wax treatments for hand therapy. Physiother 38:79, 1986.
32. Atkinson, G and Harrison, R: Implications of the health and safety at work act of relationship to hydrotherapy departments. Phys Ther 67:263, 1981.
33. Abston, S: Burns in children. Ciba Clinical Symposia 28:14, 1976.
34. Microbiologic Control Branch Bacterial Disease Division, Bureau of Epidemiology. CDC Sept 1977.
35. Ziegenfus, RW: Povidone iodine as bactericide in hydrotherapy equipment. Phys Ther 49:582, 1969.
36. McGuekin, M, Thorpe, R, and Abrutyn, E: Hydrotherapy: An outbreak of Pseudomonas aeruginosa wound infections related to Hubbard tank treatments. Arch Phys Med Rehabil 62:283, 1981.
37. Haralson, K: Therapeutic pool programs. Clinical Management 5:10.
38. Daggett, R and Gillespie, A: Pool therapy in the treatment of rheumatoid arthritis. In Lamont-Havers, RW and Hilsop, HJ (eds): Arthritis and Related Disorders. American Physical Therapy Association, 1965.
39. Golland, A: Basic hydrotherapy. Physiotherapy 67:258, 1981.
40. Roberts, P: Hydrotherapy: Its history, theory and practice. Occupational Health 235:5, 1981.
41. Harrison, RA: Tolerance of pool therapy by ankylosing spondylitis patients with low vital capacity. Physiotherapy 67:296, 1981.
42. Kirby, RL, et al.: Oxygen consumption during exercise in a heated pool. Arch Phys Med Rehabil 65:21, 1984.
43. Stewart, JB and Basmajian, JF: Exercises in water. In Basmajian, JV (ed): Therapeutic Exercise, ed 3. Williams & Wilkins, Baltimore, 1978.
44. Bickle, RJ: Swimming pool management. Physiotherapy 57:475, 1971.
45. Randt, GA: Hot tub folliculitis. Physician and Sports Medicine 11:75, 1983.

CHAPTER 7

Therapeutic Ultrasound

Marvin C. Ziskin, M.D., M.S. Bm. E.,
Theresa McDiarmid, M.Sc., R.P.T., M.C.S.P., and
Susan L. Michlovitz, M.S., P.T.

Heating agents are divided into two major types: superficial and deep. Superficial heating agents were discussed in Chapter 5. These agents produce temperature elevations in skin and underlying subcutaneous tissues to a depth of approximately 1 cm. In the next two chapters, deep heating agents are discussed. Deep heating agents are capable of causing temperature elevations in tissues to depths of 3 cm or more. Furthermore, these agents are capable of delivering the necessary energy to the deep structures without causing excessive heating of the overlying superficial tissues.

A deep heating agent is an appropriate adjunct to treatment of ailments such as those that (1) limit range of motion owing to a decrease in the extensibility of periarticular soft tissue, (2) cause skeletal muscle spasms that are not of an acute origin, or (3) produce pain secondary to chronic soft tissue dysfunction.

There are three different deep heating agents: ultrasound, shortwave diathermy, and microwave diathermy. Ultrasound is by far the most commonly used (shortwave and microwave diathermy will be discussed in the next chapter). It should also be noted that ultrasound is receiving increasingly widespread use for its nonthermal effects. These will be discussed in detail in this chapter.

Ultrasound has been employed in medicine for more than 50 years. Biologic effects in tissues exposed to ultrasound (high frequency sound waves) were first reported by Wood and Loomis[1] in 1927. They demonstrated lysis of red blood cells and decreased mobility in mice following exposure to high frequency (300 kHz), high intensity sound waves. The application of ultrasound for medical treatment was introduced in Germany in the late 1930s[2], and in the United States in the late 1940s.[3]

Ultrasound is used in medicine for diagnosis (imaging of internal structures), physical therapy (functional restoration and healing of soft tissue ailments), and tissue destruction (in surgery and hyperthermia for tumor irradiation). The intensity of ultrasound in each classification is different; the lowest intensity is used for diagnostic procedures, and the highest intensity is used for tissue destruction.

The objectives of this chapter are to (1) present the physical principles and biophysical effects of ultrasound; (2) discuss the clinical conditions for which ultrasound is effective; (3) discuss the clinical procedures for the application of ultrasound; and, (4) present guidelines for the safe use of ultrasound, including a discussion of the contraindications and precautions for treatment with this agent.

PHYSICAL PRINCIPLES

The purpose of this section is to provide a basic foundation of the physics of ultrasound for the physical therapist. For a more complete and in-depth study, the excellent textbook by Wells[4] should be consulted.

Nature of Sound

Solids and liquids consist of molecules held together by elastic forces that behave like rubberbands connecting each molecule to each of its nearest neighbors. Thus, a molecule, if set into vibration, will cause its neighbors to vibrate, and in turn their neighbors, and so on, until the vibration has propagated throughout the entire material. Each individual molecule vibrates back and forth a small distance from its initial position. The passage of vibrational energy, however, travels over millions of molecules in propagating through tissue. The propagation of this vibratory motion is precisely what is sound.

Unlike electromagnetic waves such as light and x-rays, sound cannot travel in a vacuum. Very important for the patient is the fact that sound is nonionizing radiation and, therefore, its use does not impose the hazards attributed to ionizing radiation, such as cancer production and chromosome breakage.

FREQUENCY

The number of oscillations a molecule undergoes in 1 second defines the frequency of a sound wave and is expressed in units of hertz (Hz): that is, 1 Hz = 1 cycle per second; 1 kHz = 1000 cycles per second; and 1 MHz = 1 million cycles per second. Theoretically, frequency can vary from 0 Hz to infinity, however, the human ear is sensitive only to sound frequencies between 16 Hz and 20,000 Hz. Sound with a frequency greater than 20,000 Hz is called *ultrasound*.

For a given sound source, the higher the frequency, the less the emerging sound beam diverges. Sound at audible frequencies appears to spread out in all directions, whereas ultrasound beams are well collimated, similar to a light beam leaving a flashlight (Fig. 7-1). Ultrasound beams at frequencies greater than 800 kHz are sufficiently collimated to selectively expose a limited target area for physical therapy treatment.

Attenuation

Energy contained within a sound beam is decreased as it travels through tissue. This results from two processes: scattering and absorption. *Scattering* is the deflection of sound out of the beam that results when the sound strikes a reflecting surface. *Absorption* is the transfer of energy from the sound beam to the surrounding tissues.

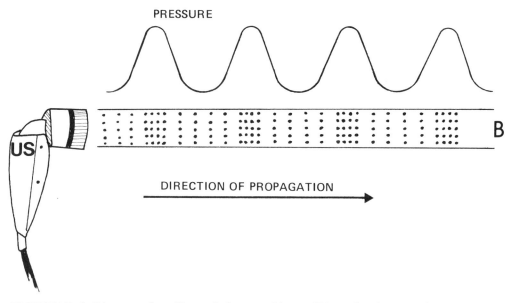

FIGURE 7–1. Diagram of a collimated ultrasound beam (*B*) coming from an ultrasound (US) applicator. The associated pressure wave is diagrammed above. Areas of increased molecular concentration (:::) are condensations. Areas of decreased molecular concentration are rarefactions (:.:).

Absorption of sound, and therefore attenuation, increases as the frequency increases. Absorption occurs in part because of the internal friction in tissue that needs to be overcome in the passage of sound. The higher the frequency, the more rapidly the molecules are forced to move against this friction. As the absorption increases, there is less sound energy available to propagate further through the tissue (Fig. 7–2). At frequencies greater than 20 MHz, superficial absorption becomes so great that less than 1 percent of the sound penetrates beyond the first centimeter.

For physical therapy applications, 1.0 MHz is the frequency most often used, because it offers a good compromise between sufficiently deep penetration and adequate heating under customary exposure levels. However, many units in the United States now also offer a 3.0 MHz frequency for the treatment of superficial tissues.

SOUND VELOCITY

Velocity is the speed at which the vibratory motion is propagated through a material. The more rigid the material, the greater the velocity of sound passing through it. Sound travels through average soft tissue at 1540 m per second, and through compact bones at 4000 meters per second. The depth of a structure beneath the skin can be determined by measuring the time required for sound to travel to the structure and return. This ability to chart the position of reflecting surfaces forms the basis of the extensive use of ultrasound in medical diagnosis.

WAVELENGTH

A finite period of time elapses before the vibration of a molecule causes its neighbor to vibrate. Because of this delay, the first molecule will reach its point of maximal excursion before its neighbor does and, as long as the two molecules continue to vibrate,

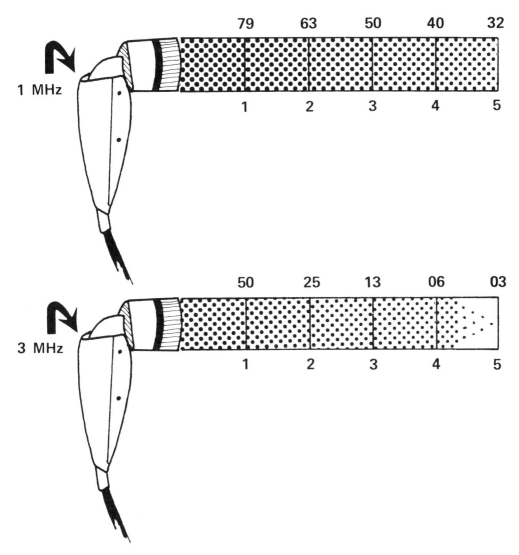

FIGURE 7 – 2. Attenuation of the sound beam in soft tissue at various frequencies, assuming that uniform attenuation is approximately 1 dB/cm/MHz.

the second molecule will lag behind the first. These molecules are said to oscillate asynchronously, or be out of phase, and the time delay is called the *phase shift*. There is an equal phase shift between each of the successive molecules in the path of sound propagation. Because of this overall asynchrony, the concentration of molecules increases in regions called *condensations* and decreases in alternating regions called *rarefactions* (see Fig. 7 – 1). The local pressure is proportional to the molecular concentration and, as shown in Figure 7 – 1, varies sinusoidally along the direction of propagation, with its peak values occurring at regions of condensations. *Wavelength* is defined as the distance between two successive peaks in the pressure wave.

Wavelength is inversely related to frequency, as indicated in the fundamental equation, velocity = frequency × wavelength. Using the value of 1540 m per second for velocity and 1 MHz for frequency, which are typical values applicable in therapeutic situations, this equation enables us to show that the corresponding wavelength of ultrasound is 1.5 mm.

Types of Waves

Sound waves are classified as longitudinal or transverse, according to the direction of motion of the molecules of the medium through which they travel. A *longitudinal wave* is one in which the direction of motion of the molecules is parallel to the direction of wave propagation (Fig. 7–3). In a *transverse wave*, the direction of molecular motion is perpendicular to the direction of wave propagation.

Since gases and liquids are not able to sustain transverse vibrations, transverse sound waves do not occur in these substances. In solids, both longitudinal and transverse waves occur. With the exception of compact bone, the tissues of the body behave acoustically as though they were liquids, and support only longitudinal waves. Within the body, therefore, transverse waves are found only in bone.

Sound waves can be produced as continuous wave (CW) or pulsed wave. A *continuous wave* is one in which the sound intensity remains constant (Fig. 7–4), whereas a *pulsed wave* is intermittently interrupted. Pulsed waves are further characterized by specifying the fraction of time the sound is present over one pulse period. This fraction is called the *duty cycle* and is calculated using the following equation:

$$\text{Duty cycle} = \frac{\text{Duration of pulse (time-on)}}{\text{Pulse period (time-on + time-off)}}$$

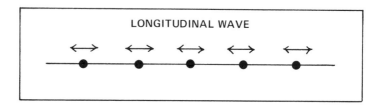

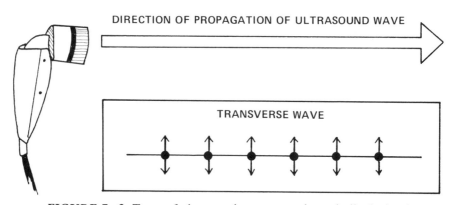

FIGURE 7–3. Types of ultrasound waves are schematically depicted.

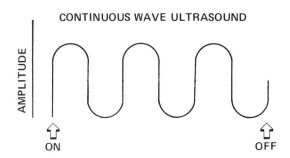

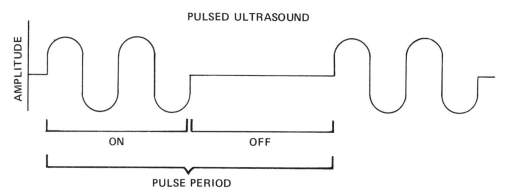

FIGURE 7-4. Continuous wave and pulsed wave ultrasound. The duty cycle of the pulsed wave mode illustrated is $\dfrac{2 \text{ msec}}{4 \text{ msec}} = 0.5 = 50$ percent.

Typical duty cycles for therapy machines, when in the pulsed mode, range from 0.05 (5 percent) to 0.5 (50 percent). The most commonly used duty cycle appears to be 20 percent.

Intensity

The strength of an ultrasound beam is determined by its intensity. *Intensity* is the rate at which energy is delivered per unit area; it is expressed in units of watts per square centimeter (W/cm^2). Intensities employed in physical therapy range from about 0.25 to 3.0 W/cm^2. With all other factors held constant, the greater the intensity, the greater the resulting temperature elevation.

The measurement of intensity is performed by measuring the total power output (in watts) of the ultrasound applicator and dividing by the area (in cm^2) of the applicator face. Because the ultrasound beam is not uniform, some regions of the beam will be more intense than other regions. The above measurement of intensity gives an average intensity and is referred to as the *spatial average intensity*. Occasionally, it is desirable to know the greatest intensity anywhere within the beam. This is called the *spatial peak intensity* (Fig. 7-5).

In the case when the sound beam is pulsed, the intensity will be zero when the

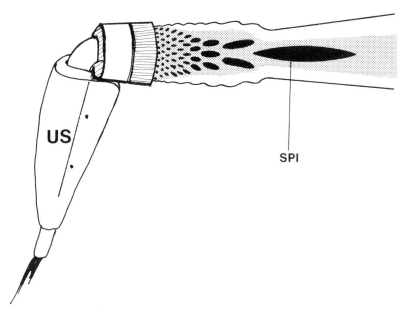

FIGURE 7–5. Schematic diagram of ultrasound beam. The darkest areas indicate more intense regions. The greatest intensity within the beam is the spatial peak intensity (SPI). (Adapted from Stewart, HF and Stratmeyer, ME (eds): An Overview of Ultrasound: Theory, Measurement, Medical Applications, and Biological Effects. HHS Publication FDA 82-8-90, 1982.)

sound is off and at its maximum during the pulse (Fig. 7–6). This maximum intensity is called the *temporal peak intensity* or the *pulse average intensity*. The temporal average intensity is obtained by averaging the intensity over both the on and off periods. For example, a pulsed sound beam with a duty cycle of 0.5 (50 percent) and a temporal peak intensity of 2.0 W/cm² would have a temporal average intensity of 1.0 W/cm² (2.0 W/cm² × 0.5 = 1.0 W/cm²); if the duty cycle had been 0.25 (25 percent), the temporal average intensity would be 0.5 W/cm². In this chapter, unless stated otherwise, all pulsed intensities quoted will be spatial average, temporal peak values, along with the duty cycle.

The amount of heating depends on the temporal average intensity rather than the temporal peak. By interrupting (pulsing) a continuous wave sound beam, the temporal average intensity is decreased proportionately to the amount of time the sound is off. Thus, less heating will occur even though the temporal peak intensity is unchanged. Pulsing would be of benefit when the desired effect is due to a nonthermal mechanism

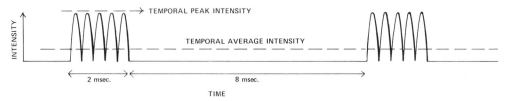

FIGURE 7–6. A typical pulsing pattern. The total pulse period is 10 msec. The pulse duration is 2 msec. The duty cycle is 0.20 (20 percent).

and when heating is to be minimized, such as in the treatment of stasis ulcers and acute soft tissue injuries.

Also, it should be noted that the ultrasonic beam is not homogeneous, resulting in high spatial peak intensities within the beam, commonly known as "hot spots." These hot spots may cause damage to the insonated tissues and, therefore, should be avoided. This is best done by always using a moving applicator technique when in direct contact to prevent any buildup of energy in any one spot. The beam nonuniformity ratio (BNR) should also be within the acceptable range. This ratio defines the maximal point intensity on the transducer to the average intensity value across the transducer surface. The BNR should be as low as possible, between 2 and 6. The lower the BNR, the more even is the distribution of energy from the transducer, and the less risk there is of damage to tissues from areas of concentrated ultrasound energy. In the United States, ultrasound units manufactured since 1979 are required by the Food and Drug Administration to have labels indicating the BNR; the therapist should be aware of the BNR of the equipment being used.

When recording the ultrasound exposure administered to a patient, it is important to specify clearly the frequency, the intensity, the duty cycle, and the total duration, for example, 3.0 MHz/0.5 W/cm^2/p20%/5 minutes. For continuous wave exposures, the frequency, the spatial average intensity, the continuous wave, and the duration are reported, for example, 3.0 MHz/0.5 W/cm^2/cw/5 minutes.

Spatial average intensities ranging from 0.25 to 2.0 W/cm^2 are used in therapeutic applications. The World Health Organization limits the spatial average intensity to a maximum of 3.0 W/cm^2.[5] Intensities greater than 10.0 W/cm^2 are used to destroy tissue surgically, and intensities (temporal average) below 0.1 W/cm^2 are used for diagnostic purposes.

When considering the intensity applied to the patient, one should also consider that ultrasound vibrations that are propagated through the housing of the applicator into the hand of the physical therapist have been termed *parasitic radiation*.[6] This radiation has been reported possibly to result in acute pain in the hand and finger joints of the therapist. The significance of, or dangers secondary to, parasitic radiation are at this time speculative at best.

Generation of Ultrasound

Sound within the audible frequency range is normally produced by vibrating membranes, such as the vocal cords or the diaphragm of a loudspeaker. Movement of these membranes sets up corresponding vibrations in the surrounding air molecules and, when this vibration pattern reaches our ears, we perceive it as sound. The frequency of the sound is precisely the frequency of the membrane vibration. Because of their inertia, these membranes cannot vibrate rapidly enough to generate ultrasonic frequencies. However, ultrasound can be generated by replacing these membranes with special crystals that are able to vibrate very rapidly and possess the property of piezoelectricity.

THE PIEZOELECTRIC EFFECT

There are two forms of the piezoelectric effect: direct and reverse (indirect) (Fig. 7–7). The direct piezoelectric effect is the generation of an electric voltage across a crystal when the crystal is compressed. If the crystal is expanded instead of compressed,

DIRECT PIEZOELECTRIC

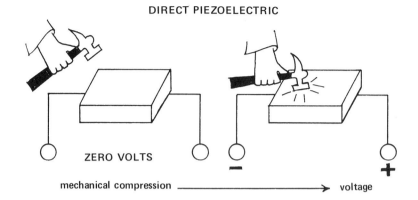

REVERSE PIEZOELECTRIC

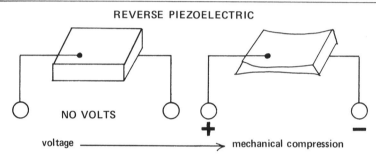

FIGURE 7–7. The direct and indirect (reverse) piezoelectric effects are shown.

a voltage of opposite polarity is induced. A sound wave impinging on a piezoelectric crystal will cause the crystal to expand and contract at the same frequency as the sound wave and, in turn, induce an oscillating voltage across the crystal face. The direct piezoelectric effect is used for converting ultrasound into an electrical signal that replicates the sound pattern and can be conveniently and accurately processed and analyzed.

The reverse piezoelectric effect is the contraction or expansion of a crystal in response to a voltage applied across its face. A change in the polarity of the applied voltage causes a contracted crystal to expand, and vice versa. An alternating voltage makes the crystal vibrate at the frequency of the electrical oscillation. In this manner, a piezoelectric crystal can be used to generate ultrasound at any desired frequency.

THE TRANSDUCER

A transducer is any device that converts one form of energy into another. The piezoelectric crystal is a transducer that converts electrical energy into sound energy, and vice versa.

Many naturally occurring crystals, such as quartz, possess the property of piezoelectricity, but synthetic ceramic crystals, such as barium titanate or lead zirconate titanate (PZT), are almost always used because of their superior mechanical and electrical properties. These crystals are sliced into wafers approximately 2 to 3 mm thick. The diameter may vary from 1 to 3 cm depending on the intended use. Because of their small size and mechanical fragility, these crystals must be mounted in an applicator to be clinically useful and durable and to facilitate electrical connections. The entire applicator is commonly referred to as the transducer.

Therapeutic Ultrasound Units

The basic components of therapeutic ultrasound units include a power supply, oscillator circuit, transformer, coaxial cable, and ultrasound applicator. The purpose of the therapeutic ultrasound unit is to produce a sound beam at a specific frequency. The frequency is generated by an oscillator circuit carefully tuned by the manufacturer to the preferred frequency for the transducer. Occasional tuning adjustments may be necessary, particularly when a transducer is replaced. These adjustments are best left to the biomedical technician. The intensity is determined by the electrical voltage applied to the transducer. The voltage is controlled by the setting of the intensity control, which adjusts a variable gain transformer.

A circuit can be added that interrupts the oscillator to produce a pulsed mode. The duty cycle control selector on the face of the machine can change the on or off times by controlling a pulse timing circuit. The treatment timer limits how long the instrument is energized. In some units, the timer also serves as the on–off switch.

To work properly, the unit is supplied with appropriate voltages obtained through a transformer to which electrical power from the wall receptacle is applied. Appropriate power can also be supplied through a battery. A coaxial cable connects the ultrasound applicator to the generator (console). The purpose of the coaxial cable is to maximize transmission of the electrical energy and to minimize frequency distortion and interference with the external environment.

All units have a power meter calibrated to read in both watts (acoustic power) and W/cm² (acoustic intensity). For any given applicator, the ratio of the acoustic power to the intensity is a constant, the effective radiating area (ERA). Some machines now also feature self-calibration testing, output power control in response to tissue loading, and automatic shut off in case of transducer overheating or inadequate coupling. A typical ultrasound unit is pictured in Figure 7–8.

QUALITY CONTROL

Surveys of ultrasound machines used in physical therapy departments[6-9] revealed that a considerable number of machines were not functioning within acceptable limits, especially with regard to the effective intensity. In light of these reports of machine inadequacies, it would appear that physical therapists should be more vigilant in ensuring that their ultrasound equipment is functioning safely and correctly. A survey of 204 hospital physical therapy departments and 109 private clinics in England and Wales[10] revealed how often the ultrasound machines were calibrated, by whom, and how many physical therapists had access to a radiation balance. To ensure that ultrasound machines are performing correctly and safely, factors such as beam shape, power, and pressure should be checked annually, as should all the electrical components. The transducer assembly, in particular, is prone to deterioration and should be frequently checked, especially for water tightness. These factors are generally checked by the manufacturers or a biomedical instrumentation service, but every ultrasound machine should be checked weekly in its department of use to ensure that it is at least transmitting the ultrasound energy correctly (see Chapter 3).

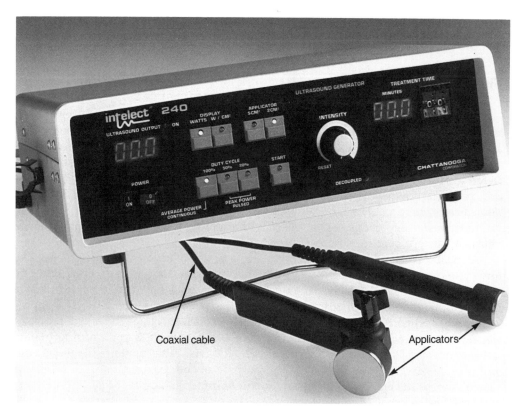

FIGURE 7–8. A therapeutic ultrasound generator is depicted. Note two different size applicators. (Photo courtesy of Chattanooga Corporation, Chattanooga, TN.)

BIOPHYSICAL EFFECTS

The biophysical effects resulting from the interaction of ultrasound with tissue can be grouped into two classifications:

1. Thermal—effects produced by the ability of ultrasound to elevate tissue temperature.
2. Nonthermal—effects attributed to a mechanism other than an increase in tissue temperature.

The mechanism of some of the biologic changes produced by ultrasound may be thermal or nonthermal, or a combination of both. For many responses, such as the pain reduction reported following insonation, the underlying physiologic or physical mechanism has not been thoroughly identified and is only speculative at this time.

Thermal Effects

The principal reason for the use of ultrasound as a therapeutic agent is that ultrasound can elevate tissue temperature to depths of 5 cm or more. The physiologic responses attributed to a thermal mechanism include increase in collagen tissue extensibility, alterations in blood flow, changes in nerve conduction velocity, increase in pain threshold, increased enzymatic activity, and changes in contractile activity of skeletal muscle. Physiologic changes such as these are reviewed in Chapter 5. Ultrasound intensities at ranges higher than those used for therapeutic application have been demonstrated to retard growth of long bones, damage spinal cord tissue, and destroy various other tissues.

Tissues of high collagen content absorb a large amount of the ultrasound beam and, thus, are affected to a greater extent by ultrasound energy. The amount of heat produced will depend on the intensity and frequency of ultrasound, the duration of exposure, and the size and type of tissue insonated. Bone and joint capsular structures have a very high collagen content and are, therefore, the structures that absorb the most ultrasound energy. Ultrasound penetrates through skin and subcutaneous fat with small to moderate attenuation (Table 7–1).

Ultrasound energy absorption and the subsequent tissue temperature elevation are frequency dependent. The higher the frequency, the greater the attentuation of energy in superficial structures. At 3.0 MHz, most of the energy is absorbed within a depth of 1 to 2 cm. At a lower frequency of 1.0 MHz, there is less attenuation in the superficial tissues, allowing more energy to be available for absorption into deeper tissues. This latter frequency is commonly used in the United States in the treatment of musculoskeletal dysfunctions, when an increased depth of penetration and subsequent absorption are desired. However, as many of the conditions commonly treated with therapeutic ultrasound involve superficial tissues (e.g., ankle sprains, tennis elbow, stasis ulcers), it is important that the appropriate frequency be used to treat the injured tissue. In general, a 3.0 MHz frequency should be used in treating tissues up to 1 to 2 cm from the skin surface, and 1.0 MHz frequency should be used in treating tissues deeper than 1 to 2 cm from the skin surface.

Ultrasound can be used as a deep heating agent to increase selectively the temperature of periarticular structures[11] and muscle at the bone–muscle interface.[12,13] Intensities required to elevate tissue temperature to a range of 40°C to 45°C vary from 1.0 to 2.0 W/cm² continuous wave for a duration of 5 to 10 minutes. A residual increase in length of tendons in amphibians has been demonstrated by elevating tissue temperature with ultrasound and then applying a stretch during the time the temperature remains elevated.[14] In mammalian preparations, similar increases were reported when tissue temperature was elevated by a water bath and a stretch was applied.[15,16] This effect has been attributed to the change in viscous properties of the tissues irradiated, which produces a change in the plastic deformation of collagen tissues. This information has

TABLE 7–1. Attenuation of a 1 MHz Ultrasound Beam

Tissue	Attenuation (%/cm)
Blood	3
Fat	13
Muscle	24
Blood vessel	32
Skin	39
Tendon	59
Cartilage	68
Bone	96

been applied clinically to increase range of motion of contracted joints (see section on clinical application).

With an increase in tissue temperature, a mild inflammatory response and an increase in blood flow would be expected. Numerous investigators have measured blood flow in limbs following ultrasound irradiation, some reporting an increase in flow, some a decrease, and some no changes. Intensities, frequencies, duty cycles, and exposure durations of ultrasound application and the methods of measuring changes in blood flow were not consistent among the experimenters. Drawing clinically useful conclusions, therefore, is difficult. However, the following statements appear to summarize this information accurately. Following 10 to 20 minutes of ultrasound, at intensities greater than 2.0 W/cm^2, 1.0 MHz frequency, continuous wave, skeletal muscle temperature and blood flow increases have been found.[17-19] At lower intensities and for shorter durations, either no change or inconsistent changes in blood flow were noted.[19-21]

Changes in motor and sensory nerve conduction velocity after ultrasound exposure have been reported. Five minutes of ultrasound at 1.5 W/cm^2, 1.0 MHz frequency, continuous wave over the lateral cutaneous branch of the radial[22] and superficial cutaneous branch of radial nerves[23] decreased latency. No changes were found in the amplitude or duration of the nerve action potential. When sensory nerve latency is decreased, an increase in conduction velocity is implicit. In a similar experimental setup, latency was decreased in the superficial radial nerve following 1.0 W/cm^2, varying from 5 to 20 minutes.[24] Two groups of investigators compared ultrasound with infrared heating.[23,24] Because latencies were reduced with both agents, and temperature increases were similar, the investigators attributed their findings to thermal mechanisms.

Ulnar motor nerve conduction velocity (NCV) increased 3.0 m per second with continuous wave ultrasound at 1.5 W/cm^2 for 5 minutes, and with infrared radiation.[25] Placebo ultrasound and pulsed ultrasound at 1.5 W/cm^2 (1 : 5 pulse ratio) for 25 minutes caused a decrease in NCV. The decrease was proposed to be correlated with the reduction of temperature caused by a cool coupling medium. The thermal effects, rather than the nonthermal effects, were thought to produce the increased NCV.

Pain threshold was elevated following increases in tissue temperature with 0.8 MHz frequency continuous wave ultrasound at 1.5 W/cm^2.[26] These findings are consistent with what is expected when tissue temperature is elevated by a thermal agent.

Nonthermal Effects

Some effects of ultrasound cannot be explained by a thermal mechanism. These nonthermal effects include cavitation and mechanical and chemical alterations. *Cavitation* is the vibrational effect on gas bubbles by an ultrasound beam. Changes in local pressure produced by ultrasound can cause the expansion and compression of small gas bubbles that may be present in the blood or tissue fluids. During the period of rarefaction, the small bubbles will expand; during condensations, these bubbles will be compressed. The pulsation of the bubbles in the ultrasound field, if sufficiently intense, can cause changes in cellular activity and tissue damage. If the bubbles in the field pulse, but do not increase much in overall amplitude, stable cavities result. These stable cavities can result in diffusional changes along cell membranes and, thus, alter cell function.[22] Unstable or transient cavitation refers to the violent collapse of bubbles within the sound field, resulting in tissue destruction. Transient cavitation may be responsible for blood vessel damage.[28] The threshold intensity for unstable cavitation is higher than for stable cavitation. The intensity threshold for cavitation may be within the intensity range used in therapy and, although many questions remain, there is some evidence that cavitation may occur in therapeutic applications. We do not know which, if any, of the beneficial nonthermal effects are due to stable cavitation.

Acoustic streaming refers to the movement of fluids along the boundaries of cell membranes as a result of the mechanical pressure wave. This streaming has been implicated in the changes in ion fluxes and subsequent changes in cellular activity found with ultrasound application. Increases in cell membrane and vascular wall permeability have been found within the range of therapeutic intensities. Potassium leakage from red blood cells in vitro resulted following insonation at ranges from 0.5 to 3.0 W/cm^2.[29] Increases in fibroblastic activity (for example, protein synthesis)[30] and increases in calcium fluxes across smooth muscle membranes of the mouse uterus were found using pulsed ultrasound.[31] These changes may be a result of the mechanical action of ultrasound on cell membranes, rather than of a thermal mechanism.

On the other hand, changes in the diffusion of ions across epithelial cells in isolated frog skin have been attributed to both thermal and mechanical components.[32] Using a stationary applicator, ultrasound at 1.5 W/cm^2 applied to the small blood vessels in the hamster cheek pouch resulted in areas of petechiae and demonstrable increases in vascular permeability at the level of the postcapillary venules.[33] The results could have been due to thermally induced changes in permeability or to cavitation resulting in damage to vessel endothelial cells. Petechiae in mice were also found after abdominal exposure to ultrasound.[28] Cavitation was implicated as the mechanism producing the observed results.

Other adverse reactions, including stasis of blood flow and endothelial damage, have been demonstrated in chick embryos.[34] Platelet aggregation in blood vessels was shown to occur in guinea pig ears.[35] These responses were attributed to nonthermal mechanisms, because either pulsed ultrasound or very low intensity continuous wave ultrasound was administered. A stationary transducer was used for all applications. The investigators speculated that such results would not be produced with a moving sound head.

To further elucidate the effects of ultrasound on the microcirculation, Hogan and associates[36,37] recently have studied the effects of ultrasound on circulation in the rat in an ischemic muscle preparation. When pulsed ultrasound was applied at a frequency of 1.0 MHz at 2.5 W/cm^2 for 5 minutes on alternating days, an increase in capillary density and improved blood flow to medium-sized arterioles was found. At higher intensities of pulsed ultrasound, increased vasomotion of small arterioles and decreased flow was found. Although the underlying mechanisms for all the changes seen were not known, they probably were not thermal in origin, because similar findings were not observed when the skeletal muscle was heated in the absence of ultrasound.

In summary, a review of the literature shows that ultrasound can cause many effects, most of which are intensity dependent. With appropriate care to control intensities, ultrasound can be applied to patients in a safe and effective manner.

CLINICAL APPLICATIONS OF ULTRASOUND AT THERAPEUTIC INTENSITIES

Ultrasound is commonly used in rehabilitation as an adjunct in the management of various soft tissue dysfunctions, including joint contracture, scar tissue, tendinitis, bursitis, skeletal muscle spasms, and pain. In addition, ultrasound at therapeutic intensities has been included in treatment regimens for the management of stasis ulcers, pressure sores, and plantar warts and as a noninvasive technique to drive medication through the skin (phonophoresis). The basis for the clinical application of ultrasound as a therapeutic agent was developed in the previous section. Although there is now an abundance of laboratory and clinical reports on the effects and applications of therapeutic ultrasound, much of the material lacks full description of the treatment regimens, and many of the results present contradictory conclusions.[38] In this section, the procedures and rationale for the clinical use of ultrasound will be discussed.

Joint Contracture and Scar Tissue

Joint contracture is a debilitating consequence of immobilization or trauma. If range of motion is limited owing to periarticular connective tissue changes, stretching exercises are usually employed to increase motion. Elevation of tissue temperature to 45°C, preceding or during a gentle passive or active stretch, will be more effective in gaining motion than when either is done in isolation. The concept of "heat and stretch" has been demonstrated in well-designed in vitro laboratory studies.[15,16,39] A greater residual increase in tissue length with less potential damage is produced when preheating or simultaneous heating is employed. Length–tension analyses revealed that tissue extensibility was increased when Gersten[14] applied ultrasound at intensities of 1.0 to 3.0 W/cm^2, resulting in tissue temperatures ranging from 30°C to 47°C.

Heating has been postulated to alter the viscoelastic properties of collagen tissue and collagen molecular bonding, thus facilitating ease of stretch. Deep tissues responsible for decreasing the range of motion at a joint are rich in collagen. Therefore, ultrasound is a logically chosen thermal agent to selectively heat these deep structures.

Lehmann and associates[40] demonstrated that ultrasound was effective in increasing the temperature of the hip joint when applied within therapeutic intensities for at least 5 minutes. A combination of ultrasound and exercise was compared with infrared and exercise for increasing range of motion of the hips of elderly patients following internal fixation of fractures.[41] Ultrasound was applied to the anterior, lateral, and posterior hip joint at intensities of 1.0 to 2.5 W/cm^2 for 5 minutes per field. The other group received infrared heating for 30 minutes. Results of treatment were evaluated by range of motion measurements. Individuals receiving ultrasound improved in range of motion. Those receiving infrared showed less or no gain when compared with those receiving ultrasound. Information obtained from these studies can certainly be applied to the treatment of joint contracture in other areas of the body. Joints with a smaller amount of soft tissue coverage, such as the elbow, wrist, or ankle, are usually treated at intensities averaging 1.0 W/cm^2 or less.

Ice and ultrasound applications were compared for the treatment of painful "frozen shoulder."[42] Ultrasound therapy was administered to one group at an intensity of 0.5 W/cm^2 for 5 to 8 minutes, 3 times a week for a total of 15 treatments. Iced towels were applied to the other group for 15 minutes 3 times a week for a total of 12 treatments. Both groups were placed on a program of passive and active range of motion exercises following thermal agent application. All patients reported a decrease in pain and had an increased range of motion that was attributed to their treatment with no apparent differences between the groups. The intensity of ultrasound used for treatment, however, was less than that which has been demonstrated to elevate joint structure temperature at the knee,[11] a joint with approximately as much soft tissue coverage as the shoulder. This observation points out that unless a sufficient intensity is used, one should not expect any greater benefit from the use of ultrasound than from superficial heating or cooling.

Scar tissue is more dense than surrounding tissue and can be selectively heated by ultrasound energy before friction massage and range of motion exercises. Bierman[43] reported successfully increasing the range of motion in a small series of patients who had scar tissue secondary to lacerations, x-ray burns, and Dupuytren's contracture. Continuous wave ultrasound was administered at intensities of 1.0 to 2.0 W/cm² for 6 to 8 minutes every other day. On the other hand, Wright and Haase[44] found that ultrasound at a lower intensity than used by Bierman was not effective in reducing the size of keloids. The low intensity used may have accounted for the unsuccessful treatment they reported.

Ultrasound has a definite role in the treatment of joint contractures and scar tissue. To be used effectively, however, more work is needed to determine what intensities and durations should be used to obtain the possible beneficial effects of ultrasound.

Reduction of Pain and Muscle Spasm

Following ultrasound application, pain threshold is usually increased. Although the mechanism of pain reduction is not clear, the heat produced by ultrasound could result in counterirritation, heat activation of large diameter fibers, or an altering of the response to stimulation of the pain receptors (free nerve endings). Pain threshold was elevated following ultrasound application to the arm at 1.5 W/cm² for 2 minutes.[26] Because similar changes were found with infrared and microwave diathermy applications (both surface heating and deep heating agents), the implicated mechanism of action is through the ability of all three agents to elevate the threshold for activation of the free nerve endings through thermal effects. Williams and coworkers[45] measured a significant decrease in the perception threshold for electrical pain after exposure to ultrasound. This effect developed within 30 to 60 seconds and was increased both with increasing intensity at constant frequency and with increasing frequency at constant intensity. When the same amount of ultrasound energy was delivered using a variety of pulsed regimens, exactly the same reduction in pain threshold was obtained. The authors concluded that this indicated a thermal interaction mechanism.

Munting[46] compared ultrasound combined with exercise with exercise alone for the treatment of patients with shoulder pain. The patients included in the study had no evidence of tendinitis, fracture, or degenerative joint changes. During a 3-week period, ultrasound was applied for a total of 10 treatments each — at an intensity of 1.5 W/cm² for 3 to 5 minutes — to the anterior, inferior, and posterior aspects of the shoulder. The patients who received ultrasound reported a higher percentage of pain relief (81%) than those who received only exercise (44%). In addition, the gains in active and passive range of motion were greater in the ultrasound-treated groups. At 3-month followup, 73 percent of the patients who had received ultrasound reported no pain, compared with 55 percent of the exercise-only group. Similar results were obtained by Middlemast and Chatterjee,[47] who treated a variety of acute soft tissue injuries at 1.5 MHz, pulsed wave, for 4 to 10 minutes, at intensities varying from 0.5 to 1.0 W/cm² for superficial tissues and 1 to 2 W/cm² for deeply placed structures. They assessed spontaneous pain, tenderness, erythema, restriction of active movement and swelling and found that, after 10 treatments during a 12-day period, the patients treated with ultrasound showed a significantly better overall response than the patients treated with infrared, short-wave diathermy, or wax bath.

Patients with hemiplegia who had painful shoulders were treated using three different regimens: (1) range of motion exercises, positioning, and ultrasound at 0.5 to 2.0 W/cm²; (2) range of motion exercises, positioning, and sham ultrasound; or, (3) only range of motion exercises and positioning.[48] No statistically significant difference in range of motion was reported among the groups. The authors concluded that, in this patient sample, ultrasound was probably not a useful adjunct to treatment with the dosages they administered.

Neuromas in amputation stumps can be sources of pain and can delay the rehabilitation process. Ultrasound has been used in the conservative management of neuromas. When Soren[49] applied ultrasound to patients' painful neuromas at intensities averaging 1.5 W/cm², five of the six patients studied had decreased pain and improved function.

Ultrasound therapy is often included in the care of patients with low-back dysfunction of various etiologies. Considering the extent of use, little had appeared in the literature to support or refute its efficacy in the management of this clinical condition. The technique that is generally employed is paravertebral application, with or without insonation along the involved nerve trunk(s). There appear to be only three reports on such application, two from the 1950s and one from the 1980s. Kuitert[50] described six patients with referred pain secondary to osteoarthritis of the spine, damage to vertebral bodies, or herniated intervertebral discs. Doses of 0.5 to 1.5 W/cm² were applied paravertebrally on a daily basis for 6 to 12 sessions, averaging 10 minutes per session. Five patients reported decreased pain and muscle spasm and improved motion. One patient had no change. No other treatments were compared with ultrasound.

Two hundred and nine cases of low back pain secondary to herniated intervertebral disc syndrome were reported by Aldes and Grabin.[51] Symptoms were relieved in 86 percent of the patients when treated with a 12-session course of ultrasound at intensities ranging from 0.3 to 0.8 W/cm². Ultrasound was administered paravertebrally and along the gluteus maximus, the hamstring, and the gastrocnemius muscles in patients with radiculitis. Since hot packs and massage were also included in treatment regimens, the relief experienced by the patients may have been produced by these superficial heating agents rather than by the ultrasound. The ultrasound intensities used by the investigators were lower than those customarily used for an area with such a large amount of soft tissue.

Low back pain resulting from herniated intervertebral discs from L-4 to S-2 were treated by Nwuga[52], using three different protocols. All patients were seen within 2 weeks after onset of pain. The three groups designated received: (1) analgesics and bed rest; (2) sham ultrasound and bed rest; and, (3) ultrasound at 1.0 to 2.0 W/cm² for 10 minutes and bed rest. Ultrasound and sham ultrasound were given 3 times a week during a 4-week period. Straight leg raising (Lasèque test) and lumbar spinal flexion, extension, side flexion, and rotation were measured. Subjective assessments of pain were made. The group treated with ultrasound obtained the best results, with the greatest improvement in flexion, extension, and straight leg raising, and a reduction in pain.

The use of ultrasound combined with high voltage pulsed current in the treatment of long-standing low back pain (mean = 5 years) was found to be effective in locating and treating trigger points.[53] The ultrasound transducer was used as the active electrode and, when trigger points in the area insonated were identified by increased pain, they were treated by a stationary technique until the pain decreased (average, 5 seconds). All patients reported an analgesic effect, but no attempt was made in this study to differentiate the specific effects of the two modalities.

Skeletal muscle temperature can be elevated by ultrasound. Temperature measurements of thighs were made, using implanted thermistors.[13] Ultrasound produced temperature elevations at the bone–muscle interface. The ability of ultrasound to elevated tissue temperature may partially explain the basis for the use of this agent in treating skeletal muscle spasm. Ultrasound did seem to reduce muscle spasms in patients with neck dysfunction and with muscle spasms of the lower extremity secondary to poliomyelitis.[54] It also was found to produce a marked reduction of pain, muscle tenderness, and temporomandibular joint (TMJ) clicking when compared to short wave diathermy (SWD) in the treatment of myofascial joint dysfunction.[55] The authors felt that ultrasound deeper penetration to muscle tissue accounted for its superiority over SWD.

The mechanism of action for reduction of skeletal muscle spasm with ultrasound is not clear, but it may be due to thermal effects that alter the skeletal muscle contractile process directly, reduce muscle spindle activity, or reduce pain resulting in a break in the pain–spasm–pain cycle.

Ultrasound used alone was not as effective as ultrasound used in conjunction with occlusive splint therapy, acupuncture, and muscle-conditioning exercises in patients with TMJ dysfunction and associated muscle spasms. When administered for TMJ dysfunction, coupling was achieved through a small water-filled plastic bag. Intensities were kept below 0.6 W/cm^2.[56] Of interest is the suggestion that a higher intensity of ultrasound may have produced even more beneficial results.

The mechanical effect of ultrasound over the affected dermatome in cases of herpes zoster (shingles) is considered responsible for its pain-relieving effects.[57] This mechanical action is thought to increase the activity of the larger nerve fibers, thereby closing the pain gate at the substantia gelatinosa, and so reintroducing normal inhibition of the smaller unmyelinated fibers. In Payne's study of post-herpetic neuralgia, ultrasound was not found to be effective in decreasing pain. In studies by Garrett and Garrett[58] and Jones,[59] however, patients suffering with acute herpes zoster showed good pain relief from treatment. The duration of the condition might help to explain the different results, as well as the use of pulsed ultrasound by Jones,[59] especially if the mechanical effects of ultrasound are responsible for its benefits.

The effects of ultrasound on peripheral sympathetic nerve fibers, as well as increased blood flow, are cited as possible explanations for the dramatically beneficial effects produced by the daily use of low dose ultrasound (0.5W/cm^2 for 5 minutes) in the treatment of lower extremity reflex sympathetic dystrophy.[60]

Bursitis and Tendinitis

Another common use of ultrasound is with patients having bursitis and tendinitis. There is little statistically significant supportive documentation that demonstrates the efficacy of this modality for patients with these problems. A study by Binder and colleagues,[61] however, found that ultrasound applied at a frequency of 1.0 MHz, with a duty cycle of 20 percent, an intensity of 1.0 to 2.0 W/cm^2, and a duration of 5 to 10 minutes for 12 treatments during 4 to 6 weeks significantly enhanced recovery in 63 percent of patients with lateral epicondylitis. Lundeberg and coworkers[62] found, in a similar study using continuous ultrasound at 1.0 W/cm^2 for 10 treatments of 10 minutes, that there was only a significant difference in improvement of epicondylalgia between the insonated and the rest groups, with no significant difference between the insonated and the mock-insonated groups. Decreased pain, increased range of motion, and decreased tenderness have been reported in patients receiving ultrasound therapy for subacromial bursitis.[63-65] Similar success was found in patients with bicipital tendinitis.[65] None of these reports, though, compared ultrasound with other forms of therapy.

In a recent study,[66] the combination of sham ultrasound and exercise was compared with real ultrasound and exercise in patients with subacromial bursitis of greater than 1 month's duration. Ultrasound was administered at an intensity averaging 1.0 to 2.0 W/cm^2 for 6 minutes, 3 times a week for 4 weeks. Intensity levels were determined by increasing power until the patient reported a dull aching or pricking sensation, then reducing the ultrasonic intensity by 10 percent. Therefore, intensity was determined individually for each case. All medications were held constant during the time of the study. No differences between the groups could be found in pain relief, range of motion of the shoulder, or overall condition. The authors concluded that ultrasound was probably not a useful adjunct in the conservative management of subacromial bursitis.

There also have been recent comparative studies of the therapeutic benefits of ultrasound compared to ice massage, iontophoresis, and phonophoresis in the treatment of shin splints;[67] ultrasound compared to phonophoresis, transcutaneous nerve stimulation, and steroid injection in the treatment of lateral epicondylitis of the elbow;[68] and ultrasound and ice compared to ice, phonophoresis, and iontophoresis in the treatment of knee extensor mechanism disorders.[69] All the treatments studied were found to be superior to control groups, but only ice and ultrasound contrast treatments were found to offer any great improvement over the other treatments.

The rationale for the treatment of tendinitis and bursitis with ultrasound appears to lie in ultrasound's effects of increased blood flow to aid healing, increased tissue temperature to reduce perceived pain, and its phonophoretic effect.

Calcium Deposits

Some clinicians have stated that ultrasound can be a valuable agent in assisting the reabsorption of calcium deposits in soft tissue. Although case reports[70] have concluded that ultrasound facilitates calcium reabsorption and may increase the perfusion of a calcified bursa and affect the integrity of the bursal sac,[71] no controlled studies or followup studies using radiographic analysis have appeared in the literature. Therefore, statements that ultrasound exposure results in calcium reabsorption may be incorrect. Ultrasound may nevertheless help relieve the inflammation around a calcium deposit, thus relieving a patient's pain and improving function.

Phonophoresis

Ultrasound energy has been used to drive anti-inflammatory drugs (cortisol, dexamethasone, salicylates) and local analgesics (lidocaine) through the skin to underlying tissue. The technique of delivering medication by ultrasound has been termed *phonophoresis*. The rationale for this technique is that it delivers the drug directly to the site where the effect is sought. Cortisol has been driven to depths of 5 to 6 cm subcutaneously into skeletal muscle and peripheral nerve following phonophoresis.[72] More lidocaine was extracted from rabbit tissue following ultrasound than when the lidocaine was applied topically and not followed by ultrasound.[73]

The implicated mechanism that allows the medication to be driven across the skin to underlying tissues could be due to the changes in tissue permeability following heating with ultrasound. Furthermore, the radiation pressure of the ultrasound beam could force the medication away from the transducer into the body. Diffusion rates possibly could be enhanced by acoustic streaming. Thus, the medication can follow the well-focused pattern of the ultrasound beam.

Ultrasound also has been used to enhance the effects of hydrocortisone injection.[74] Griffin and associates[75] studied the effects of ultrasound and a placebo cream versus the effects of ultrasound and hydrocortisone ointment on patients with osteoarthritis, periarticular arthritis, and rheumatoid arthritis. Sixty-eight percent of the group treated with hydrocortisone and ultrasound (at less than 1.5 W/cm² for 5 minutes, once a week) had improved range of motion and decreased pain. Of those treated with placebo cream and ultrasound at the same dosage, only 25 percent had marked improvement in the measured characteristics. All patients received other forms of therapy during the experimental period. The results of phonophoresis, however, were not shown to be superior to that of ultrasound alone in the treatment of lateral epicondylitis[68] or in the treatment of extensor carpi radialis brevis tendinitis.[76]

Moll[77] treated a series of trigger points comparing three groups treated with: (1) a placebo solution and sham ultrasound; (2) a water-based solution and ultrasound, or (3) a decadron–lidocaine solution and ultrasound. The ultrasound dosage was less than 1.5 W/cm² for 5 minutes, twice a week for 3 weeks. While greatest improvement was found in those patients receiving the phonophoresis with decadron–lidocaine solution, the number of subjects in the study was too small to show a statistically significant difference.

More well-controlled studies on the efficacy of phonophoresis are warranted. When considering the use of phonophoresis, the transmission of the ultrasound energy through the pharmaceutical product should also be considered. Benson and McElnay[78] found that relatively few of the products commonly used for phonophoresis had good transmission characteristics. Considering that such products are usually applied directly onto the skin, it is likely that the effectiveness of the insonation itself is decreased. It would appear, however, that this technique may provide the clinician with a means of administering medication locally in a relatively easy and painless fashion. Phonophoresis may be the method of choice in patients who are apprehensive about receiving injections with hypodermic needles.

Tissue Healing

Low intensity continuous wave or pulsed wave modes have been used in the treatment of acute and chronic wounds to enhance the reparative process. During the first 24 to 48 hours following trauma, edema prevention or reduction is an important goal. Persistent edema can prolong the inflammatory process and increase pain, thereby reducing function. Recently, attention has been given to the anti-inflammatory effects of therapeutic ultrasound. El Hag and coworkers[79] reported that ultrasound reduced facial swelling and trismus following removal of lower third molars. The authors could not clarify why the nonthermal effects produced by their use of low intensity pulsed ultrasound (i.e., increased protein synthesis, increased mast cell production) should lead to decreased swelling, as these changes would be likely to lead to increased vascular permeability. They did feel, however, that the massaging and placebo effects of ultrasound treatment could contribute to its anti-inflammatory effect. The placebo effect was further supported by Hashish and colleagues[80] when they reported little difference between the anti-inflammatory effects of ultrasound and mock ultrasound, as measured by changes in facial swelling, trismus, pain, and serum C-reactive protein levels following removal of impacted lower third molars. The authors reported that although the majority of the anti-inflammatory action appeared to be a placebo effect, increasing the intensity of ultrasound was counterproductive, and the most beneficial intensity was 0.1 W/cm². The authors suggest that higher intensities might produce more pro-inflammatory changes, such as increased cell membrane permeability and mast cell degranulation, which might explain the partial reversal of anti-inflammatory activity seen in their study. They concluded that low intensity ultrasound might inhibit the release of inflammatory mediators from cells. In a study designed to assess the effect of ultrasound on acute inflammation, as measured by temperature differences between inflamed and normal surrounding skin, Snow and Johnson[81] also found little difference between the insonated and mock-insonated groups.

Using an animal model to look particularly at plasma extravasation following soft tissue damage, Fyfe and Chahl[82] induced edema in abdominal tissue with an intracutaneous injection of silver nitrate. (The release of histamine, prostaglandins, and other chemical mediators of inflammation can be induced by silver nitrate). The animals treated for 2 to 4 minutes with pulsed ultrasound, 0.5 W/cm², at a 20 percent or 50 percent duty cycle at 0.79 MHz, had less leakage from the capillaries into the interstitial space than did untreated animals.

In a further study,[83] the investigators found that ultrasound treatment increased plasma extravasation during the first 24 hours, but later reduced it significantly compared to controls. The effects of ultrasound on plasma extravasation were found to vary according to both the duration of insonation and the number of insonations. Although early extravasation might result in increased delivery of oxygen and nutrients to enhance tissue repair, the authors questioned whether this early increase represents an advantageous effect in terms of enhancing tissue repair.

To further understand the effects of ultrasound on tissue repair, Dyson and Luke[84] considered many variables in an attempt to determine the effect of ultrasound on mast cell degranulation. Mast cell degranulation induces inflammation, so stimulation of this degranulation should be expected to increase physiologic changes necessary for wound healing. The authors suggest that, as the induction of mast cell degranulation by low intensities of therapeutic ultrasound in injured tissues may be of significance in the acceleration of tissue repair, it is apparent that the effects of ultrasound on such tissues should be carefully monitored to prevent the possibility of further damage. They conclude that much more research into the mechanisms of ultrasound is needed before the effects of ultrasound therapy on human tissues can be "adequately predicted and its safe and efficient use optimized."[84]

Dyson and associates[85] reported that ultrasound facilitated a greater increase in growth of tissue in experimentally wounded rabbit ears, compared with that in untreated control subjects, following excision of a small amount of tissue. Ultrasound was initiated 2 weeks after the wound occurred, and was continued 3 times a week. The dosages found to be most effective were 0.25 and 0.5 W/cm² pulsed (20% duty cycle) and 0.1 W/cm² continuous wave at 3.5 MHz for 5 minutes. With higher intensities— 4.0 to 8.0 W/cm² pulsed (25% duty cycle)—swelling resulted. Because tissue temperature increases were only 0.53°C to 1.35°C in the successfully treated wounds, the investigators suggested that acoustic streaming may have been part of the mechanism that facilitated repair. Streaming may in fact alter ion fluxes across membranes.

This work of Dyson and associates[85] on tissue regeneration has served as an impetus for further studies on the use of ultrasound for fresh-wound healing. Roberts[86] applied ultrasound through a "window" in the casts of animals with surgically repaired tendons. The dosage given was 1.1 MHz frequency, 0.8 W/cm² pulsed for 5 minutes, 5 days a week for 6 weeks. The control animals with tendon repairs were treated only by cast immobilization for 6 weeks. In the casted-only group, tensile strength of the tendons (as measured by breaking strength) at 6 weeks was within the range of values reported by Lundborg and Rank[87] following tendon repair. In the ultrasound group, none of the tendons showed evidence of healing; the breaking strength was less than that of the casted-only group. Therefore, the use of ultrasound in the early period after tendon repair was considered to be detrimental to healing. The investigators stated that the intensity of ultrasound chosen for the experiment was similar to that which would be administered to the human hand.

A study of the effects of ultrasound following partial rupture of Achilles tendons in rats was carried out in light of Roberts' results.[88] This study found that the tensile strength of the insonated tendons seemed to be greater and that the insonated tissue appeared to be at a more advanced stage of healing. Treatment in this study was only 3 times a week for 3 weeks. Stevenson and colleagues[89] also found that ultrasound enhanced the functional return of repaired flexor tendons in the hen. They used ultrasound at a frequency of 3.0 MHz, intensity of 0.75 W/cm² for 5 minutes, for 20 consecutive treatments, with treatment starting after 4 weeks of immobilization post-surgical repair of the profundus tendon. They also reported, however, that ultrasound had no effect on gap formation or tensile strength of the repaired tendons.

These preliminary studies on wound healing suggest that the point at which ultrasound therapy is administered in the course of healing is important. The total amount of ultrasound energy delivered into the tissues also may determine the positive or negative effects on healing. When therapy is initiated during the early stages of wound healing, within the first week, repair may be hindered. On the other hand, if therapy at low intensities is initiated after 2 weeks, during the proliferative phase (fibroblastic infiltration and collagen formation) and early into the remodeling phase, ultrasound at low intensities may be beneficial. In contrast to this, it was found that the higher intensity of 1.5 W/cm² was highly significant in the healing of traumatized soft tissue of experimental animals when compared to the lower intensity of 0.5 W/cm².[90] It is clear that further well-designed and well-controlled investigations are needed to determine the efficacy of ultrasound in facilitating wound repair.

Clinically, ultrasound has been employed in the treatment of chronic skin ulcers, especially when other methods of therapy have failed. Paul and associates[91] used dosages of 0.5 to 1.0 W/cm² 3 times a week in managing pressure sores in patients with spinal cord injuries. Thirteen of the 23 ulcers treated with ultrasound healed, 5 improved, and the remainder did not benefit from the treatment. Previous methods of treatment had failed.

McDiarmid and associates[92] found that, although no effect of ultrasound was observed on the healing rate of clean pressure sores, ultrasound therapy appeared to improve the healing rate of dirty sores. It was postulated that such an effect might be due to the stimulation of the production of wound factors by ultrasound.[93]

Dyson and Suckling[94] reported on a series of patients with chronic varicose ulcerations. Sham ultrasound was compared with ultrasound at 1.0 W/cm², pulsed at a 20 percent duty cycle, for 5 to 10 minutes 3 times a week. The frequency of the ultrasound generator used was 3.0 MHz. At 28 days after the initiation of treatment, the average size of the ultrasound-treated ulcers was 66 percent smaller compared with only a 10 percent reduction in the sham-ultrasound group. Ultrasound treatment to chronic leg ulcers was also given just once a week, at 1.0 MHz frequency, 0.5 W/cm² for 1 minute per applicator area by Callam and colleagues.[95] A 20 percent positive difference in ulcer area between the control and treatment groups was apparent at 4 weeks and was maintained for the 12-week duration of the study.

If ultrasound is chosen as an adjunct treatment in ulcer care, coupling can be direct or indirect in water, depending on the location of the ulcer. Another agent, Geliperm, has also been described as a sterile coupling agent particularly suitable in the treatment of broken skin by ultrasound.[96] The ultrasound energy can be applied around the periphery of the ulcer for 5 minutes, or it can be increased to 10 minutes in ulcers greater than 2.5 cm² in size. It is important to emphasize that other aspects of ulcer care should not be ignored. Before ultrasound application, the wound should be cleansed and debrided, if necessary. Between ultrasound treatments, the wound should be kept clean and moist, with all pressure kept off the area. All of these measures should aid in preventing further skin breakdown and facilitate healing.

Also, there have been several reports of the effectiveness of ultrasound therapy at low doses in decreasing pain and increasing the dispersal of bruising following childbirth,[97,98] surgery, and episiotomies,[99] as well as in pain relief of indurated episiotomy scars of long standing.[100]

Plantar Warts

Plantar warts (verruca plantaris) are skin lesions containing thrombosed capillaries in a soft whitish core covered by hyperkeratotic epithelial tissue.[101] They occur most often in children and young adults and are usually found on the weightbearing areas of the feet. These often painful lesions are probably of viral origin, but traumatic and psychogenic etiologies also have been proposed. A multitude of treatments, including electrodesiccation and curettage, surgical excision, x-ray, and cryosurgery with liquid nitrogen or dry ice, have been performed to eradicate plantar warts. Ultrasound has also been employed in the management of these lesions by some clinicians during the past 25 years. The proponents of such treatment feel that ultrasound causes no discomfort during application, leaves the patient more comfortable between treatment sessions than other forms of treatment, and is less likely to result in scar formation.

Ultrasound, at intensities averaging 0.6 W/cm² for 7 to 15 minutes, has been recommended most commonly for wart removal.[102] The suggested number of treatment sessions has ranged from 2 to 15. Both direct and indirect contact methods have been suggested.

The reported efficacy of treatment has varied. In a preliminary report, Kent[103] had a 90 percent success rate, as measured by pain relief and necrosis of the warts, using ultrasound at 0.6 W/cm² for 15 minutes 2 times a week. Quade and Radzyminski[106] felt the best results were in patients who had no previous treatment and had lesions of the shortest duration.

The direct method versus the indirect method of coupling were compared by Vaughn.[107] With the direct technique, at 0.69 W/cm² for 15 minutes, an 83 percent success rate was found with an average of 7.8 treatment sessions. A lower percentage of success, 51 percent, was reported with the underwater coupling method at an intensity of 0.75 W/cm².

Only one double-blind study using ultrasound to treat plantar warts has been reported. Braatz and coworkers[108] compared sham ultrasound with actual ultrasound, at an intensity of 0.8 W/cm² for 12 minutes, with underwater coupling. Both groups demonstrated disappearance of the plantar warts, after an average of 9.7 weeks (85% of the patients) for the sham-ultrasound-treated group and after 7.6 weeks (82% of the patients) for the ultrasound-treated group. Braatz and associates[108] concluded that ultrasound was probably of little benefit in the care of plantar warts.

None of the investigators reported an exacerbation of pain, an increase in size of the lesion, or any other adverse reactions, when ultrasound was given for the conservative management of plantar warts. Additional studies (for instance, those that use control subjects and those that compare ultrasound with other methods of care) are warranted, to demonstrate the role of ultrasound in the treatment of plantar warts.

GUIDELINES FOR CLINICAL ADMINISTRATION

The therapeutic goal with continuous wave ultrasound is to elevate the tissue temperature for a given duration at a specific anatomic location. The pulsed wave mode, or a continuous wave mode of very low intensity, can be chosen if the goal of treatment is to facilitate soft tissue healing, and when a significant increase in tissue temperature is not desired (for example, in the case of stasis ulcers). The average intensity for a given power output machine setting is less with the pulsed wave mode than with the continuous wave mode.

To achieve the therapeutic goal that has been delineated, certain protocols should be followed when applying ultrasound. The ultrasound generators for patient care should be properly calibrated and electrically safe (see Chapter 3). Even though the operation of all units is similar, the instructions provided by the manufacturer should be carefully reviewed before the use of a machine. The therapist should be present during treatment. Having patients administer their own ultrasound should be discouraged.

Coupling Techniques

Unlike electromagnetic energy, which can travel well through air, ultrasound energy is markedly attenuated in air and is totally reflected at air–tissue interfaces. A coupling medium must be used, therefore, to transmit ultrasound energy from the transducer to the irradiated surface. When the surface area being treated is larger than the applicator surface and is relatively regular or flat in contour, a direct method of coupling can be employed. With this technique, a thin layer of water-soluble gel is spread over the area to be treated, and the sound head is placed in contact with the gel. The objective of coupling is to eliminate as much air as possible between the transducer and the skin, thereby maximizing the amount of sound entering the body. The choice of a coupling agent for the direct contact technique is based on transmission characteristics, viscosity, ease of application, cost, and therapist preference.

Impedance match between the transducer and the coupling medium also should be considered.[109] Substances that may irritate or be driven through the skin should be avoided. The viscosity of the gel should be high enough to prevent any "run off" during treatment and low enough to permit ease of movement of the transducer across the skin surface. The gel can feel very cold to the patient as it comes directly out of its storage container and, therefore, some therapists preheat the gel for patient comfort. Overzealous heating of the gel, however, will decrease viscosity and often make the gel "runny." Lehmann and coworkers[110] have suggested that coupling agents such as mineral oil, when applied at a temperature of 18°C to 20°C, will be more effective in transmitting ultrasound energy to deeper tissues without heating superficial tissues than they will be at a temperature of 24°C. However, the differences produced in deep tissue temperature elevation were found to be minimal. In the interest of patient comfort, therefore, it may be best to preheat the gel slightly.

Although a number of agents have been suggested in the past, commercially available gels for ultrasound therapy are usually more practical to use in a busy clinic. The salt found in gels used for electrocardiograms (ECG) or surface electromyograms (EMG) may damage transducer faces, so if these gels are used, they should be cleaned from transducer faces very carefully, using tap water, after treatment is completed.

If there are bony prominences in the area (for example, over the lateral epicondyle of the humerus in a small-framed person), or if the surface is small and irregular in contour (for example, a distal extremity), one of the more recently available small-sized applicators should be used in direct contact. If such an applicator is not available, however, other methods of coupling may be selected.

For treatment of the hand and wrist or foot and ankle areas, a basin can be filled with room temperature water, and the part can be immersed in the bath. Ideally, degassed water is the medium of choice, but its preparation and maintenance render it impractical for clinical use. In the study previously described, Fyfe and Chahl[83] found no significant difference between responses of controls and treated groups when tap water was used compared to degassed, deionized water. Forrest and Rosen,[111] however, found that temperature elevations in the extensor tendons of the lateral epicondyles of pigs failed to reach therapeutic levels when treatment was given under water, but did reach such levels when the same treatment parameters (1 MHz, 2.0 W/cm²) were used in direct contact. As these results have not been confirmed by other studies, tap water should be considered a reasonable alternative, especially when an uneven surface would make treatment with direct contact extremely difficult.

If treatment is given in a metal basin or whirlpool, some of the ultrasound energy will be reflected off the metal, thus increasing intensity in certain areas near the metal. A plastic or rubber basin will not cause as much reflection. In addition, water in a whirlpool often has a large number of air bubbles, which tend to reduce the transmission of ultrasound. This situation can be particularly troublesome if the turbine has been used before the ultrasound is to be given.

Both mineral oil and glycerin have been tested as couplants for the immersion technique. The use of either can result in greater surface heating and an increase in couplant temperature, compared with a water medium.[112] When coupling is done with the immersion technique, the recommended medium for the bath is water.

When the immersion technique is employed, the transducer should be held 0.5 to 3.0 cm from the body surface area to be treated. Small air bubbles tend to accumulate on the face of the applicator and the skin surface when this method is used. The operator can wipe off the accumulated bubbles during exposure, however, as long as this is done quickly to prevent the therapist's being unduly exposed to the ultrasound energy.

Another alternative for the irradiation of an irregular surface has been suggested.[113] A rubber balloon or condom is filled with water and the entry is closed. The sac is then placed between the skin surface and the transducer, with layers of coupling gel between the transducer and the balloon and the balloon and the skin surface. Another choice is to secure the open end of the water-filled balloon to the transducer and put a layer of coupling gel between the balloon and the skin surface.

MOVING VERSUS STATIONARY APPLICATOR

Two treatment methods have been used to deliver ultrasound energy to the tissue to be irradiated—a stationary applicator and a moving applicator.

Some clinicians have preferred to hold the transducer stationary over the area to be irradiated. This technique has usually been done when the treated area was very small (e.g., over a plantar wart) or when the intensity delivered was very low (less than 0.5 W/cm^2). Because of the nonuniformity of the sound beam, the distribution of energy to the tissue is uneven. Therefore, some areas within the beam may receive a large amount of energy and other areas effectively may receive none. This situation predisposes the patient to "hot spots" and potential tissue damage. Various effects due to a stationary sound beam have been noted in laboratory studies using animal models. In particular, stasis of blood flow,[34] venular endothelial damage, and platelet aggregation[35] have occurred at therapeutic intensities. This stationary technique, therefore, should be avoided. It could be safely used in underwater applications, however, because hot spots occur in the near field of an ultrasound beam, which can be kept in the water if sufficient distance from the tissue is maintained (e.g., with a 5 cm treatment head, the near field is about 10 cm long).

With the moving technique, the transducer is slowly moved over the underlying tissue at approximately 4 cm per second.[25] (Many clinicians move the transducer too rapidly, thus decreasing the amount of energy absorbed by tissue.) The purpose of the motion is to distribute the energy as evenly as possible throughout the tissue. Longitudinal stroking or overlapping circular movements can be used. The total area covered is usually 2 to 3 times the size of the irradiating crystal for every 5 minutes of exposure.[114] If a larger area is covered, the effective dosage delivered to any one region is decreased, and the tissue temperature rise will be less. With the moving technique, the energy delivered to the target tissue should be evenly distributed, causing no hot spots within the sound field. For this reason, the moving technique is preferred over the stationary technique.

EXPOSURE FACTORS

Although the dosage delivered to the patient cannot be precisely controlled or calculated, an estimate can be made and duplicated for subsequent treatments, if the exposure factors are recorded. These factors include the power output of the ultrasound beam, the effective radiating area (ERA) of the crystal, the ultrasound frequency, and the duration of exposure. The surface area of the body that is irradiated should also be reported.

As mentioned earlier, the intensity is recorded in watts per square centimeter, or W/cm^2 (power per effective radiating area of the crystal). With the continuous wave mode, the usual method of recording intensity is by the spatial average (the average power across the beam per ERA). With pulsed wave ultrasound, the duty cycle also should be included.

The intensity selected for ultrasound therapy is based upon the objective of the treatment and the amount of soft tissue being treated. When vigorous heating is desired, Lehmann and de Lateur[115] recommend increasing the ultrasound power to the maximally tolerated level to the first dull ache, then reducing the power slightly to just below pain threshold. A mild sensation of warmth may be felt by the patient during the treatment. When using the continuous-wave mode to elevate tissue temperature over an area such as the hip or low back—where there is a large quantity of soft tissue— intensities as high as 1.5 to 2.0 W/cm² typically are used. This intensity should be effective in increasing tissue temperature and should result in the desired physiologic response.

A lower intensity, of the order of 0.5 to 1.0 W/cm², and a higher frequency are employed over areas where there is less soft tissue coverage and where bone is closer to the skin surface (e.g., over the wrist). At tissue–bone interfaces, about 35 percent of the ultrasound beam is reflected, resulting in increased intensity in the soft tissue overlying the bone, specifically the periosteum.

Higher intensities are usually chosen when the purpose of treatment is to elevate tissue temperature of periarticular structures during or preceding a slow, sustained stretch with limited range of motion. A lower intensity can be employed when the desired temperature rise is not as high, for pain reduction, and for relief of muscle-guarding spasms. The best guideline for determining a maximal, tolerated intensity that will not produce a burn or other tissue damage, however, is patient tolerance or the patient's report of a feeling of deep warmth underlying the transducer. When ultrasound is used for heating, therefore, it is important that the patient's pain and temperature sensations be intact. Furthermore, patients should be instructed not to "rough it." Should the patient report deep aching (periosteal pain), either the power can be reduced or a larger area can be covered.

Occasionally, a patient will report an increase in temperature of the transducer, a feeling of surface heating. This sensation can be indicative of inadequate coupling, of loosening of the crystal in its mounting, or of hot spots due to a high beam nonuniformity ratio (BNR). If coupling appears to be adequate, the transducer should be tested by a qualified service technician.

The aforementioned intensities are appropriate for typically sized transducers, but they would need to be modified if transducers with smaller or larger effective radiating areas were used. For example, suppose we wish to heat a 10 cm² tissue area using a transducer with an effective radiating area of 10 cm² and emitting ultrasound at an intensity of 1 W/cm². If the transducer is held stationary, the 10-cm² area of skin immediately beneath the transducer crystal would receive a total exposure of 10 W (1 W/cm² × 10 cm²). In contrast, a transducer with a smaller effective radiating area, say 5 cm², emitting the same ultrasonic intensity would have to be applied with a moving technique in order to cover the 10-cm² area of skin. In this latter case, the total exposure would be 5 W (1 W/cm² × 5 cm²). Consequently, heating of this area of skin would be reduced by a factor of 2. Thus, to produce the same therapeutic effect, the intensity of the smaller transducer would have to be raised to 2 W/cm², or exposure time would have to be doubled over the same area.

When pulsed wave ultrasound is applied, the spatial average intensity read from the meter will appear to be the same as with the continuous wave mode. But the time averaged intensity will be less, because the energy is delivered in periodic bursts, with the power on for a fixed duration, and then off for a fixed duration. The time the power is on sometimes is referred to as the "mark," and the time off as the "space." Thus a mark:space ratio can be reported. Both time on and time off are measured in milliseconds. A more common way of providing the same information is by reporting the duty cycle. As defined previously, the duty cycle is the percentage of time the power is on during one pulse period (time on + time off). Some generators are equipped with variable duty cycles. As duty cycle increases (for example, from 20% to 50%), the time averaged intensity will increase. With a low duty cycle, there will be minimal, if any, detectable rise in tissue temperature. As duty cycle increases, a rise in tissue temperature can be expected.

If the desired response from the treatment is nonthermal, a small duty cycle should be chosen. There is increasing evidence that nonthermal effects of ultrasound may be important in enhancing tissue repair (see Tissue Healing). Although there are conflicting recommendations about treatment regimens for specific conditions, in general, it would be best to use the appropriate frequency for the depth of tissue to be treated, to use a continuous or pulsed wave, according to the aims of treatment, and to use the lowest intensity and duration that will achieve the desired result, in order to avoid the risk of tissue damage that may or may not be apparent to the treating therapist.

TECHNIQUE OF PHONOPHORESIS

When performing phonophoresis, coupling can be direct or indirect using water. The medication (such as hydrocortisone ointment) is rubbed directly onto the surface of the skin. Coupling gel then is spread over the medication, and sonation is initiated. With the indirect technique, the ointment is spread over the area to be treated, then the part is placed in a water bath.

A 10-percent hydrocortisone ointment is preferred by some clinicians, rather than a 1-percent ointment. Results obtained in treating humeral epicondylitis and subdeltoid bursitis were better with the 10-percent ointment than with the 1-percent ointment.[116] The 10-percent hydrocortisone ointment should be prepared by a pharmacist.

When hydrocortisone is prepared pharmaceutically, it may have air trapped in it; massaging the ointment into the skin may reduce air bubbles and improve transmissivity. In fact, it has been demonstrated in laboratory studies that the transmission of ultrasound energy through hydrocortisone ointments is less than through other coupling media.[117]

Patient Positioning and Field Selection

Because ultrasound energy can be well focused at a delineated target, careful patient positioning and determination of areas to be treated are often critically important in producing an effective treatment. The anatomic structures to be treated and the treatment goal should be well delineated by careful evaluation. The site of soft tissue involvement, whether muscle, joint capsule, tendon, or bursa, should be determined. Depending on the particular pathology, the position of the patient can vary for each joint or body surface area affected.

As a representative example, dysfunction about the shoulder will be discussed. Three different examples of shoulder dysfunctions are: (1) capsular shortening or contracture; (2) supraspinatus tendinitis, and (3) muscle-guarding spasm and pain secondary to degenerative joint disease. In the first case, the area of the joint capsule around the glenohumeral joint, which is likely to shorten or develop tightness, is the anterior–inferior aspect. The resulting limitations in motion affect predominantly abduction and external rotation. To facilitate an increase in range of motion, while elevating joint capsular temperature with ultrasound, the therapist can externally rotate and abduct the

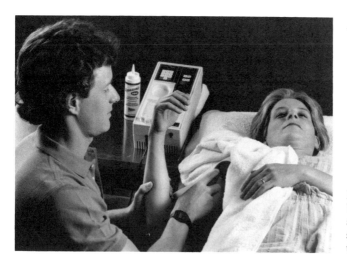

FIGURE 7–9. Ultrasound being applied to a patient with adhesive capsulitis of the shoulder. Note the position of the arm in abduction.

patient's shoulder and simultaneously apply ultrasound over the anterior and inferior axillary areas (Fig. 7–9).

If the intention is to elevate temperature at the site of the insertion of the supraspinatus, as in the second example, the position of choice for ultrasound application would be with the arm abducted and internally rotated. This position is chosen in order to expose the supraspinatus tendon from under the acromion process (Fig. 7–10).

In the third case, the patient with muscle spasm is in pain and is therefore guarding motion. The position of choice would be that in which the patient is comfortable and as relaxed as possible.

In all of these examples, the patients have shoulder dysfunction, but in each case a different anatomic site has been delineated as being problematic. Ultrasound can be well focused over an area to achieve a particular therapeutic goal, therefore, if anatomic relationships are appreciated.

TREATMENT PRECAUTIONS

Therapeutic ultrasound should not be applied over the eye. The blood supply to the lens is poor, so that heat applied to that area is not dissipated adequately. Temperature elevations can result in cataract production.[118] Most of the sound entering the eye will reach the retina, because the aqueous humor and the vitreous humor minimally attenuate the ultrasound energy. Local destruction of areas of the retina can result.

Irradiation over the heart should be avoided. In preliminary laboratory experimentation, one of this chapter's authors (MZ) found ECG changes (ST segment elevation) in dogs following direct exposure at 2.5 W/cm^2 to the heart. At all costs, cardiac pacemakers should be protected from direct ultrasound exposure because of the possibility of the sound's interference with the electrical circuitry of the pacemaker.

One should not apply therapeutic ultrasound over the pregnant uterus. The fetus should not be exposed to the therapeutic ultrasound beam, because temperature elevation of the fetus has been shown to cause abnormalities such as low birth weight, brain size reduction, and various orthopedic deformities in experimental animals.[119] Unless reassured by the patient that she is not pregnant, it is probably prudent to avoid

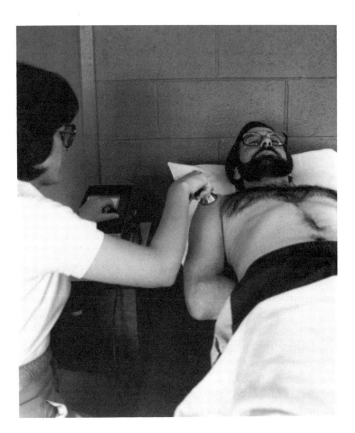

FIGURE 7-10. Ultrasound being applied to a patient with supraspinatus tendinitis. Note the position of the arm in adduction and internal rotation.

exposing a woman over the abdominal region or low back during the reproductive years except during the first 10 days following onset of menses.[120]

Ultrasound should not be applied over the testes. Prolonged temperature elevation in this area can produce temporary sterility.

Except in the special case of treatment for cancer (hyperthermia), ultrasonic irradiation to malignant tissue should be avoided. Research done under in vitro conditions has suggested that this may increase cellular detachment and the possibility of metastasis.[121,122]

A major safeguard for patients undergoing therapeutic ultrasound is their ability to perceive accurately any changes in pain and temperature. For this reason, the therapist must be very cautious when applying ultrasound over areas of impaired pain or temperature sensation. This concern is particularly pertinent in areas where sensory nerves may have been severed immediately following surgery (for instance, on the extremities or spine).

Caution also should be used in applying ultrasound over areas with reduced circulation, because of possible excessive temperature elevation. Owing to the reduced circulation, the heat generated cannot be adequately dissipated. Ultrasound should not be administered over areas of thrombophlebitis, because the possibility of clotting, or of dislodging a thrombus, could be increased.

Epiphyseal areas (growth areas of bone) in children should be exposed to ultrasound only minimally. Literature in the field suggests that intensities used therapeutically would be safe.[123] But at intensities greater than 3.0 W/cm^2, there is some evidence of demineralization of bone, damage to epiphyseal plates, and retardation of bone growth when using a stationary transducer for periods of 3 minutes or more.[124-126]

There are no reasons to avoid ultrasound application over fracture sites, unless sensation to the area is impaired. In fact, recent animal studies by Dyson and Brookes[127] have demonstrated that pulsed ultrasound may accelerate fracture healing. Certainly, this subject warrants further investigation.

CLINICAL DECISION MAKING

Ultrasound has become one of the most prevalent treatments in physical therapy clinics. Considering the foregoing material, it should be clear to clinicians that its effects are complex and generally not immediately apparent to the practicing clinician. In order to use this modality efficiently, and to avoid any possibility of increasing tissue damage, one must consider the aims of treatment and then choose the treatment parameters that would be most likely to achieve those aims. The choice of ultrasound as the preferred treatment should also be made with consideration of any other modalities available.

After treatment goals and plans have been established, if a heating agent is desired, the choice of which one to use can depend on a number of factors. These factors include: (1) stage of inflammation and repair; (2) site of pathology, including depth and anatomic location; (3) total amount of tissue to be heated; and, (4) presence or absence of orthopedic metal implants.

During the subacute stages of healing, a mild heat would be the logical choice. Surface heating agents, such as hot packs or infrared, may provide the desired response. If the site of pathology is in deep-seated structures, such as the hip joint, then low intensity ultrasound at less than 1.0 W/cm^2 may be best. With a chronic condition, in which pain and limited range of motion are the key problems, a deep heat-like ultrasound treatment at a higher intensity may be used.

The site of pathology is also important. If the goal of application is to deliver a deep heat to a well-defined area, ultrasound should be the therapeutic agent of choice. For example, a knee flexion contracture secondary to capsular tightness may respond best to ultrasound followed by a slow, gentle stretch. If a larger area with a large muscle mass is to be heated, then the agent chosen should be shortwave diathermy. For example, limited motion and pain secondary to chronic hamstring strain may be best heat treated by an agent that can apply heat to the entire muscle belly in the most efficient manner. Of course, ultrasound is capable of elevating hamstring temperature, but only a small area at a time can be heated using ultrasound.

Many patients seen for rehabilitation have surgical metal implants, either for stabilization of fractures or replacement of damaged joint surfaces. In these cases, ultrasound can be safely employed over the area of the metal implant using the moving technique.[128,129] Shortwave and microwave diathermy, however, may not be given over areas of metal implants. Many of the implants used for prosthetic joint replacements have high-density polyethylene components and are fixed in place by methylmethacro-

TABLE 7–2. Clinical Decision Making: Ultrasound
vs. Diathermy for Deep Heating

Note: Case examples are provided with supporting rationale for treatment with the
chosen deep heat agent. (Readers should cover the authors' decision and rationale while
formulating their own, then uncover and compare with their own decision.)

Case Problem	Decision	Rationale
70-yr-old women, 2 mo postopen reduction and internal fixation of intertrochanteric hip fracture with a nail and plate; now has pain on hip flexion and abduction; muscle-guarding spasms contribute to decreased ROM	Continuous ultrasound	Pain reduction; able to increase temperature of joint structures and overlying muscle; can focus energy to target areas; can apply over metal implant
45-yr-old bricklayer 1 mo postlumbar injury; L-5 to S-1 herniated intervertebral disk with paravertebral muscle-guarding spasms	Shortwave diathermy with induction drum	Capable of increasing temperature of paravertebral musculature; can cover a relatively large area

late cement. Lehmann and de Lateur[115] suggest the need for more studies determining the effects of ultrasound around these implants prior to determining if ultrasound at heating doses can be safely used over them.

Often ultrasound is used in conjunction with other physical agents, such as hot packs, cold packs, and electrical stimulation. Hot packs may provide additional pain relief and encourage relaxation of the patient. Cold packs should not be given before ultrasound, because cold alters the patient's perception of pain and temperature, which thereby limits the patients' ability to tell the therapist if the ultrasound intensity is too high.

Also, it is clear that ultrasound is likely to have a beneficial effect on the healing of soft tissue. However, as apparent from the literature reviewed, the effects of ultrasound at different stages of healing and with different treatment parameters are not well understood. Therefore, although the use of ultrasound to enhance soft tissue repair generally appears to be recommended, the clinician should be alert for any negative effects and should use the minimal dosage necessary to produce a beneficial effect.

There is also evidence that ultrasound is effective as a pain-relieving modality due to other than its thermal effects.[50,51,59,60,80,98] As early as 1953, Kuitert[50] suggested that mechanical stimulation of the neural pathways may be the reason for the relief of radicular pain. Investigation of the mechanical effects of ultrasound (i.e., cavitation, microstreaming) on the pain gate might yield information that would alter our explanation of its analgesic benefits.

In conclusion, although the effects and mechanics of ultrasound are still not freely understood, its use in physical therapy practice is well established. Therapeutic ultrasound should be used for a specific physiologic effect on a specific part of the body, only for as long as there is evidence of benefit from its application.

Clinical decision-making examples are provided in Table 7–2.

SUMMARY

Ultrasound high frequency acoustic energy, can be employed in a physical rehabilitation program to increase tissue temperature to depths of up to 5 cm. The physiologic effects of ultrasound, including increasing collagen tissue extensibility, decreasing pain and muscle spasm, and facilitating tissue healing, serve as rationales for its use as a therapeutic agent. To maximize effectiveness and appropriateness of treatment with ultrasound, the therapist should be knowledgeable about the physics, biophysical effects, and possible adverse consequences of the use of ultrasonic energy at therapeutic intensities.

REFERENCES

 1. Wood, RW and Loomis, AL: The physical and biological effects of high frequency waves of great intensity. Philosoph Mag 4:417, 1927.
 2. Buchtala, V: The present state of ultrasonic therapy. Br J Phys Med 15:3, 1952.
 3. Kuitert, JH and Harr, ET: Introduction to clinical application of ultrasound. Phys Ther Rev 35:19, 1955.
 4. Wells, PNT: Biomedical Ultrasonics. Academic Press, London, 1977.
 5. Hill, CR and ter Haar, G: Ultrasound and non-ionising radiation protection. In Suess, MJ (ed): WHO Regional Publication, European Series No. 10. World Health Organization, Copenhagen, 1981.
 6. Hekkenberg, RT, Oosterbaan, WA, and van Beekum, WT: Evaluation of ultrasound therapy devices. Physiotherapy 72:390, 1986.
 7. Stewart, HF, et al: Survey of use and performance of ultrasonic therapy equipment in Pinelles County. Physical Therapy 54:707, 1974.
 8. Burns, PN and Pitcher, EM: Calibration of physiotherapy ultrasound generators. Clinical Physics and Physiological Measurement 5:37 (abstract), 1984.
 9. Docker, MF: A review of instrumentation available for therapeutic ultrasound. Physiotherapy 73:154, 1987.
10. ter Haar, G, Dyson, M, and Oakley, EM: The use of ultrasound by physiotherapists in Britain, 1985. Ultrasound in Medicine and Biology 13:659, 1987.
11. Lehmann, JF, et al: Heating of joint structures by ultrasound. Arch Phys Med Rehabil 49:28, 1968.
12. Lehmann, JF, et al: Heating produced by ultrasound in bone and soft tissue. Arch Phys Med Rehabil 48:397, 1967.
13. Lehmann, JF, et al: Therapeutic temperature distribution produced by ultrasound as modified by dosage and volume of tissue exposed. Arch Phys Med Rehabil 48:662, 1967.
14. Gersten, JW: Effect of ultrasound on tendon extensibility. Am J Phys Med 34:662, 1955.
15. Lehmann, JF, et al: Effect of therapeutic temperatures on tendon extensibility. Arch Phys Med Rehabil 51:481, 1970.
16. Warren, CG, Lehmann, JF, and Koblanski, JN: Heat and stretch procedures: An evaluation using rat tail tendon. Arch Phys Med Rehabil 57:122, 1976.
17. Paul, ED and Imig, CJ: Temperature and blood flow studies after ultrasonic irradiation. Am J Phys Med 34:370, 1955.
18. Abramson, DI, et al: Changes in blood flow, oxygen uptake and tissue temperatures produced by therapeutic physical agents. I. Effect of ultrasound. Am J Phys Med 39:51, 1960.
19. Bickford, RH and Duff, RS: Influence of ultrasonic irradiation on temperature and blood flow in human skeletal muscle. Circ Res 1:534, 1953.
20. Wyper, DJ, McNiven, DR, and Donnelly, TJ: Therapeutic ultrasound and muscle blood flow. Physiotherapy 64:321, 1978.
21. Paaske, WP, Hovind, H, and Seyerson, P: Influence of therapeutic ultrasonic irradiation on blood flow in human cutaneous, subcutaneous and muscular tissues. Scand J Clin Lab Invest 31:389, 1973.
22. Currier, DP, Greathouse, D, and Swift, T: Sensory nerve conduction: Effect of ultrasound. Arch Phys Med Rehabil 59:181, 1978.
23. Currier, DP and Kramer, JF: Sensory nerve conduction: Heating effects of ultrasound and infrared. Physiotherapy Canada 34:241, 1982.
24. Halle, JS, Scoville, CR, and Greathouse, DG: Ultrasound's effect on the conduction latency of superficial radial nerve in man. Phys Ther 61:345, 1981.
25. Kramer, JF: Ultrasound: Evaluation of its mechanical and thermal effects. Arch Phys Med Rehabil 65:223, 1984.
26. Lehmann, JF, Brunner, GD, and Stow, RW: Pain threshold measurements after therapeutic application of ultrasound, microwaves and infrared. Arch Phys Med Rehabil 39:560, 1958.

27. Lehmann, JF and Guy, AW: Ultrasound therapy. In Reid, J and Sikov, MR (eds): Interaction of Ultrasound and Biological Tissues. DHEW Pub (FDA) 73-8008, Session 3(8):141, 1971.
28. Lehmann, JR and Herrick, JF: Biologic reactions to cavitation: A consideration for ultrasonic therapy. Arch Phys Med Rehabil 34:86, 1953.
29. Lota, MJ and Darling, RC: Change in permeability of the red blood cell membrane in a homogeneous ultrasonic field. Arch Phys Med Rehabil 36:282, 1955.
30. Harvey, W, et al: The simulation of protein synthesis in human fibroblasts by therapeutic ultrasound. Rheumatol Rehabil 14:237, 1975.
31. Dyson, M and ter Haar, GR: The response of smooth muscle to ultrasound (abstr). In Proceedings from an International Symposium on Therapeutic Ultrasound. Winnipeg, Manitoba, September 10, 1981.
32. Lehmann, JF and Biegler, R: Changes of potentials and temperature gradients in membranes caused by ultrasound. Arch Phys Med Rehabil 35:287, 1954.
33. Michlovitz, SL, Lynch, PR, and Tuma, RF: Therapeutic ultrasound: Its effects on vascular permeability (abstr). Fed Proc 41:1761, 1982.
34. Dyson, M, et al: The production of blood cell stasis and endothelial damage in the blood vessels of chick embryos treated with ultrasound in a stationary wave field. Ultrasound Med Biol 11:133, 1974.
35. Zarod, AP and Williams, AR: Platelet aggregation in vivo by therapeutic ultrasound. Lancet 1:1266, 1977.
36. Hogan, RD, Burke, KM, and Franklin, TD: The effect of ultrasound on microvascular hemodynamics in skeletal muscle: Effects during ischemia. Microvasc Res 23:370, 1982.
37. Hogan, RD, et al: The effect of ultrasound on microvascular hemodynamics in skeletal muscle: Effect on arterioles. Ultrasound Med Biol 8:45, 1982.
38. McDiarmid, T and Burns, PN: Clinical applications of therapeutic ultrasound. Physiotherapy 73:155, 1987.
39. LaBan, MM: Collagen tissue: Implications of its response to stress in vitro. Arch Phys Med Rehabil 43:461, 1962.
40. Lehmann, JF, et al: Comparative study of the efficiency of shortwave, microwave and ultrasonic diathermy in heating the hip joint. Arch Phys Med Rehabil 40:510, 1959.
41. Lehmann, JF, et al: Clinical evaluation of a new approach in the treatment of contracture associated with hip fracture after internal fixation. Arch Phys Med Rehabil 42:95, 1961.
42. Hamer, J and Kirk, JA: Physiotherapy and the frozen shoulder: A comparative trial of ice and ultrasonic therapy. NZ Med J 83:191, 1972.
43. Bierman, W: Ultrasound in the treatment of scars. Arch Phys Med Rehabil 35:209, 1954.
44. Wright, ET and Haase, KH: Keloids and ultrasound. Arch Phys Med Rehabil 52:280, 1971.
45. Williams, AR, McHale, J, Bowditch, M, et al: Effects of MHz ultrasound on electrical pain threshold perception in humans. Ultrasound in Medicine and Biology 13:249, 1987.
46. Munting, E: Ultrasonic therapy for painful shoulders. Physiotherapy 64:180, 1978.
47. Middlemast, S and Chatterjee, DS: Comparison of ultrasound and thermotherapy for soft tissue injuries. Physiotherapy 64:331, 1978.
48. Inaba, MK and Piorkowski, M: Ultrasound in treatment of painful shoulders in patients with hemiplegia. Phys Ther 52:737, 1972.
49. Soren, A: Nature and biophysical effects of ultrasound. J Occup Med 7:375, 1965.
50. Kuitert, JH: Ultrasonic energy as an adjunct in the management of radiculitis and similar referred pain. Am J Phys Med 33:61, 1954.
51. Aldes, JH and Grabin, S: Ultrasound in the treatment of intervertebral disc syndrome. Am J Phys Med 37:199, 1958.
52. Nwuga, VCB: Ultrasound in treatment of back pain resulting from prolapsed intervertebral disc. Arch Phys Med Rehabil 64:88, 1983.
53. Quirion-de Girardi, C, et al: The analgesic effect of high voltage galvanic stimulation combined with ultrasound in the treatment of low back pain: A one-group pretest/post-test study. Physiotherapy Canada 36:327, 1984.
54. Fountain, FP, Gersten, JW, and Sengu, O: Decrease in muscle spasm produced by ultrasound, hot packs and IR. Arch Phys Med Rehabil 41:293, 1960.
55. Talaat, AM, El-Dibany, MM, and El-Garf, A: Physical therapy in the management of myofacial pain dysfunction syndrome. Am Otol Rhinol Laryngol 95:225, 1986.
56. Grieder, A, et al: An evaluation of ultrasonic therapy for temperomandibular joint dysfunction. Oral Surg 31:25, 1971.
57. Payne, C: Ultrasound for post-herpetic neuralgia. Physiotherapy 70:96, 1984.
58. Garrett, AS and Garrett, M: Letters: Ultrasound for herpes zoster pain. Journal of the Royal College of General Practice, Nov, 709, 1982.
59. Jones, RJ: Treatment of acute herpes zoster using ultrasonic therapy. Physiotherapy 70:94, 1984.
60. Portwood, MM, Lieberman, SS, and Taylor, RG: Ultrasound treatment of reflex sympathetic dystrophy. Arch Phys Med Rehabil 68:116, 1987.
61. Binder, A, et al: Is therapeutic ultrasound effective in treating soft tissue lesions? Br Med J 290:512, 1985.
62. Lundeberg T, Abrahamsson, P, and Haker, E: A comparative study of continuous ultrasound, placebo ultrasound and rest in epicondylalgia. Scand J Rehab Med 20:99, 1988.

63. Bearzy, HJ: Clinical applications of ultrasonic energy in the treatment of acute and chronic subacromial bursitis. Arch Phys Med Rehabil 34:228, 1953.
64. Bundt, FB: Ultrasound therapy in supraspinatus bursitis. Phys Ther Rev 38:826, 1958.
65. Echternach, JL: Ultrasound: An adjunct treatment for shoulder disability. Phys Ther 45:865, 1965.
66. Downing, DS and Weinstein, A: Ultrasound therapy of subacromial bursitis (abstr). Phys Ther 66:194, 1986.
67. Smith, W, Winn, F, and Parette, R: Comparative study using four modalities in shinsplint treatments. Journal of Orthopaedic and Sports Physical Therapy 8:77, 1986.
68. Halle, JS, Franklin, RJ, and Karalfa, BL: Comparison of four treatment approaches for lateral epicondylitis of the elbow. Journal of Orthopaedic and Sports Physical Therapy 8:62, 1986.
69. Antich, TJ, et al: Physical therapy treatment of knee extensor mechanism disorders: Comparison of four treatment modalities. Journal of Orthopaedic and Sports Physical Therapy 8:255, 1986.
70. Cline, PD: Radiographic follow-up of ultrasound therapy in calcific bursitis. Phys Ther 43:16, 1963.
71. Gorkiewicz, R: Ultrasound for subacromial bursitis. Phys Ther 64:46, 1984.
72. Griffin, JE, Touchstone, JC, and Liu, A: Ultrasonic movement of cortisol into pig tissues: II. Peripheral nerve. Am J Phys Med 44:20, 1965.
73. Novak, EJ: Experimental transmission of lidocaine through intact skin by ultrasound. Arch Phys Med Rehabil 45:231, 1964.
74. Newman, MK, Kill, M, and Frampton, G: Effects of ultrasound alone and combined with hydrocortisone injections by needle or hydrospray. Am J Phys Med 37:206, 1958.
75. Griffin, JE, et al: Patients treated with ultrasonic driven cortisone and with ultrasound alone. Phys Ther 47:594, 1967.
76. Stratford, PW, et al: The evaluation of phonophoresis and friction massage as treatments for extensor carpi radialis tendinitis: A randomized controlled trial. Physiotherapy Canada 41:93, 1989.
77. Moll, MJ: A new approach to pain: Lidocaine and decadron with ultrasound. USAF Medical Service Digest, May–June, 8, 1977.
78. Benson, HAE and McElnay, JC: Transmission of ultrasound energy through topical pharmaceutical products. Physiotherapy 74:587, 1988.
79. El Hag, et al: The anti-inflammatory effects of dexamethasone and therapeutic ultrasound in oral surgery. British Journal of Oral and Maxillofacial Surgery 23:17, 1985.
80. Hashish, I, Harvey, W, and Harris, M: Anti-inflammatory effects of ultrasound therapy: Evidence for a major placebo effect. British Journal of Rheumatology 25:77, 1986.
81. Snow, CJ and Johnson, KA: Effect of therapeutic ultrasound on acute inflammation. Physiotherapy Canada 40:162, 1988.
82. Fyfe, MC and Chahl, LA: The effect of ultrasound on experimental oedema in rats. Ultrasound Med Biol 6:107, 1980.
83. Fyfe, MC and Chahl, LA: The effect of single or repeated applications of "therapeutic" ultrasound on plasma extravasation during silver nitrate induced inflammation of the rat hindpaw ankle joint "in vivo." Ultrasound in Medicine and Biology 11:273, 1985.
84. Dyson, M and Luke, DA: Induction of mast cell degranulation in skin by ultrasound. IEEE Transactions and Ultrasonics, Ferroelectrics, and Frequency Control UFFC-33:194, 1986.
85. Dyson, M, et al: The stimulation of tissue regeneration by means of ultrasound. Clin Sci 35:273, 1968.
86. Roberts, M, Rutherford, JH, and Harris, D: The effect of ultrasound on flexor tendon repairs in the rabbit. Hand 14:17, 1982.
87. Lundborg, G and Rank, F: Experimental intrinsic healing of flexor tendons based upon synovial fluid nutrition. J Hand Surg 3:21, 1978.
88. Friedar, S, et al: A pilot study: The therapeutic effect of ultrasound following partial rupture of achilles tendons in male rats. Journal of Orthopaedic and Sports Physical Therapy 10:39, 1988.
89. Stevenson, JH, et al: Functional, mechanical, and biochemical assessment of ultrasound therapy on tendon healing in chicken toe. Plastic and Reconstructive Surgery 77:965, 1986.
90. Stratton, SA, Heckmann, R, and Francis, RS: Therapeutic ultrasound: Its effect on the integrity of a nonpenetrating wound. Journal of Orthopaedic and Sports Physical Therapy 5:278, 1984.
91. Paul, BJ, et al: Use of ultrasound in the treatment of pressure sores in patients with spinal cord injury. Arch Phys Med Rehabil 41:438, 1960.
92. McDiarmid, T, et al: Ultrasound and the treatment of pressure sores. Physiotherapy 71:66, 1985.
93. Dyson, M: Therapeutic applications of ultrasound. In Nyborg, WL and Ziskin, MC (ed): Biological Effects of Ultrasound. Churchill-Livingstone, Edinburgh, pp 121–133, 1985.
94. Dyson, M and Suckling, J: Stimulation of tissue repair by ultrasound: A survey of mechanisms involved. Physiotherapy 64:105, 1978.
95. Callam, MJ, et al: A controlled trial of weekly ultrasound therapy in chronic leg ulceration. Lancet 2(8552):204, 1987.
96. Brueton, RN and Campbell, B: The use of geliperm as a sterile coupling agent for therapeutic ultrasound. Physiotherapy 73:653, 1987.
97. McLaren, J: Randomised controlled trial of ultrasound therapy for the damaged perineum. Clinical Physics and Physiological Measurement 5:40 (abstract), 1984.
98. Creates, V: A study of ultrasound treatment to the painful perineum after childbirth. Physiotherapy 73:162, 1987.

99. Ferguson, HN: Ultrasound in the treatment of surgical wounds. Physiotherapy 67:12, 1981.
100. Fieldhouse, C: Ultrasound for relief of painful episiotomy scars. Physiotherapy 65:217, 1979.
101. Isselbacher, KJ: Harrison's Principles of Internal Medicine, ed 9. McGraw-Hill, New York, 1980.
102. Delacerda, FG: Ultrasonic techniques for treatment of plantar warts in athletes. Journal of Orthopedics and Sports Physical Therapy 1:100, 1979.
103. Kent, H: Plantar wart treatment with ultrasound. Arch Phys Med Rehabil 40:15, 1959.
104. Rowe, RJ and Gray, JM: Ultrasound treatment of plantar warts. Arch Phys Med Rehabil 46:273, 1965.
105. Cherup, N, Urben, J, and Bender, LF: The treatment of plantar warts with ultrasound. Arch Phys Med Rehabil 44:602, 1963.
106. Quade, AG and Radzyminski, SF: Ultrasound in verruca plantaris. J Am Podiatry Assoc 56:503, 1966.
107. Vaughn, DT: Direct method versus underwater method in treatment of plantar warts with ultrasound. Phys Ther 53:396, 1973.
108. Braatz, JH, McAlistar, BF, and Broaddus, MD: Ultrasound and plantar warts: A double blind study. Milit Med 139:199, 1974.
109. Balmaseda, MT, et al: Ultrasound therapy: A comparative study of different coupling medium. Arch Phys Med Rehabil 67:147, 1986.
110. Lehmann, JF, de Lateur, BJ, and Silverman, DR: Selective heating effects of ultrasound in human beings. Arch Phys Med Rehabil 46:331, 1966.
111. Forrest, G and Rosen, K: Ultrasound: Effectiveness of treatments given under water. Arch Phys Med Rehabil 70:28, 1989.
112. Griffin JE: Transmissiveness of ultrasound through tap water, glycerin, and mineral oil. Phys Ther 60:1010, 1980.
113. Summer, W and Patrick, MK: Ultrasonic Therapy. American Elsevier, New York, 1964.
114. Reid, DC and Cummings, GE: Factors in selecting the dosage of ultrasound with particular reference to the use of various coupling agents. Physiotherapy Canada 63:255, 1973.
115. Lehmann, JF and de Lateur, BJ: Therapeutic heat. In Lehmann, JF (ed): Therapeutic Heat and Cold, ed 4. Williams & Wilkins, Baltimore, 1990.
116. Kleinkort, JA and Wood, F: Phonophoresis with 1 percent versus 10 percent hydrocortisone. Phys Ther 55:1320, 1975.
117. Warren, CG, Koblanski, JN, and Sigelmann, RA: Ultrasound coupling media: Their relative transmissivity. Arch Phys Med Rehabil 57:218, 1976.
118. Sokoliu, A: Destructive effect of ultrasound on ocular tissues. In Reid, JM and Sikov, MR: Interaction of Ultrasound and Biological Tissues. DHEW Pub (FDA) 73-8008, 1972.
119. Edwards, MJ: Congenital defects in guinea pigs: Prenatal retardation of brain growth of guinea pigs following hyperthermia during gestation. Teratology 2:329, 1969.
120. NCRP Report No. 74: Effects of Ultrasound: Mechanisms and Clinical Implications. National Council on Radiation Protection and Measurements, Bethesda, MD, 1983, p 197.
121. Conger, AD, Ziskin, MC, and Wittels, H: Ultrasonic effects on mammalian multicellular tumor spheroids. J Clin Ultrasound 9:167, 1981.
122. Siegel, E, et al: Cellular attachment as a sensitive indicator of the effects of diagnostic ultrasound exposure on cultured human cells. Radiology 133:175, 1979.
123. Vaughen, JL and Bender, LF: Effects of ultrasound on growing bone. Arch Phys Med Rehabil 40:158, 1959.
124. Bender, LF, Janes, JM, and Herrick, JR: Histologic studies following exposure of bone to ultrasound. Arch Phys Med Rehabil 35:555, 1954.
125. Cerino, LE, Ackerman, E, and Janes, JM: Effects of ultrasound on experimental bone tumor. Surg Forum 16:466, 1965.
126. DeForest, RE, Herrick, JF, and Janes, JM: Effects of ultrasound on growing bone: An experimental study. Arch Phys Med Rehabil 34:21, 1953.
127. Dyson, M and Brookes, M: Stimulation of bone repair by ultrasound (abstr). Ultrasound Med Biol 8(Suppl 50):50, 1982.
128. Gersten, JW: Effect of metallic objects on temperature rises produced in tissues by ultrasound. Am J Phys Med 37:75, 1958.
129. Lehmann, JF, et al: Ultrasound effects as demonstrated in live pigs with surgical metallic implants. Arch Phys Med Rehabil 40:483, 1959.

CHAPTER 8

Diathermy and Pulsed Electromagnetic Fields

Luther C. Kloth, M.S., P.T.
Marvin C. Ziskin, M.D., M.S., Bm.E

The application of electromagnetic energy (EM) to the body from the radio frequency (RF) part of the spectrum involves transmission and absorption of nonionizing radiation by the body. Ultrasound is also nonionizing, but it introduces acoustic, not electromagnetic, energy into the tissue. In the cases of shortwave diathermy (SWD) and microwave diathermy (MWD), continuous waves of EM radiation are absorbed by the body and are converted into heat by the resisting tissues.[1,2] When the continuously propagated SWD energy is periodically interrupted at regular intervals, pulses or bursts of EM energy are delivered to the tissues. These pulses of electromagnetic energy are referred to as pulsed electromagnetic fields (PEMFs or pulsed SWD). Depending on the total energy delivered by PEMFs, tissue temperature may or may not increase.

Therapeutic devices that deliver continuous SWD and those that deliver PEMFs use high-frequency alternating currents that oscillate at specified frequencies between 10 and 50 MHz. SWD and PEMFs[2] are most commonly used for physical therapy applications at a frequency of 27.12 MHz. MWD, another form of EM radiation, has qualities that allow it to be beamed or directed toward the body and reflected from the skin, owing to its ultra-high frequency (UHF). The frequency most commonly used with therapeutic microwave is 2450 MHz. MWD is used clinically today much less than SWD is used.

Clinical application of SWD for its thermal effects was introduced in Germany in the late 1920s. Therapeutic applications of microwave heating began in the United States in the late 1940s. The clinical use of diathermy in the health professions may be divided into three categories: (1) functional restoration and analgesia; (2) facilitation of healing of recently injured soft tissue; and, (3) hyperthermia for tumor eradication. Clinical effectiveness in therapeutic applications of SWD and PEMFs is dependent upon the intensity and duration of exposure and the production of thermal or non-thermal physiologic effects in the target tissue.

The objectives of this chapter are to: (1) Provide a basic understanding of the physical principles and effects of diathermy (SWD and MWD) and pulsed electromagnetic fields (PEMFs); (2) discuss the clinical methods for applying SWD, MWD, and PEMFs; (3) discuss the clinical conditions for which SWD, MWD, and PEMFs are suggested to be effective; and, (4) discuss potential hazards related to the use of these forms of EM energy.

PHYSICAL PRINCIPLES OF ELECTROMAGNETIC RADIATION

The term *diathermy* literally means to heat through. Diathermy is applied to a patient using electromagnetic waves that produce heat, but are nonionizing. Electromagnetic waves cover a tremendously wide range of frequencies and corresponding wavelengths (see Fig. 3–1). Electromagnetic wavelengths range from one billionth of a meter up to miles. All of these wavelengths do not pass through the body with equal ease; in fact, there is no simple relationship between wavelength and the ability of these electromagnetic waves to travel through the body. For example, very long waves, such as RF waves, travel through the body almost unimpeded. This explains why you can listen to a radio, whether or not a person is standing in front of you, blocking the radio.

Wavelengths within the visible part of the spectrum, that is light, cannot penetrate more than a few fractions of a millimeter into the skin. A region of wavelengths that comprise the RF part of the spectrum, however, can travel through the body reasonably well, and these are the shortwave and the microwave radiations. It is these latter two regions that are used in physical therapy applications of SWD, MWD and PEMFs.

Because of the great demands of the use of various frequencies for communication, the Federal Communications Commission (FCC) has very carefully regulated what frequencies can be used in television and radio transmissions, radar, and medical applications. Consequently, all of the medical applications of diathermy are limited to those frequencies listed in Table 8–1.

Electromagnetic waves, regardless of wavelength, possess certain properties, which will now be enumerated. First, they transport electrical and magnetic energy through space (hence, they are called *electromagnetic* waves). Unlike soundwaves, they do not require a medium through which to travel. They can travel through a vacuum unimpeded. They do not have mass, and they are composed of pure energy. Although the electromagnetic waves themselves do not contain matter, they do have an effect on the matter through which they travel. This occurs because matter contains electrical charges, which are interacted with, and influenced by, electromagnetic waves.

Regardless of the type of wave propagation, there is a fundamental relationship between frequency and wavelength, which is given by the equation:

$$\text{velocity of light} = \text{frequency} \times \text{wavelength}.$$

The velocity of light is a constant and equal to three hundred thousand million meters per second (3×10^8 m/sec.). If either the wavelength or the frequency is known, the other can be calculated. Because the product of the wavelength and the frequency is constant, a higher frequency will automatically lessen the wavelength, as seen in Table 8–1.

Whenever a therapist applies any form of energy to the body, safety is a concern. (See Chapter 3, for more details pertaining to the biologic effects of electrical current

TABLE 8–1. Frequencies Approved by the FCC for
Shortwave/Microwave Diathermy and Pulsed Electromagnetic Fields

Frequency (MHz)	Wavelength	Type of Diathermy
13.56	22 m	SWD
27.12*	11 m	SWD
40.68	7.5 m	SWD
915.00	33 cm	MWD
2450.00*	12 cm	MWD

*Most widely used frequency.

flowing through the body.) With one exception, diathermy is not a source of electrical shock. The one exception is when a person has direct contact with a metallic portion of the machine, and there happens to be an excess of what is referred to as leakage current (see Chapter 3).

The harmful effect of current is dependent upon the magnitude of the current and the frequency of the energy. Figure 8–1 illustrates a curve of the amount of current required to produce a "can't let go" effect, as a function of frequency. If current exceeds a certain threshold, muscular contraction is so severe and so persistent that a person is not able to let go voluntarily. This is particularly dangerous, because the person is not able to remove himself from the source of a dangerous electrical shock. This is most dangerous in the range of approximately 40 to 100 Hertz, which is the frequency range in which ordinary household electrical supply lies. The threshold increases significantly, however, with increases in frequency. Consequently, at sufficiently high frequencies, we do not have to worry about currents causing a persistent muscular contraction.

The frequencies used for SWD and MWD are not capable of depolarizing motor nerves or eliciting a contractile response from innervated or denervated skeletal muscle. Excitation of these tissues, resulting in depolarization, does not occur with diathermy because the wavelength (duration) of the high-frequency alternating current does not last sufficiently long to cause migration of ions through cellular membranes of nerve or

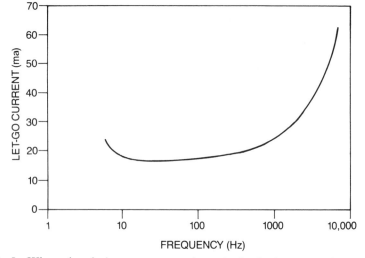

FIGURE 8–1. When electrical currents pass through the body at certain frequencies and amplitudes, muscular contraction is so strong that one is not able to let go.

muscle. This is an important reason why such high frequencies are used in diathermy applications. Another important reason for using these frequencies is that they are nonionizing, which means that there is insufficient energy concentration to dislodge orbiting electrons from atoms. Therefore, no mutations are induced, as could occur with ionizing radiations, such as x-ray.

Shortwave Diathermy

ELECTRICAL CHARGES

Electrical charges exist in either a positive or a negative state. The characterization of charges actually stems from Benjamin Franklin, who decided to call one type of charge positive and the other negative. Other than the fact that oppositely charged particles attract, and similarly charged particles repel each other, not much about these charges is known. It is not clear why there should be any attraction between them. Nevertheless, a great deal is known about how charges behave. The forces of attraction and acceleration can be precisely quantified. The same is true of quantifying effects of how charged particles behave when electromagnetic waves pass in their vicinity.

Within molecules, charges can exist in both free and fixed forms, depending on how tightly they are bound to the nucleus. Free charges are so loosely bound that they can readily leave the molecule when an electrical voltage is applied. Fixed charges, on the other hand, are confined within the boundaries of the molecule and can only move within that molecule.

In order to explain and quantitatively predict the behavior of charges, physicists have found it convenient to define an electrical field, which relates the force that will be exerted on a charged particle when it is brought into a particular region of space. In this context, surrounding any charged particle is an electrical field (Fig. 8–2). When a charge of the same polarity is brought within this field, the charge will experience a repulsive force. If the particles are oppositely charged, there will be an equal force, but one of attraction. The mechanism by which this force acts over a distance to cause attraction or repulsion is not understood.

Because of forces of attraction and repulsion, the following situation develops when electrically charged metal plates are placed in close proximity to living tissue. The positively charged plate tends to push positive charges away from it, whereas the negatively charged plate tends to attract the positively charged particles. Inside the body, within the tissues, there are many free ions, which are negatively or positively charged. These ions will travel toward the plate of the opposite polarity, inducing a

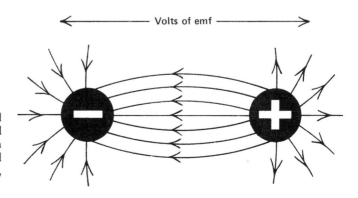

FIGURE 8–2. The electrical field pattern around charged particles. (Adapted from Grob, B: Basic Electronics, ed 4. McGraw-Hill, New York, 1977, p 289.)

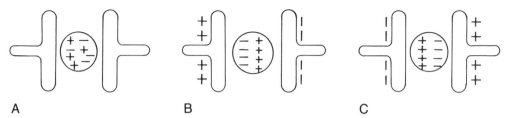

A   B   C

FIGURE 8–3. Displacement current or the net transfer of charge over a short distance (*A*) Molecule containing fixed charges. (*B*) Dipole molecule resulting from an applied voltage across the plates of a capacitor. (*C*) Reversal of polarity of dipole molecule occurs each time polarity is altered, which causes the fixed charges to move. At MHz frequencies, this results in tissue heating produced by overcoming the internal friction.

current. There are many molecules within the body that do not possess free ions. These molecules contain electrical charges that are not free to move, or at least do not move any significant distance. Under the electrical field imposed by the charged plates (i.e., diathermy treatment applicators), however, the positive charges tend to congregate at the end of the molecules closest to the negative plate, and the negative charges within the molecules tend to accumulate at the end of the molecule closest to the positive plate. (Fig. 8–3). This causes an effect called a dipole action, which is often referred to as a displacement current (because charges are being displaced). Displacement current is not the same as conduction current, which is the movement of free electrons (e.g., ions in tissues) over significant distances. In the body, we can have both types of current.

Figure 8–4 illustrates the basic components of a SWD device, which include the: (1) Power supply that converts AC wall current to DC current for the power amplifier and high-frequency oscillator circuits; (2) oscillator that produces the high-frequency (27.12 MHz) AC current; (3) power amplifier that amplifies AC current produced by the oscillator circuit to give adequate power output for therapeutic applications; and, (4) patient-tuning circuit with treatment applicators that allow delivery of EM energy from the device to the patient.

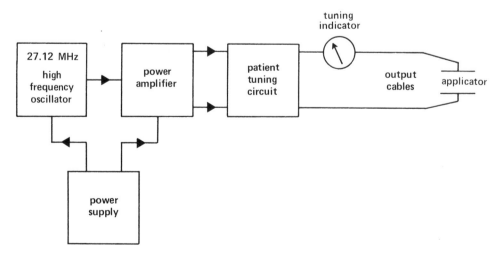

FIGURE 8–4. Basic components in a shortwave device showing a capacitor-type applicator in the patient circuit.

TABLE 8–2. Dielectric Constants of Select Tissues and Materials.*

Tissues/Materials	Dielectric Constants (ϵ)
0.9% saline	80
Muscle	85–100
Kidney	120–130
Bone marrow	7–8
Fat tissue	11–13
Distilled water	80
Oil	2
Metals	—

*Values are given for tissues and materials at 37°C and 50 MHz. The values are temperature and frequency dependent.

DIELECTRIC CONSTANT

Materials can be characterized by the number of polarizable molecules that can be forced to go into a dipole motion. The amount of this depolarization capability is characterized by a constant called the dielectric constant. The greater the number of dipoles within the material, the higher the dielectric constant (Table 8–2). The importance of this is that the greater the number of dipoles, the more charge the tissue can hold for a given imposed voltage across the treatment applicator plates. It is possible, however, to speak instead of the capacity. The dielectric constant is nothing more than the ratio of the capacity of this material to that of free space. Capacity is perhaps more easily understood, and it is simply defined as the amount of charge that the material can hold for a given voltage imposed upon it. In using the capacitance-application technique (i.e., air-space plates) to deliver EM energy to the body from a SWD device, tissues with large capacitance (and dielectric constant) will be most affected and will be the sites at which the greatest heat production will occur.

CONDUCTIVITY

Probably more important for understanding how electromagnetic waves affect the body is the conductivity of tissue. This is a measure of how readily electrical currents can be forced to travel within tissues in the body. Conductivity is defined as the amount of current generated by a given voltage difference across the tissue. Blood is a reasonably good conductor of electricity and has a conductivity of 0.7 siemens per meter. Other tissues of the body that are well perfused by blood have similarly high conductivity values. Tissues with lesser water content, such as fatty tissues, will have a lower conductivity. Metals, on the other hand, with a large percentage of free electrons, are superb conductors, and have extremely high conductivities (Table 8–3).

The importance of the differential conductivities of tissue is that the amount of current passing through any region depends upon the conductivity, and it is the current density that is responsible for heating within any tissue. The higher the current density, the greater the heating that will occur.[3] When we apply electrical voltage across the body, therefore, the greatest currents occur in those tissues that have the greatest conductivity, and these tissues will be the areas that are heated the most. Conductivity and dielectric, or capacitance, properties are not directly related.

Materials can be categorized as conductors and nonconductors. Only the nonconductors have capacitance. Conductivity has to do with the fundamental chemical nature

TABLE 8–3. Conductivities of Select Tissues and Materials*

Tissues/Materials	Conductivity (σ)
Blood	11.7
Muscle	0.7–0.9
Lung	0.1
Bone	0.01
Bone marrow	0.02–0.04
Fat tissue	0.04–0.06
Distilled water	2×10^4
Oil	10^{11}
Metals	10^4–10^7

*Values are given for tissues and materials at 37°C and 50 MHz. The values are temperature and frequency dependent. The unit for conductivity is siemens per meter, s/m.

of the material in which there are excess electrons that are not tied to the atoms. These electrons are able to move freely through the material. Whenever a voltage is applied across the material, these electrons move very readily, as in good metal conductors. In the body, the charges may be ions in solution as well as free ions. On the other hand, nonconductors or, as they are frequently called, dielectric materials possess molecules in which electrons are not free, but are bound to the nucleus. Voltages applied across nonconductors are not able to dislodge the electrons to move them over any great distance.

ELECTRIC FIELDS

The force generated by an electric field that exists between two charged plates is somewhat complicated. In those regions in which the plates are very close to each other, the electrical field is most intense. The intensity is represented by the number and closeness of "lines of force"[3] (Fig. 8–5). The influence of the electrical field on the tissue will be greater in the central region than when it is close to the ends of these plates. In

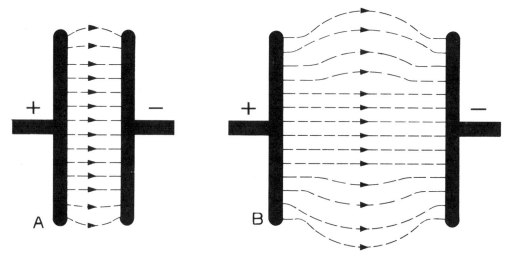

FIGURE 8–5. Lines of force of the electric field created between parallel, equal-sized capacitor plates with narrow spacing (A) and wide spacing (B). (Adapted from Ward,[3] p 115.)

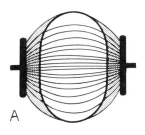 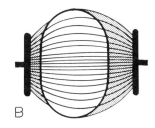

A. Even distribution of the lines of force in electrodes of equal size and equal electrode-skin distance.

B. Stronger heating with an electrode located closer to the body.

FIGURE 8–6. Concentration of electric field lines of force on a body part placed within the field. (*A*) Even distribution of the lines of force between applicators of equal size and equal distance between them. (*B*) More intense electric field at the more closely spaced applicator, resulting in greater heating at that applicator. (Adapted from Thom,[4] pp 46, 48.)

other words, the electrical field is most intense where lines of force are most concentrated. When a part of the body is placed midway between two electrically charged plates, this region of the body becomes centrally located and experiences the same concentration of lines of force throughout both sides (Fig. 8–6A). In Figure 8–6B, however, a body part is placed closer to one plate than to the other, and the closer proximity to one plate encounters a higher concentration of lines of force. This results in a more intense electrical field on the side closest to the near plate and, consequently, any effects from the diathermy will be more pronounced on this side. If plates are not applied properly, and their orientation is not parallel to the body part being treated, it is possible to create a very nonuniform electrical field.[4] Then some parts of the body will experience very large field strengths, and other parts of the body will experience very low field strengths. If the plates are improperly positioned, it is possible to unintentionally cause excessive heating, which may be perceived as hot spots or even result in burning of tissues.

When the skin surface is very close to the plate, electrical field lines are more intense at the skin than in the more central regions of the body part. If the plates are backed away, the high concentration of field lines at the body surface is reduced, thus allowing for more uniform energy distribution throughout the tissues. Figure 8–6, however, also illustrates the fact that the mere presence of an object in an electrical field alters the field to some extent. This is particularly important whenever there is a material of high conductivity within the field, as it tends to concentrate electrical lines of force (Fig. 8–7). The clinical implications of this occur whenever there is sweat on the surface

FIGURE 8–7. More intense concentration of electric field lines of force on materials of high conductivity that are either on the surface or within the patient's tissues. (Adapted from Ward,[3] p 129.)

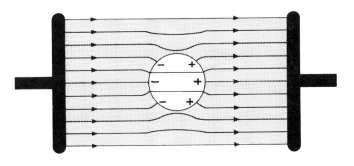

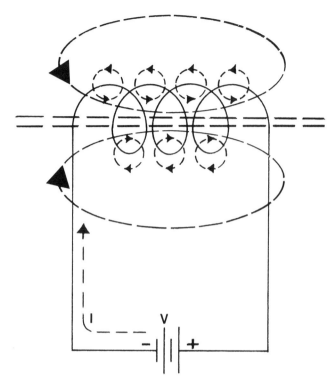

FIGURE 8–8. Current passed through a coiled cable produces a total field pattern consisting of an electrostatic field (large dashed lines and circles) and an electromagnetic field (small circles). (Adapted from Grob, B: *Basic Electronics*, ed 4. McGraw-Hill, New York, 1977, p 297.)

of the skin, or a metallic object is present inside, or on the surface of, the body. Unless caution is taken in these cases, it is possible to do considerable harm to a patient by causing excessive heating around implanted metal objects and by potential thermal necrosis of the tissues in contact with the metal. This is also true for external devices made of metallic materials and other materials, such as jewelry, metal chairs, and tables patients may be lying upon.

MAGNETIC FIELDS

Shortwave diathermy is delivered to the body by one of two techniques — by either capacitance or inductance applicators. Capacitance was described in the preceding section. The second type of shortwave application is that of the inductive technique. The nature of the inductive technique arises from the observation that whenever an electrical current flows in a material, a magnetic field is generated that influences surrounding tissue and, in turn, can induce secondary currents in the tissue (Fig. 8–8).

When a conductor is configured into a coil and made to encircle a conductor, the magnetic field induced by this coil causes a secondary electrical current to flow in the conductor. This is the approach taken when applying the inductive technique to the body. A wire or cable is wrapped into the shape of a coil or, as is more frequently done, the wire is coiled within a plastic housing, which serves as the applicator.

Energizing the cable with an appropriate frequency induces a magnetic field that actually causes a current to flow within the part of the body. Certain local currents are generated, such as eddy currents (Fig. 8–9). Regardless of the type of current, frictional forces must be overcome in order for charges to flow. The amount of heating resulting

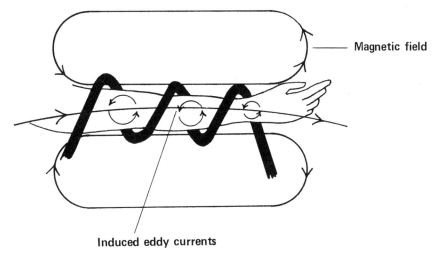

FIGURE 8-9. Eddy currents are induced in tissues by the magnetic field produced by inductive applicators.

from overcoming the internal resistance of the tissues depends on the amount of current passing through the tissue and the resistance of the tissue. The inductive technique is particularly effective for heating tissues with high conductivities, and particularly those well perfused with blood, such as muscle. High temperatures are also produced in areas surrounding joints. This method of application does not cause as much heating in fat as the capacitive technique, because fat is not a good conductor. This technique is also inappropriate whenever there is a metallic implant present in the field of application because of the concern of excessive heating.

Figure 8-10 shows the cross-section of a limb, around which is placed an electromagnetic coil. This figure shows the various tissue layers of the body and illustrates fairly well that a region such as skeletal muscle, which possesses the greatest conductivity, could be heated the most evenly, even though it is located deep within the limb.

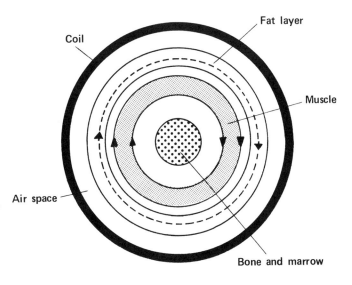

FIGURE 8-10. An inductive (coil) applicator may provide the most even heating of tissues that possess the highest conductivity, such as muscle. (Adapted from Ward,[3] p 159.)

TABLE 8–4. Relative Conductivities of Various Tissues

High Conductivity*	Low Conductivity
Blood	Fat
Muscle	Ligament
Sweat	Tendons
	Cartilage

*Conductivity = water content
Heating = current² × resistance × time

The amount of heating occurring within a tissue is given in the following equation:

$$\text{heating} = \text{current}^2 \times \text{resistance}.$$

This is helpful, because it shows us that the amount of heating depends most importantly on the current density, and this in turn is affected by the conductivity of the tissue. The above computation also requires knowing the resistance, if the amount of heating is to be calculated. In general, the longer the heating, the greater will be the temperature elevation, until the maximum temperature is achieved (see Chapter 5).

It is helpful to characterize tissues according to whether they are high-conducting tissues or low-conducting tissues (Table 8–4). In general, tissue conductivity depends in large measure upon the water content. High-conductivity tissues, for example, are blood, muscle, and sweat; low-conductivity tissues include fat, ligaments, tendons, and cartilage. High-conductivity tissues are affected most by the inductive application technique, whereas low-conductive tissues will be affected more by the capacitance technique.

Microwave Diathermy

An alternate method of applying electromagnetic energy is the MWD application. In this method, the electrical field predominates and very little magnetic field is generated or transmitted. MWD devices rely on a specialized amplifying component called the magnetron, which applies a high-oscillating voltage at the appropriate frequency to an antenna (Fig. 8–11). The advantage of microwaves are that they have sufficiently small wavelengths and can be well focused and guided into the patient with convenient antenna (treatment applicator) arrangements. In the interaction of microwaves with tissue, the heating mechanism relates to the fact that in the body are polar molecules, such as described before. Polar molecules possess asymmetrically located charges, so that one end of the molecule will be positive, and the other end will be negative. The electromagnetic radiation in the microwave wavelengths interacts with these polar molecules, causing them to rotate. The rotation that occurs is hindered by internal resistance. Overcoming the internal friction causes heat formation and, thus, a temperature elevation.

A major concern of microwave radiation is penetration. Because of relatively high attenuation, the amount of microwave radiation reaching deep structures is progressively diminished with increasing depth. A special concern related to microwave radiation is that there can be excessive radiation of superficial structures, which may cause blistering of the skin or fat-layer burns. (A general discussion of special conditions requiring special precautions appears later in this chapter.)

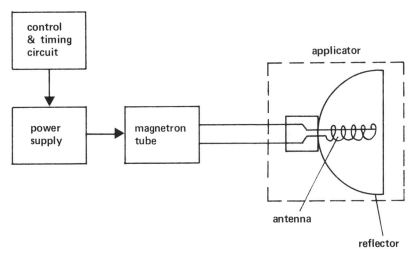

FIGURE 8–11. A schematic diagram of microwave diathermy components. (Adapted from Ward,[4] p 232.)

Because of their small wavelengths, microwaves have properties similar to light. They are reflected and refracted, for example, when they strike a boundary between two materials having different electrical properties. When microwaves cross tissue boundaries within the body, some of the energy is reflected. The more that neighboring tissues differ in their electrical properties, the greater will be the amount of energy reflected. Most soft tissues have similar electrical properties, and reflections from soft-tissue interfaces will be very small. However, considerable energy will be reflected at soft-tissue–bone interfaces. The reflected microwaves can interact with the incident microwaves to produce standing waves. Standing waves occur when two waves travelling in opposite directions combine to form a pattern of alternating nodes (points at which the electrical energy is minimal) and antinodes (points at which the energy is maximal). Heating by microwaves will be maximal at antinodes and minimal at nodes. For microwaves with wavelengths of 12 cm, the distance between antinodes is 6 cm. Although the theoretical maximal amplitude of a standing wave is twice that of the incident wave, values actually occurring in the body will be considerably less because of attenuation, and because only a portion of the total energy will be reflected at any surface.

Microwave energy not reflected at a tissue boundary is transmitted through to the next deeper tissue. However, the direction of the transmitted microwave may be bent away from its original direction. This bending in direction is called *refraction*. The greater the difference in electrical properties between two tissues, the greater will be the amount of refraction.

Pulsed Electromagnetic Field (PEMFs)

Time varying or pulsed electromagnetic fields (PEMFs) are derived from the radio frequency (RF) part of the electromagnetic (EM) spectrum. *RF radiation* is the term generally applied to propagating EM waves between 10 kilohertz (KHz) and 300 Gigahertz (GHz) (one KHz is 1×10^3 cycles per second; one GHz is 1×10^9 cycles per second). Microwaves, which lie in the 300 MHz to 300 GHz frequency range, are included in RF radiation (one MHz is 1×10^6 cycles per second). When photons from RF radiation are absorbed by body tissues, they cause atoms and molecules to vibrate and rotate, which in turn causes heat to be generated in the tissues. The induction of increased temperature in biologic tissues by RF radiation is the primary basis for RF diathermy. These heat-induced changes were long thought to be the principal, if not the only, biologic effect of RF radiation. However, preliminary studies that will be discussed later suggest that perhaps nonthermal effects also occur, especially when PEMFs are absorbed by the tissues.

PEMFs are created by interrupting the output of continuous RF waves at regular intervals. When the continuous high-frequency wave output from a shortwave device is interrupted at regular intervals, bursts of energy are delivered in pulse trains during successive "on times," usually separated by longer-lasting "off times" (Fig. 8–12). When the commonly used frequency for SWD (27.12 MHz) is considered, one finds that the duration of 1 complete cycle at this frequency lasts a very short time (i.e., approximately 36 nanoseconds [36×10^{-9} sec]). If, as is true of some pulsed shortwave devices, the pulse or burst on time (duration) lasts 65 microseconds (μ sec [65×10^{-6} sec]), then there will be about 1800 complete sine-wave cycles delivered as a pulse train to the treatment applicator before the off time begins. Some other pulsed shortwave devices produce pulses, or bursts, having durations as short as 8 or as long as 400 μsec.

The duration of the off time depends on the pulse- or burst-repetition rate which, depending on the device, ranges from 1 to 7000 pulses per second[6] (pps) and is selected with a pulse-frequency control on the equipment-operation panel. The primary technical difference between pulsed shortwave therapy and continuous shortwave thermotherapy may be attributed to the brief on time to off time ratio that characterizes pulsed shortwave output. With a pulse duration of 65 microseconds, and a pulse repetition rate of 400 pps, the pulse off time is 2,435 μsec ($2,435 \times 10^{-6}$ sec). In this example, the on time to off time ratio is approximately one to 37.[7] Thus, the application of PEMFs, in the form of pulsed shortwave, to the body may produce some transient heat buildup in the tissue during the short on time period of the pulse. However, owing to the relatively long off time that follows successive pulses at low pulse-repetition frequencies, (for example, 15 to 35 pps) the heat dissipates, and the tissue may cool before the next pulse arrives. Thus, with low-frequency pulsed shortwave there is no perception of heat, because the tissue temperature does not increase significantly.

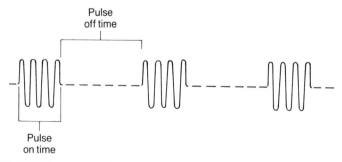

FIGURE 8–12. PEMFs are created by interrupting the RF wave output at regular intervals to deliver pulse trains or bursts of energy during successive "on times" separated by longer lasting "off times."

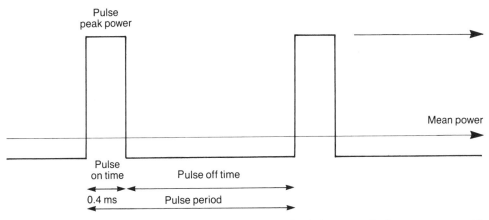

FIGURE 8–13. A measure of heat production with pulsed shortwave is the mean power. The highest mean power produced by pulsed SW devices is always lower than the power produced by most continuous SW devices. (In van den Bouwhuijsen, F, et al,[7] p 20.)

With an increase in the pulse repetition frequency, from 90 to 200 pps, the heat produced in the tissues may summate, causing the sensation of heat to be just barely perceptible.

In most applications of PEMFs with shortwave devices, the proposed goal is to select the highest possible pulse power while generating the least amount of heat possible. A measure of heat production with pulsed shortwave therapy is the mean power. For most pulsed shortwave devices, the peak pulse power (the power in watts delivered during a pulse) ranges between 100 and 1000 watts. If the pulse duration is 400 microseconds (0.4 millisecond), and the peak pulse power and pulse repetition frequency are known, the mean power may be easily calculated. For example, at a peak pulse power of 1000 watts, if the pulse repetition frequency is 35 pps then the pulse period (the pulse on time plus the pulse off time) is $1000 \div 35 = 28.57$ milliseconds (Fig. 8–13). In this example, therefore, the percentage of time during which the pulsed shortwave output is delivered is $0.4 \div 28.57 = 1.4$ percent. Consequently, the mean power is 1.4 percent of 1000 W or 14 W. Generally, with most pulsed shortwave devices, the highest mean power output that can be delivered is always lower than the power delivered (80 to 120 W) during most continuous shortwave thermotherapy treatments.

THERMAL EFFECTS OF DIATHERMY

The ability of a SWD device to induce a heating effect in tissues depends largely on the power output of the device. For continuous SWD devices, the power output range is 55 to 500 W.[6] This power range is usually more than adequate, because for most SWD applications, in which the goal is to raise the tissue temperature to within the physiologically effective range of 40°C to 44°C, a power output of between 80 and 120 W is required. Although the range of peak (instantaneous) pulse power for most pulsed shortwave devices is 100 to 1000 W, the potential for producing a heating effect with these devices is dependent on the mean power delivered to the tissues with successive bursts of pulse trains. As mentioned earlier, the highest mean power that can be delivered with pulsed shortwave devices (80 W) is lower than the usual power output delivered during continuous SWD treatments.[7]

The effects of SWD heating on skin bloodflow in humans was studied by Millard,[8] who showed that clearance of radioactive sodium increased nearly 150 percent after exposure, resulting in an average temperature rise of 5.3°C. In the same study, muscle-clearance rates increased by 36 percent, with a muscle temperature rise of 5.2°C. Using 2450 MHz microwave diathermy, McNiven and Wyper[9] produced a 400 percent increase in vastus lateralis muscle bloodflow in five subjects. This occurred after an 8-minute exposure at a power output adjusted to a "comfortable" level.

The effect of SWD application on the circulation of knees resulted in a 100 percent increase, according to Harris[10] in a study of radio-sodium clearance from the knee joint. Similar SWD treatment of chronic (quiescent) rheumatoid knees showed a circulation increase of 60 percent, whereas with most acute rheumatoid knees treated there was a resultant decrease in circulation. This decrease was comparable to decreases found with intra-articular hydrocortisone. Harris[10] suggests that this provides some rationale for using mild local heat therapy in rheumatoid arthritis with acutely inflamed joints.

The physiologic effects obtained with other forms of therapeutic heat are also produced with SWD and MWD. Generally, the power of EM fields from continuous wave diathermy devices allows greater depth of heating than occurs with superficial heating agents. Logically, then, the selection of SWD or MWD is correct when the desired treatment outcome is to increase extensibility of deep collagen tissue, decrease joint stiffness, relieve deep pain and muscle spasm, increase blood flow, and assist in resolution of inflammation.

MODE OF ACTION OF PEMFs ON TISSUE: THEORETICAL CONSIDERATIONS

Most of the clinical reports related to PEMFs address their use in treatment of wounds and soft-tissue injuries. Although reports on the efficacy of PEMFs in promoting tissue repair and resolution of the inflammatory reaction are conflicting, it nevertheless seems that *in theory*, the explanation for the reported effects may occur at the cellular level, specifically as relates to the cell-membrane potential. When cell injury occurs, there is some depolarization associated with cell dysfunction. It has been suggested that PEMFs may help healing by repolarizing damaged cells. In addition, based on the proposition that the cell-membrane potential is involved in the control of cell division and cell proliferation, and the neurons and muscle cells — which have relatively high, stable membrane potentials — do not regenerate, perhaps such mechanisms could be favorably influenced by PEMFs.[11] Barnothy[12] has noted that reactions of biologic materials following exposure to PEMFs are delayed and, therefore, perhaps biologic changes are triggered. Another theory suggests that, during the inflammatory state, the action of the sodium pump is reduced, causing sodium to build up in the cell, which in turn causes a decrease in cell negativity. In this situation, it may be possible that under the influence of a magnetic field, the sodium pump is reactivated, which allows the cell to restore its own ionic balance.[13]

INSTRUMENTATION AND METHODS OF APPLICATION

Continuous Shortwave Diathermy (SWD)

The patient-tuning circuit shown in Figure 8–4 is either a manually or an automatically controlled component of a shortwave device. Some shortwave devices are made to give only continuous, or only pulsed, shortwave electromagnetic radiation, whereas others allow the operator to select either the continuous or the pulsed mode.

Two types of fields associated with shortwave and microwave therapeutic devices were discussed earlier, namely electric and magnetic fields. Various types of applicators may be used to deliver to the body the energy associated with these fields. Although each type of applicator delivers both types of fields simultaneously, some applicators deliver more electric field energy, and others deliver more magnetic field energy. Applicators designed to deliver more electric field energy are called electric-field or capacitive applicators. This type of applicator consists of 2 metal plates, varying in diameter from 7.5 to 17.5 cm, which are mounted at the ends of separate adjustable arms that extend from the console of the shortwave device. When the capacitive applicators are applied to a patient for tissue heating, the plates, plus the intervening air and the patient's tissues placed between the plates form a capacitor. Thus, with air-spaced plates, the high-frequency electric field oscillates from one plate to the other, with the intervening body part of the patient playing an integral part of the system.

With air-spaced plates, a glass or plastic plate guard surrounds each plate to prevent contact between the plate and the patient's skin. A severe electrical burn may occur if either the therapist's or the patient's skin contacts the bare metal plate with the diathermy device in operation. To prevent concentration of the electric field on moisture that may accumulate on the skin from perspiration, a single layer of terrycloth toweling should be placed between the plate guards and the patient's skin to absorb the moisture. Most plates are manually movable through a distance of about 3 cm within the guard. In some older models, the plate is not movable, but the plate guard can be manually adjusted so the plate to skin distance is 2 to 3 cm. For optimal heating, the guard should be as close to the towel on the skin as possible, and the plate should be as far away from the skin as the plate guard allows. This positioning of the plate and guard, with reference to the skin, provides for increased relative heating depth of the tissues absorbing the energy.[14] In fact, when applied correctly and to patients whose subcutaneous fat layer is less than 1 cm thick, the capacitive-field technique may be capable of delivering energy into tissue depths that correspond to the depths heated with inductive applicators.[15] This is achieved with shortwave devices engineered with deep-field-efficient circuitry that automatically increases wattage (power) output as the plate–skin distance increases, and decreases output as plate–skin distance decreases. In practice, most SWD devices maintain constant power output with changes in plate–skin distance. Thus, power will be high when the plate–skin distance is small, which may lead to selective, and even deleterious, heating of skin and subcutaneous fat. Air-spaced plates should always be positioned so that the distance between any part of the two plates is at least as great as the diameter of the plate.

Magnetic field or inductive shortwave applicators are available in two forms—the more widely and frequently used drum and the cable. The drum shown in Figure 8–14 may be a single or a multiple unit. The single-drum unit is intended to treat only one surface. A smaller version of the single-drum unit, called the "minode," and a larger version, called the "monode," consist primarily of an induction coil arranged in either a

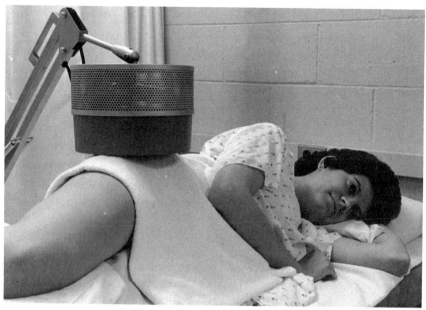

FIGURE 8–14. Magnetic field (inductive) shortwave applicator. In this illustration, a single-drum unit is applied to the lateral hip. Note layer of toweling for spacing.

monoplanar or a multiplanar configuration contained within a rigid insulator housing. This applicator allows delivery of predominantly magnetic field energy only from the applicator treatment surface, which is placed in contact with a single layer of terrycloth toweling on the patient's skin. The treatment surface of the applicator housing, therefore, serves the same function as the plate guard in the air-spaced applicator—to space the inductive coil away from the skin.

The multiple-unit drum, called a *diplode*, is hinged so that one or more body-part surfaces can be treated simultaneously. The diplode consists of a rectangularly arranged induction coil contained within an insulator housing, which also serves to space the coil away from the patient's skin. Because of the coil's closer proximity to the treatment surface within the diplode, approximately 1 cm of terrycloth toweling must be used to separate the applicator from the patient's skin to prevent excessive surface heating.

The cable electrode may vary in length from 2 to 5 meters and may be wound in a monoplanar (pancake) or helical fashion around the body part. Hence, the cable electrode may be used to treat one or more surfaces simultaneously, although its greater flexibility compared with that of the drum requires more time to position the cable properly for each treatment. Because there is no rigid housing, as there is with the drum, the user must always add a dielectric material such as terrycloth between the cable insulation and the patient's skin. This dielectric is needed to absorb perspiration, which could cause a superficial skin burn. For ideal energy transfer to the patient, the intervening dielectric material should be 1 to 2 cm thick, except when the body weight is resting on the cable, when a dielectric 2 to 3 cm thick is required. The radiated energy can travel from coil to coil along the surface of the skin. When the cable turns are less than 3 cm apart, therefore, there is increased energy exchange between adjacent coil turns. This causes inefficiency and a decrease in deep-tissue temperature because of an undesired loss of energy between cable turns.

All shortwave devices have external cables that connect the applicator to the console and deliver the EM energy from the high-frequency oscillating circuit to the applicator. Because these cables are usually rubber-insulated and may emit radiation in all directions when the applicators are energized, care must be taken to prevent them from directly contacting the patient or any metal or synthetic materials.

Pulsed Shortwave (PEMFs)

Shortwave devices that are designed to transmit PEMFs most commonly deliver them with the drum type of applicator. Within the outer casing of the applicator is usually a metal coil wound in the form of a flat spiral. The high-frequency pulsed EM waves generated by the device are made to flow around the coil, which then radiates EM energy through the air to the patient.[16] Recall that the application of pulsed shortwave to the body will cause little heat to be generated in the tissues because of short on time of the pulse period. Furthermore, owing to the relatively long off time that follows, the tissue is allowed to cool before another pulse arrives. In most treatments with pulsed shortwave, there is no detectable temperature increase.

Microwave Diathermy (MWD)

Several applicators may be used to transmit MWD into the body. They are classified as either spaced or direct-contact applicators. Spaced applicators generally allow more of the microwave radiation to be reflected when it arrives at the skin than direct-contact applicators allow. Spaced applicators are either rectangular or hemispheric and come in four different sizes and shapes. The area and pattern of heating are dictated by the type of applicator used and by the distance between the applicator and the patient's skin. When these applicators are positioned further from the skin, the area that can be treated increases in size proportionately (inverse square law). Although the term *direct-contact applicator* suggests that these applicators are placed in direct contact with the patient's skin, this is not so. Usually they are positioned about 1 cm from the skin. Even though these applicators have been shown to be more efficient than spaced applicators at delivering MW radiation, they are not sold in the United States.

Dosage Considerations for Applying SWD, MWD, and PEMFs

Because it is clinically impractical to measure the quantity of electromagnetic energy actually transferred from SWD or MWD devices to the tissue without invasive temperature probes, therapists must use the patient's subjective heat-sensation response as a guide for dosage. A significant problem often encountered with patients who do not have normal heat sensation is the difficulty they may have in making reliable verbal responses about what they feel. Individuals should be tested for pain and temperature sensation before beginning treatment to determine if they have any cutaneous (sensory) nerve deficit.

In evaluating the patient, the therapist should determine whether the stage of the condition to be treated is acute, subacute, or chronic. Having identified the stage of the condition, the extent of involvement (that is, volume of involved tissue) should be determined. This will allow selection of a SWD or MWD device with applicator appropriate for delivering energy that produces either thermal or nonthermal changes in the involved tissues.

The evaluation should also establish whether there are any bony prominences, metal implants, shrapnel, or surface metal in the area to be treated. Direct application of continuous SWD over bony prominences or metal may result in tissue destruction. Following the evaluation, the patient should be positioned comfortably for treatment. Clothing, dressings, and bandaging should be removed from the body surface to be treated.

When using continuous SWD or MWD, therapists should always keep in mind that the extent of biologic reactions elicited depends on the tissue temperature reached at the end of treatment. Since the therapeutic range for increasing tissue temperature is between 40°C and 44°C, it is imperative that the therapist know how intensely, how long, and how frequently the treatment should be applied, based on the stage of the condition. According to Thom,[4] a lower dose of continuous SWD administered over a longer period of time is more effective therapeutically than a more intense dose given over a shorter time.

Heat dosage, or the amount of thermal energy delivered to the tissues per unit time, is very important when specific treatment outcomes are desired. Lehmann's[17] definitions of mild and vigorous heating discussed in Chapter 5 may be used in conjunction with the doses described by Schliephake[18] for continuous SWD application. The following dosage scheme may also be used for pulsed SW and for MWD application:

Dose I. Lowest — just below the point of any sensation of heat (acute inflammatory process).
Dose II. Low — mild heat sensation, barely felt (subacute, resolving inflammatory process).
Dose III. Medium — moderate, but pleasant, heat sensation (subacute, resolving inflammatory process).
Dose IV Heavy — vigorous heating that produces a well-tolerated sensation (chronic conditions). The pain threshold may be reached, but the output is immediately lowered to just below maximal toleration.

It has been suggested that acute conditions like soft-tissue trauma should be treated 2 or 3 times daily, with either dose I or II, for 15 minutes.[19] The acute condition will not require the deep-tissue temperature rise that results from longer, more intense applications (vigorous heating). Chronic conditions (for instance, contracture) call for either dose III or dose IV and longer treatment periods of 15 to 30 minutes. Remember that the electrical properties of tissues are much higher than they are for air. Applicators that are larger than the body part (such as a limb) to be treated, therefore, should be used so that field lines bend toward the part, and spreading of the field in minimized. It is also very important for the therapist to assess the relative thickness of the patient's subcutaneous fat layer before electric field applicators are used.

Inductive (magnetic field) SWD applicators include the minode, the monode, the diplode, and the cable. Generally, these applicators provide more uniform heating of superficial and deep musculature without as much risk of overheating skin and subcutaneous fat. Cable turns should never be allowed to touch one another and should be insulated from the patient with terrycloth toweling of appropriate thickness.

Because of the size of microwave applicators, the use of MWD is more appropriate when smaller body areas or smaller tissue volumes require deep heating. (The spaced, conventional MWD applicators and the direct-contact applicators were described earlier in this chapter.)

For moderate to vigorous heating effects, a comfortable feeling of warmth perceived by the patient is the best available guide for adjusting the dosage of either continuous SWD or MWD.

Pulsed SW devices do not emit a continuous flow of energy to the tissues, therefore, because any heat buildup that occurs is rapidly dissipated by the circulating blood, patients normally do not experience any sensation of heat unless maximal-pulse-frequency settings are used in conjunction with shorter pulse off times. Thus, the quantity of energy delivered can be influenced by altering the pulse repetition frequency. In acute cases, a low pulse frequency is recommended, since the tissues may be adversely affected by heat. This would correspond to dose I. As the inflammatory reaction resolves, a slightly higher pulse frequency may be used (dose II). Later, when the inflammatory response has resolved or the condition is chronic and heat is indicated, either continuous SWD or MWD would be appropriate at dosage levels III or IV.

TREATMENT INDICATIONS

Indications for Diathermy

All of the common indications for thermotherapy are also indications for treatment with continuous SWD and MWD. In fibrous muscular or joint capsular contractures, prior heating of the shortened tissues may enhance collagen extensibility[20] when followed by stretching done manually, with continuous passive-motion devices or with neuromuscular electrical-stimulation devices. Either continuous SWD or MWD may be used, since both are able to heat superficial to deep muscle layers. When contracted structures are deep to thick layers of soft tissues, microwave will not significantly heat the target tissues.[21]

Muscle guarding and pain, which occur as a result of injury to tendons and joint structures, degenerative joint disease, bursitis, sacroiliac strains, and ankylosing spondylitis, may be relieved by continuous SWD or MWD applications to the muscles in spasm.[21]

Joint structures may be selectively heated by continuous SWD when the joint is covered by a thin layer of soft tissue (such as the elbow). Vigorous heating of a synovial joint should only be done in chronic disease conditions, such as contracture or the advanced degenerative (quiescent) stage of rheumatoid arthritis. The purpose of such treatment is to improve joint range of motion by decreasing stiffness and improving resilience of contracted soft tissues. In the subacute stage of traumatic arthritis, continuous SWD at dose level II or pulsed SW at dose levels III or IV may be beneficial in joints with a thin soft-tissue cover to improve blood circulation, thereby aiding in the resolution of edema and hemorrhage. This concept may also apply to acute or subacute epicondylitis, for which mild heating from continuous SWD or pulsed SW may help in reabsorption of inflammatory exudates.

Very mild heating, at dosage level I from continuous SWD, may be used in recurring inflammatory conditions to improve blood flow and facilitate diffusion of oxygen and metabolite clearance.[21] Lehmann[21,22] advocates the use of continuous SWD to induce mild heating, which produces a mild physiologic response, in the later stages of traumatic arthritis, chronic pelvic inflammatory disease, epicondylitis, degenerative joint disease, ankylosing spondylitis, and other chronic arthritic conditions.

A reflex or consensual mild heating response of a body part (such as an extremity) is achieved by applying the source of heat proximal to the site of vascular occlusion. If this approach is used in treating peripheral arterial insufficiency, it avoids the potential for overheating tissues that are poorly vasculated and are, therefore, incapable of adequately dissipating direct applications of heat. It is not known whether improved deep collateral circulation occurs with this method, in addition to the reflex dilation of skin blood vessels that is evoked.[9] Additional research is needed to establish the efficacy of this technique.

Continuous shortwave techniques may be used for selective heating of pelvic organs in chronic inflammatory pelvic diseases. According to Lehmann,[21] this treatment produces a significant increase in vascularity and blood flow, with the result that cardiac output is increased in women. As a result of the improved vascularity, antibiotic levels to inflamed tissues may be enhanced.

Allberry[23] and Barnett[24] have reported positive results with continuous SWD in enhancing the drying up of blisters from herpes zoster and in alleviating the associated pain. Both reports emphasized the importance of applying mild heating within a few days of the onset of rash, or on the first day if possible. Treatment consists of daily 20-minute applications at the level of the involved dorsal root ganglia until pain is decreased or the scabs fall off.

Proposed Indications for Pulsed SW, SWD, and PEMFs

Many scientific attempts have been made to demonstrate the efficacy of pulsed SW for therapeutic purposes. Some studies[25,26] have shown that the benefits of heat produced in deep tissues with pulsed and continuous SWD have similar therapeutic value. In one of these, Pasila and associates[25] compared two pulsating SW devices (1 hour per day for 3 days) with a placebo in the treatment of 300 ankle and foot sprains. In measurements of strength, joint range of motion, swelling, impairment of gait, and function of disability, they found little significant difference between the placebo group and those treated with pulsed SW. Barker and associates[27] also reported no significant differences between two groups of patients following pulsed SW treatment or placebo applications to acute ankle sprains with respect to range of motion, gait, pain, or swelling.

Wilson,[28,29] on the other hand, has demonstrated that pulsed SW reduced pain and disability in several acute ankle sprains significantly better than did continuous SWD treatment. In one study, Wilson[28] compared the nonthermal effects of pulsed SW with placebo effects of pulsed SW. He assigned patients with recent inversion ankle sprains to two match-paired groups of 20. The treatment group received a 1-hour treatment of pulsed shortwave daily for 3 days. For these treatments, a pulsed shortwave device with a frequency of 27.12 MHz was adjusted to provide an output of 975 watts for each 65 microsecond pulse. The off-time interval between successive pulses was 1600 microseconds. The control group received a 1-hour placebo treatment of pulsed shortwave daily for 3 days. Wilson reported that, statistically, symptoms of pain and disability were relieved more rapidly in the treatment than in the control group, however, there was no significant difference between the two groups regarding improvement in swelling. To assess the possibility that the beneficial effects observed in the treatment group might have resulted from an increase in blood flow owing to some small, transient degree of heating (which is the mode of action attributed to continuous shortwave diathermy) a second clinical study was conducted to compare the effects of pulsed shortwave with continuous shortwave diathermy.[29] The same number of patients with recent inversion ankle injuries were assigned in matched pairs to 2 groups and, depending on the group, received either a 1-hour treatment of pulsed shortwave or 2 15-minute treatments within 1 hour of continuous inductive shortwave diathermy daily for 3 days.

Analysis of the data revealed statistically significant differences—at the 1.0 percent level of confidence in reduction of swelling and at the 0.1 percent level in reduction of pain and disability—by pulsed shortwave compared with continuous shortwave. In comparing total energy delivered to patients in the two groups, it was found that those treated with continuous SWD received approximately 22.5 watt hours compared to 15 watt hours received by patients treated with pulsed shortwave. The fact that better clinical responses were produced with less energy was interpreted by Wilson[28] as support for the idea that beneficial results were due to specific nonthermal effects. It is widely accepted, however, that heat applied in the early stages following soft-tissue trauma may exacerbate the inflammatory response to injury. Thus, it is possible that patients in this study who were treated with heat either did not improve or got worse, whereas those who received athermic pulsed shortwave would have improved spontaneously without any treatment. This question could have been resolved if the design of the study had included a control group.

An improvement in the rate of soft-tissue healing has also been reported following studies with pulsed shortwave in the treatment of surgical wounds from dental and podiatric procedures. In 90 patients who had had dental surgery, Aronofsky[30] treated 30 with pulsed shortwave pre- and postoperatively, 30 others only postoperatively, and 30 served as controls. Patients in both treatment groups reportedly exhibited substantially less time for their wounds to heal compared to wounds of patients in the control group. In a double-blind study on 100 patients who received a variety of podiatric surgical procedures, Kaplan and Weinstock[31] randomly applied placebo or actual pulsed short-wave treatments to the surgical site. They anecdotally reported significant reductions in postoperative edema, erythema, and pain in patients who received actual pulsed short-wave treatments, compared to those who received placebo shortwave treatments.

Golden and associates[32] conducted a controlled double-blind clinical study, which compared treatment of donor sites of medium-thickness-split grafts with pulsed short-wave versus control-donor sites treated with a placebo of pulsed shortwave. Patients in both groups received one 30-minute treatment before receiving medication before surgery and then received a 1-hour treatment daily for 7 days after surgery. The treatment group received pulsed shortwave at a peak output of 975 watts and a frequency of 400 pps. With a pulse duration of 65 microseconds, the mean power output was 25.3 watts. Wounds were evaluated daily by medical staff who were unaware of the patients' grouping. On the seventh postoperative day, dressings were removed and the percent of wound area healed was determined. In the treatment group, 17 of 29 patients had wounds that were healed 90 percent or more, compared with only 11 of 38 patients in the placebo group. Data analysis revealed that this difference was statistically significant. Cameron[33] also reported favorable results in surgical wound healing during a double-blind clinical study in which 100 surgical patients were assigned either to a pulsed shortwave placebo group or to a pulsed shortwave treatment group. In addition, the effects of PEMFs on healing of induced wounds in animals reportedly reduced edema faster in treated than control wounds[34] and significantly accelerated reabsorption of hematomas.[35] Other studies in which PEMFs was used to treat induced full-thickness skin wounds or burn wounds in an animal model showed no significant difference in healing time or tissue tensile strength between treatment and control wounds.[34]

Other studies related to pulsed SW have been published, especially those done with animal models.[36,37] Pulsed electromagnetic energy to nerve-damaged rats resulted in quicker regeneration, as well as earlier wound healing, compared with results from a control group, according to Wilson and associates.[36] They also noted considerably more scarring and fibrosis around the nerve-suture site in the control group. Following injections of a myotoxic drug into the gastrocnemius muscle in rabbits, Brown and Baker[37] found no significant differences between a control group and a group treated with pulsed shortwave radiation.

Despite the positive clinical outcomes reported in the literature for pulsed SW, additional controlled clinical studies are needed to establish the efficacy and effectiveness of this modality before it can be considered as a viable treatment for managing soft-tissue injury or enhancing pain relief.

HYPERTHERMIA IN ONCOLOGY

Hyperthermia induced by diathermy for treatment of cancer is undergoing clinical investigation at present. Moderate elevation of tissue temperature surrounding a tumor may accelerate the rate of growth of the tumor[38] and cause metastasis. At higher temperatures, malignant cells are thermolabile, and they are killed when exposed to temperatures greater than 42°C.[38] Continuous SWD and MWD are effective in treating certain human neoplasms (with hyperthermia), either as single agents or synergistically with ionizing radiation.[39-41] Several investigators[42-44] have successfully used the microwave frequency of 433.92 MHz in oncologic hyperthermia studies because of its ability to penetrate fat and muscle and heat at depths of 10 cm.[43-45]

Unfortunately, treatment of cancer with microwave or continuous SWD is not without iatrogenic side effects, which may manifest as blistering of skin, fat-layer burns, and tumor necrosis.[39] The prevention of complications such as these requires coordinated health-team care and careful planning in selecting diathermy for treatment of the cancer patient. Because physical therapists are familiar with the thermal effects produced by SWD and MWD, they may be valuable resources to oncologists who perform hyperthermia therapy.

PRECAUTIONS AND CONTRAINDICATIONS

The literature cites numerous potential hazards of nonionizing radiation from continuous SWD or MWD. Hazards may result from high levels of unintended exposures to tissues or materials inside the patient's body, adjacent to the patient, or adjacent to the therapist applying the treatment.

Foremost among the potential hazards to be considered with both SWD and MWD are internal and externally worn metallic objects and electromedical devices. Neither continuous SWD nor MWD should be applied over surgical metal implants or tissues containing other foreign metallic objects, because focusing of field lines causes excessive current density within the metal and raises its surface temperature, resulting in transfer of excessive heat that may burn adjacent tissues.[3,21,46] Women with metallic intrauterine devices should not receive continuous SWD or MWD to the lumbar, pelvic, or abdominal areas.[47,48] Likewise, externally worn metallic items (jewelry and zippers, for instance) should be removed and placed outside the electromagnetic field during continuous SWD or MWD treatment.[14] Metal objects within the immediate treatment area (such as metal in the treatment table, chairs, or swivel stools) should be removed.

In addition to biologic hazards, electromagnetic interference (EMI) may cause disturbances in the function of electromedical or other devices. Wristwatches, other RF devices, diagnostic medical equipment (that is, electroencephalographs, electrocardiographs, and electromyographs), unshielded cardiac pacemakers, transcutaneous electrical nerve or muscle stimulators, electrophrenic pacers, and cerebellar and urinary bladder stimulators[21,49,50] may malfunction when either continuous SWD, MWD, or PEMFs are applied in their immediate vicinity. Unpleasant paresthesias or burning sensations may occur beneath transcutaneous electrodes that connect the device to the patient, whether or not the device is in operation. Therefore, therapists should avoid directing electromagnetic fields over or near externally worn or implanted electronic devices, their lead wires, or their electrodes.

Of prime concern regarding EMI are devices that transmit high-frequency, high-voltage electric and magnetic field energy into, and in the vicinity of, the patient. EMI may cause an unshielded cardiac pacemaker to stop pacing, revert to a prefixed rate, or to pace rapidly and erratically, if the unshielded pacemaker comes within 4.5 meters of an operational device.[3] Secondary to the induced malfunction, the patient's cardiac rhythm may revert to asystole or ventricular fibrillation. Improvements in pacemaker engineering and design have reduced their susceptibility to electromagnetic fields and have even eliminated this problem in some pacemakers.[50] However, it behooves the therapist to place adequate warning signs outside the area where devices with EM fields are being used and to select another nonelectromagnetic thermal agent to treat the patient who is equipped with an unshielded cardiac pacemaker.

Specific tissues or anatomic structures that may be adversely affected by the thermal effects of continuous SWD or MWD include: high-fluid volume areas, such as the eyes[15,22,51–56] and fluid-filled joints,[57] testes; space-occupying lesions; ischemic, hemorrhagic, malignant, and acutely inflamed tissues, as well as sensory-impaired skin. Moist wound dressings, moist clothing,[21] or accumulations of excessive perspiration[14] also will focus field lines, because of the higher dielectric constant and conductivity of isolated body fluids in comparison to surrounding tissues. The same focusing effect applies to blood vessels that run through adipose tissue. The potential for overheating of the fluids in each case from charge accumulation at the fluid-tissue interface may result in thermal necrosis of adjacent tissues. Terrycloth toweling used with all continuous SWD applicators absorbs surface perspiration, and wide spacing between skin and air-spaced applicators helps to minimize the risk of excessive heating of surface moisture.

When moisture is present in copious amounts, such as occurs in moist wounds or wounds packed with moist dressings, continuous SWD, and MWD should not be applied in a way that would allow energy absorption and selective heating of the moisture.

The high-fluid volume of the eye makes it susceptible to selective absorption of unintended or accidental doses of energy from either continuous SWD[51] or MWD.[52] Daily[52,53] and Richardson and coworkers[54,55] have demonstrated that cataracts can develop in the eyes of experimental animals exposed to microwaves. Consequently, exposure of the eye to MWD should be avoided, even though no human studies have reported cataract development or other damage due to diathermy exposure. If continuous SWD is to be applied to the maxillary sinuses of a person wearing contact lenses, the lenses should be removed before treatment to avoid a concentration of field energy that could cause excessive heating of the ciliary body.[56]

The synovial joint, as mentioned previously, that has accumulated excess fluid from effusion may also pose a hazard if the temperature of the fluid is raised a few degrees. Intra-articular temperature of normal synovial joints ranges between 30°C and 31°C.[57] Harris and McCroskery[58,59] have demonstrated in vitro that an increase of 5°C produced a fourfold increase in enzymatic lysis of human cartilage by rheumatoid synovial collagenase. Feibel and Fast[60] point out that the intra-articular temperature in knees with rheumatoid arthritis is about 36.5°C, and that a significant increase in temperature greater than this may accelerate destruction of cartilage. Based on this knowledge, therapists should use caution when considering whether mild, vigorous, or no heating from continuous or pulsed SW is appropriate for the patient who has an inflamed joint condition.

Lehmann and associates[22] suggest that exacerbation of acutely inflamed, fluid-filled joint cavities may occur as a result of selective heating by vigorous treatment using continuous SWD or MWD when the joint is covered by a thin soft-tissue layer.

Vigorous heating should be avoided in acute inflammatory processes because of the potential for causing tissue necrosis by imposing an inflammatory reaction on an existing acute inflammatory process.[22] Likewise, vigorous heating of tissue adjacent to a space-occupying lesion, such as a protruded nucleus pulposus, may exacerbate symptoms by increasing swelling and congestion of tissue surrounding the disc lesion.[21,22]

In Chapter 5, it was pointed out that a local application of heat from any source to ischemic tissue is hazardous, because the compromised blood flow may not meet the increased metabolic demand placed on the tissues by the thermal energy buildup.[61] Lehmann and colleagues[22] have indicated that the time-rate of change of temperature for vascularized tissues treated with SWD should range between 0.8°C and 2.7°C per minute, achieving a critical temperature of 44°C within 10 minutes.

To avoid rapid temperature increase in tissues with compromised blood flow, the power density and time-rate of temperature increase should be adjusted to avoid possible tissue necrosis. An alternative method using continuous SWD that avoids potential damage to tissues with arterial insufficiency is to apply the treatment proximal to the area of occluded circulation. This may evoke a consensual increase in distal blood flow owing to reflex vasodilation in the involved area.[62,63] The magnitude of the consensual effect is dependent upon the size of the local area heated. The greater the area heated, the greater the consensual response.[61]

Since an increase in tissue temperature increases blood flow owing to dilation of arterioles, neither continuous SWD nor MWD should be used to treat individuals who are predisposed to hemorrhage, such as patients with hemophilia, since the increase in blood flow secondary to the induced vasodilation would potentiate the tendency to bleed.[61-63]

Patients with pain and temperature–sensory deficits may be unable to appreciate thermal changes applied to their skin. Since dosage depends on the patient's ability to determine when heat sensation is just comfortably warm, only mild to moderate doses (based on the therapist's knowledge of previous output settings) should be applied in these situations. The patient's condition and the equipment should be checked frequently by the therapist.

Animal studies have demonstrated deleterious effects of MWD on gonad structure and function.[64-66] Although the testicles and ovaries in humans are generally considered to be sensitive to temperature rise, the testicles (because of their superficial location) are more susceptible to stray radiation than are the ovaries. Unnecessary exposure of the testes to continuous SWD and MWD, therefore, should be avoided.[67]

Continuous shortwave and MWD should not be applied to the low back, or to the abdominal or pelvic regions of pregnant women, because of the possibility of thermal damage to the fetus.[68] Studies on the effect of continuous SWD and MWD on fetal and embryonic growth and development have demonstrated that anomalies occurred in rat fetuses exposed to a frequency of 27.12 MHz,[69] and that inhibition of growth and development occurred in chick embryos exposed to 2450 MHz microwaves.[70] In both studies, the observed effects were attributed to hyperthermia. Similar effects induced by MWD and continuous SWD on human subjects have not been documented. Case-study reports by Rubin and Erdman[71] indicate that MWD exposures of 2450 MHz at 100 W output were given to four women being treated for chronic pelvic inflammatory disease. All four women were either already pregnant or became pregnant during the time of the treatment session, and none experienced any interference with ovulation, conception, or pregnancy. Daels[72] reported no adverse effects in a 1-year followup study of children whose mothers received MWD treatments during pregnancy.

Although exposure of pregnant laboratory animals to MWD[73] and continuous SWD[69] does cause fetal abnormalities, it is not known whether the fetus in the human can be reached with significant microwave radiation at clinically used intensities. Despite the possibility that amniotic fluid may selectively absorb MWD or continuous SWD energy, there are no clinical reports in the literature to substantiate whether selective heating of the pregnant uterus does or does not occur during exposure to these energies. Based on the finding that temperatures of 39.8°C or more are damaging to the human fetus,[74] Lehmann[21] advises that MWD may be hazardous if administered in a way that would allow "a significant amount of energy" to reach the pregnant uterus, and that continuous SWD should not be administered with vaginal electrodes to pregnant women for the same reason.

When diathermy has been applied to the lumbosacral region in menstruating women, clinical reports have indicated that an increase in menstrual flow occurred.[21] The low-back area of a woman may be treated during the menstrual period, but women should be forewarned that their menstrual flow may increase temporarily following treatment.

Regarding the effect of diathermy on bone, it must be emphasized that, because of the reflection properties of MWD, it should be applied with caution over bony prominences to avoid burning of tissues overlying the bone.[75] In addition, one study states that there is a potential for disturbing bone growth in children when continuous SWD creates a significant rise in temperature of the epiphyses.[44]

Animal studies have demonstrated that continuous SWD may either enhance[76] or inhibit[77] bone growth. Therapists applying continuous SWD to children should be aware, therefore, that bone is not effectively heated when covered by an adequate thickness of soft tissue,[21] and that a disturbance in bone growth will occur only at intensities that produce pain.[21] However, the size of the continuous SWD applicator relative to the size of the child may prevent application in a way that avoids superficial bone-growth centers.

Concern that the therapist who operates MWD or continuous SWD equipment may receive unintended, hazardous exposure of EM energy is not supported by published reports. Mosely and Davison[78] measured the radiation exposure to physical therapists who used MWD and concluded that exposure is not harmful if reasonable care is taken.

Unintended exposure will not occur as long as the therapist is 1 meter away from the treatment surface of an operating MWD applicator.[78] A similar study by Stuchly and colleagues[79] concurs that overexposure to the therapist from continuous SWD is possible when the distance between the therapist and the applicator is 20 cm or less.

Other materials and objects that may be hazardous during application of continuous SWD include certain synthetic substances such as nylon, foam rubber, and plastics. Objects like pillows, pillow cases, treatment tables, sandbag coverings, and clothing often contain these materials, which are nonconductive. It has been reported, however, that a pillow being used by a patient receiving continuous SWD treatment was charred at areas of contact with, or directly adjacent to, the induction power cables of the device.[80] Therapists should avoid such potential fire hazards by correct placement of equipment and by keeping cables and electrodes well away from synthetic materials.

Unlike continuous SWD, pulsed SW does not produce any significant tissue heating. Therefore, PEMFs can be safely applied to patients in spite of the presence of metal or fluid accumulation either on or within the tissues. It must be remembered, however, that PEMFs are not absolutely athermic, especially at higher pulse frequencies, and may cause the average output to approach 80 watts, which is generally the lower end of the output range for continuous SWD. Because a magnetic field is produced by pulsed shortwave equipment during operation, such devices may be dangerous to patients with unshielded cardiac pacemakers or other electronic equipment who come in close proximity to them. It is also recommended that PEMFs not be applied over neoplasms, tuberculous lesions, or to pregnant women.[7]

TREATMENT DOCUMENTATION AND DECISION MAKING

For purposes of determining whether treatment with SWD, MWD, or PEMFs has facilitated clinical improvement, and to allow replication of treatment following positive treatment outcomes, it is important that the physical therapist document the variables used in administering each treatment. The variables that should be documented include the:

1. Type of EM energy—MWD, SWD, or PEMFs.
2. Commercial model name.
3. Type of applicator(s) used.
4. Description of where on the body the applicator was applied.
5. Duration of treatment.
6. Power-output level.
7. Pulse frequency and duration, if PEMFs were used.
8. Response of the patient to treatment.

Two cases are presented here that illustrate some examples of uses of diathermy. A patient with acutely sprained lateral ankle ligaments is referred to you within 6 hours following onset. X-ray has confirmed that fracture is not present. The treatment goal is to reduce swelling and pain and to enhance tissue healing, so you elect to treat the patient's ankle with pulsed shortwave. You select a device that has a carrier frequency of 27.12 MHz, and you deliver the pulsed energy with an induction-drum applicator at a pulse frequency of 400 pps and a pulse duration of 400 μsec. At this frequency and duration, with this device, the peak pulse output is 975 W, and the mean power output is 25.3 W. Using these variables, daily treatments lasting 30 minutes for 5 days eliminated all pain and reduced swelling 50 percent without ice, elevation, or compression.

You have another patient who had repeated torn hamstring muscles, which has led to development of a 30-degree knee-flexion contracture. To reduce the contracture you use the heat-and-stretch concept, whereby you apply continuous SWD using an inductive-drum applicator with the patient prone to vigorously heat the hamstrings while you simultaneously stretch the hamstrings for 30 minutes with a 10-pound sandbag applied to the calcaneus. During the 30-minute treatment, you repeatedly check to make certain that the patient is perceiving a heat sensation barely below maximal toleration (dose IV). Maintaining this level of heating will require that you periodically decrease the power output, if the level of heat at the beginning of treatment was perceived by the patient to be just below maximal tolerance. After 30 minutes, the heat is removed from the hamstrings, but the patient remains in the prone position with the 10 pounds applied to the calcaneus to facilitate residual elongation of the tight hamstrings during a 20-minute, cool-down period. Daily measurements of knee range of motion following five consecutive treatments reduced the flexion contracture to 17 degrees.

SUMMARY

Either shortwave or microwave diathermy may be used to produce a rise in tissue temperature within the therapeutically desirable thermal range of 40°C to 44°C. The depth of penetration and extent of temperature rise depend on wave frequency, the electrical properties of the tissue(s) receiving the EM energy, and the type of applicator used. Either mild or vigorous heating may be produced. Mild heating is usually desired in acute musculoskeletal conditions, whereas vigorous heating may be needed in chronic conditions.[81] Non-thermal effects may be produced by pulsed SW when this form of EM energy is delivered to the body at low pulse frequencies and low mean power. At higher pulse frequencies, which produce higher mean power output, mild heating occurs. This means that pulsed SW may be used either in acute or in subacute conditions, where minimal heat is desirable, or in conditions that require enhancement of tissue healing by nonthermal effects.

Various conditions for which continuous SWD are beneficial and suggested uses of PEMFs are discussed. Contraindications for both types of energy are also presented.

REFERENCES

1. Schwan, HP and Piersol, GM: The absorption of electromagnetic energy in body tissues, Part I. Am J Phys Med 33:371, 1954.
2. Schwan, HP and Piersol, GM: The absorption of electromagnetic energy in body tissues, Part II. Am J Phys Med 34:425, 1955.
3. Ward, AR: Electricity Fields and Waves in Therapy. Science Press, NWS, Australia, 1980, p 166.
4. Thom, H: Introduction to Shortwave and Microwave Therapy, ed 3. Charles C Thomas, Springfield, IL, 1966, pp 46–51.
5. Erwin, DN: An overview of the biological effects of radio frequency radiation. Military Med 148:113, 1983.
6. Diathermy Units, Microwave: Diathermy Units, Shortwave. In Product Comparison System. ECRI, Plymouth Meeting, PA, March, 1988, pp 1–10.
7. van den Bouwhuijsen, F, et al: A Manual on Pulsed and Continuous Shortwave Diathermy: ENRAF-NONIUS, cat no 1419.762, Delft, Holland.
8. Millard, JB: Effect of high frequency currents and infra-red rays on the circulation of the lower limb in man. Ann Phys Med 6:45, 1961.

9. McNiven, DR and Wyper, DJ: Microwave therapy and muscle blood flow in man. J Microwave Power 11:168, 1976.
10. Harris, R: Effect of shortwave diathermy on radio-sodium clearance from the knee joint in the normal and in rheumatoid arthritis. Phys Med Rehabil 42:241, 1961.
11. Low, JL: The nature and effects of pulsed electromagnetic radiations. NZ Physiotherapy 6:18, 1978.
12. Barnothy, JM: Biological Effects of Magnetic Fields. Plenum Press, New York, 1964.
13. Sanseverino, EG: membrane phenomena and cellular processes under action of pulsating magnetic fields. Presented at the Second International Congress for Magneto Medicine, Rome, November, 1980.
14. Griffin, JE and Karselis, TC: Principles of Instrumentation. In Griffin, JE and Karselis, TC: Physical Agents for Physical Therapists, ed 2. Charles C Thomas, Springfield, IL, 1982, p 202.
15. Shortwave Diathermy Units. Health Devices, 175, June, 1979.
16. Oliver, DE: Pulsed Electro-Magnetic Energy: What is it? Physiotherapy 70:458, 1984.
17. Lehmann, JF, et al: Comparison of relative heating patterns produced in tissues by exposure to microwave energy at frequencies of 2450 and 900 megacycles. Arch Phys Med Rehabil 46:307, 1965.
18. Schliephake, E: Carrying out treatment. In Thom, H: Introduction to Shortwave and Microwave Therapy, ed 3. Charles C Thomas, Springfield, IL, 1966, p 65.
19. Hayne, CR: Pulsed high frequency energy: Its place in physiotherapy. Physiotherapy 70:459, 1984.
20. Warren CG, Lehmann, JF, and Koblanski, NJ: Heat and stretch procedures: An evaluation using rat tail tendon. Arch Phys Med Rehabil 57:122, 1976.
21. Lehmann, JF: Therapeutic Heat and Cold, ed 4. Williams & Wilkins, Baltimore, 1990, pp 470–474.
22. Lehmann, JF, Warren, CG, and Scham, SM: Therapeutic heat and cold. Clin Orthop 99:207, 1974.
23. Allberry, J: Shortwave diathermy for herpes zoster. Physiotherapy 60:386, 1974.
24. Barnett, M: SWD for herpes zoster. Physiotherapy 61:217, 1975.
25. Pasila, M, Visuri, T, and Sandholm, A: Pulsating shortwave diathermy: Value in treatment of recent ankle and foot sprains. Arch Phys Med Rehabil 59:383, 1978.
26. Silverman, DR and Pendleton, L: A comparison of the effects of continuous and pulsed short-wave diathermy on peripheral circulation. Arch Phys Med Rehabil 49:429, 1968.
27. Barker, AT, et al: A double-blind clinical trial of low power pulsed shortwave therapy in the treatment of a soft tissue injury. Physiotherapy 71(12):500, 1985.
28. Wilson, DH: Treatment of soft-tissue injuries by pulsed electrical energy. Br Med J 2:269, 1972.
29. Wilson, DH: Comparison of shortwave diathermy and pulsed electromagnetic energy in treatment of soft tissue injuries. Physiotherapy 60(10):309, 1974.
30. Aronofsky, DH: Reduction of dental post-surgical symptoms using non-thermal pulsed high-peak power electromagnetic energy. Oral Surg 32(5):688, 1971.
31. Kaplan, EG and Weinstock, RE: Clinical evaluation of Diapulse as adjunctive therapy following foot surgery. J Am Podiat Assoc 58(5):218, 1968.
32. Golden, JH, et al: The effects of Diapulse on the healing of wounds: A double-blind randomized controlled trial in man. Br J Plast Surg 34:267, 1981.
33. Cameron, BM: Experimental acceleration of wound healing: Am J Ortho 53:336, 1961.
34. Constable, JD, Scapicchio, AP, and Opitz, B: Studies of the effects of Diapulse treatment of various aspects of wound healing in experimental animals. J Surg Res 11(5):254, 1971.
35. Fenn, JE: Effect of pulsed electromagnetic energy (Diapulse) on experimental hematomas. Canadian Med Assoc J 100:251, 1969.
36. Wilson, DH, et al: The effects of pulsed electromagnetic energy on peripheral nerve regeneration. Ann NY Acad Sci 238:575, 1975.
37. Brown, M and Baker, RD: Effect of pulsed shortwave diathermy on skeletal muscle injury in rabbits. Phys Ther 67:208, 1987.
38. Overgaard, J: Effects of hyperthermia on malignant cells in vivo: A review and hypothesis. Cancer 39:2637, 1977.
39. Luk, KH, et al: The use of 2450 megahertz of microwave in cancer therapy. Phys Ther 59:405, 1979.
40. Antich, PP, et al: Selective heating of cancerous tumors at 27.12 MHz. IEEE Trans Microwave Theory Tech 26:569, 1978.
41. Kim JH, et al: Local tumor hyperthermia in combination with radiation therapy. Cancer 40:161, 1977.
42. Petrowicz, O, et al: Experimental studies on the use of microwaves for the localized heat treatment of the prostate. J Microwave Power 14(2):167, 1979.
43. Hornback, NB, et al: Radiation and microwave therapy in the treatment of advanced cancer. Radiology 130:459, 1979.
44. Paliwal, BR, et al: Heating patterns produced by 434 MHz erbotherm UHF69. Radiology 135:511, 1980.
45. Holt, JAG: The use of V.H.F. radiowaves in cancer therapy. Australasian Radiology 19:1975.
46. Lehmann, JF, et al: Review of evidence for indications, techniques of application, contraindications, hazards and clinical effectiveness for shortwave diathermy. DHEW/FDA HFA-510, Rockville, MD, 1974.
47. Sandler, B: Heat and the U.U.C.D. Br Med J 25:458, 1973.
48. Nielsen, NC, et al: Heat induction in copper-bearing IUD's during shortwave diathermy. Acta Obstet Gynecol Scand 58:495, 1979.
49. Jones, SL: Electromagnetic field interference and cardiac pacemakers. Phys Ther 56:1013, 1976.
50. Smyth, H: The pacemaker patient and the electromagnetic environment. JAMA 227:1412, 1974.

51. Konarska, I and Michniewicz, L: Shortwave therapy of diseases of the anterior portion of the eye. Klin Oczna 25:185, 1955.
52. Daily, L, et al: The effects of microwave diathermy on the eye. Am J Ophthalmol 33:1241, 1950.
53. Daily, L Jr, et al: Influence of microwaves on certain enzyme systems in the eye. Am J Ophthalmol 34:1301, 1951.
54. Richardson, AW, Duane, TH, and Haines, HM: Experimental lenticular opacities produced by microwave irradiation. Arch Phys Med 29:765, 1948.
55. Richardson, AW, et al: The role of energy, pupilary diameter and alloxan diabetes in the production of ocular damage by microwave irradiations. Am J Ophthalmol 35:993, 1952.
56. Scott, BO: Effect of contact lenses on shortwave field distribution. Br J Ophthalmol 40:696, 1956.
57. Hollander, JL, et al: Joint temperature measurement in evaluation of antiarthritic agents. J Clin Invest 30:701, 1951.
58. Harris, E, Jr and McCroskery, PA: Influence of temperature and fibril stability on degradation of cartilage collagen by rheumatoid synovial collagenase. N Engl J Med 290:1, 1974.
59. Harris, ED (ed): Rheumatoid Arthritis. MEDCOM Press, New York, 1974.
60. Feibel, H and Fast, H: Deepheating of joints: A reconsideration. Arch Phys Med Rehabil 57:513, 1976.
61. Fischer, C and Solomon, S: Physiological responses to heat and cold. In Licht, S (ed): Therapeutic Heat and Cold. Elizabeth Licht, New Haven, 1965, p 127.
62. Abramson, DI: Physiologic basis for the use of physical agents in peripheral vascular disorders. Arch Phys Med Rehabil 46:216, 1965.
63. Wise, CS: The effect of diathermy on blood blow. Arch Phys Med Rehabil 29:17, 1948.
64. Ely, TS, et al: Heating characteristics of laboratory animals exposed to ten centimeter microwaves. US Navy Med Res Inst (Res Rep Proj NM 001-156.1302) IEEE Tran Biomed Eng 11:123, 1964.
65. Gorodetskaya, SF: The effect of centimeter radio waves on mouse fertility. Fiziol Zh 9:394, 1963.
66. Imig, CJ and Free, JR: Testicular degeneration as a result of microwave irradiation. Proc Soc Exp Biol Med 69:382, 1948.
67. Van Demark, NL and Free, MJ: Temperature effects. In Johnson, AD, et al (eds): The Testis, Vol 3. Academic Press, New York, 1973, p 254–257.
68. Smith, DW, Clarren, SK, and Harvey, MAS: Hyperthermia as a possible teratogenic agent. J Pediatr 92:878, 1978.
69. Dietzel, F: Effects of non-ionizing electromagnetic radiation on the development and intrauterine implantation of the rat. In Tyler, AE (ed): Biological Effects of Nonionizing Radiation. Ann NY Acad Sci 247:367, 1975.
70. Van Ummersen, CA: The effect of 2450 mc radiation on the development of the chick embryo. Proceedings of the Fourth Annual Tri-Service Conference on the Biological Effects of Microwave Radiation. 1:201–221, 1961.
71. Rubin, A and Erdman, WJ: Microwave exposure of the human female pelvis during early pregnancy and prior to conception. Am J Phys Med 38:219, 1959.
72. Daels, J: Microwave heating of the uterine wall during parturition. J Microwave Power 11:166, 1976.
73. Rugh, R, et al: Are microwaves teratongenic? In Czerski, P, et al (eds): Biological Effects and Health Hazards of Microwave Radiation. Polish Med Pub, Warsaw, 1974.
74. Havey, MAS, McRorie, MM, and Smith, DW: Suggested limits of exposure in the hot tub and sauna for the pregnant woman. Canadian Med Assoc 125:50, 1981.
75. Lehmann, JR: Diathermy. In Krusen, FH (ed): Handbook of Physical Medicine and Rehabilitation. WB Saunders, Philadelphia, 1965, pp 308–311.
76. Doyle, JR and Smart, BW: Stimulation of bone growth by shortwave diathermy. J Bone Joint Surg 45-A:15, 1963.
77. Hutchinson, WJ and Burdeaux, BD: The effects of shortwave diathermy on bone repair. J Bone Joint Surg 33-A:155, 1951.
78. Mosely, H and Davison, M: Exposure of physiotherapists to microwave radiation during microwave diathermy treatment. Clinical Physics and Physiological Measurement 3, 2:217, 1981.
79. Stuchly, MA, et al: Exposure to the operator and patient during shortwave diathermy treatments. Health Physics 42:341, 1982.
80. Progress Report. American Physical Therapy Association, June, 1980.
81. Kloth, LC, Morrison, M, and Ferguson, B: Therapeutic microwave and shortwave diathermy: A review of thermal effectiveness, safe use, and state-of-the-art, 1984. Center for Devices and Radiological Health, DHHS, FDA 85-8237, December, 1984.

CHAPTER 9

Therapeutic Uses of Light in Rehabilitation

Lynn Snyder-Mackler, Sc.D., P.T., S.C.S.
Laurence Seitz, M.S., P.T.

The healing properties of light have been described since ancient Roman times. Light has been used in physical therapy to treat many disorders. This chapter will discuss the use of two forms of light in rehabilitation: low-power laser and ultraviolet light.

LASER

Laser is an acronym for *l*ight *a*mplification by *s*timulated *e*mission of *r*adiation.[1] Radiation is the process by which energy is propagated through space.[2] The common characteristics of all forms of radiant energy are as follows: (1) They are produced by applying electrical or other forces to various forms of matter; (2) they all may be transmitted without the support of a sensible medium; and, (3) their velocity of travel is equal in a vacuum, but may vary within different media. The direction of propagation is normally a straight line; they undergo reflection, deflection, and absorption by the media through which they travel. They are designated collectively as electromagnetic radiations. A laser is generally used as a source or generator of radiation.[3] Low-power laser is used in physical rehabilitation for pain control and soft-tissue healing.

The objectives of this section are to: (1) Establish a basic understanding of the physical principles of therapeutic laser; (2) delineate the differences between low- and high-power laser as therapeutic modalities; (3) present the clinical application of laser in physical therapy for wound healing and pain management; and, (4) discuss the con-traindications, precautions, and guidelines for the safe and proposed use of laser in physical therapy.

BACKGROUND ON LASER

The reader should understand how laser is produced and what makes it unique from other forms of light before its use as a therapeutic agent is discussed. Einstein proposed the concept of stimulated emission as it related to the atom and its component parts.[4,5] Einstein reasoned that a stimulus can cause the electron configuration of an atom to be momentarily rearranged. In returning to its original configuration, surplus energy will be released in the form of a photon, the basic unit of light. This massless particle, in turn, can release a photon from every pre-excited atom or molecule with which it collides. A chain reaction is initiated, and the stimulated emission of radiation occurs.[4]

Beginning in 1953, an interest in stimulated emission reappeared with the advent of microwave amplification.[5,6] Microwave radiations are wavelengths that possess optic properties; that is, they can be refracted, diffracted, and reflected, and can be focused by suitable lenses.[2] With the development of masers (*m*icrowave *a*mplifiers by the *s*timu-lated *e*mission of *r*adiation), speculation arose concerning the possibility of extending this principle into amplification and generation in the region of visible radiation.

Schawlow and Townes reportedly presented the feasibility of producing stimulated emission in the microwave wavelength area near the optic regions of the spectrum.[7] Their work, considered to be the impetus for the initial discoveries of all types of lasers, turned out to be surprisingly accurate in predicting the size, wavelength range, and output power for typical gas lasers having moderate input-power-excitation require-ments.[8] (However, it did not propose the use of a gas discharge for excitation of atomic components.[9])

Two years later, Maiman successfully produced the first working model of the ruby laser.[6] Javan, Bennett, and Herriott discovered the helium–neon (HeNe) laser in the fall of 1960.[6] The discovery of visible red laser output at 623.8 nanometers (nm) by White and Rigden occurred in early 1962.[10] This work generated interest in other possible applications for the laser that were in the infrared, noninvisible emission range.[9]

PHYSICAL PRINCIPLES OF LASER

When a photon, or energy particle of light, is directed at an atom, it may be absorbed, reflected, or transmitted. If the particle is reflected or transmitted, no light-energy change occurs. If the photon is absorbed, however, energy in the orbital elec-trons is increased. One or more electrons undergo a positional change from an inner orbit to a more peripheral orbit. The affected atom will have gained energy and is then said to be "excited."[9]

Excited atoms are unstable and will seek their ground state in random fashion, after a short time, without further external stimulation. This phenomenon produces sponta-neous emission of light. This process, if allowed to reach its end, will prevent the energy-transfer level necessary for laser radiation. If, however, a photon of appropriate energy strikes an atom while it is maintained in an excited state, the atom is immediately stimulated to emit its excess energy and make its transition to the ground state. This process is called *stimulated emission*. The emitted photon is an amplification of stimulat-

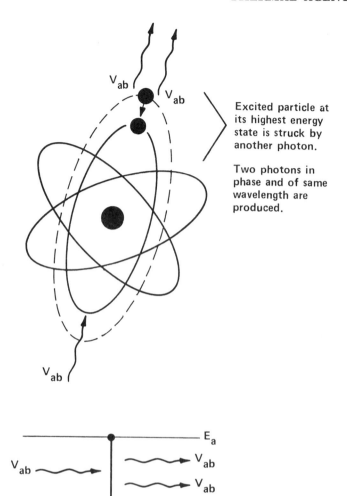

Excited particle at
its highest energy
state is struck by
another photon.

Two photons in
phase and of same
wavelength are
produced.

FIGURE 9–1. The principle of stimulated emission. Two photons are emitted from orbit when another photon strikes. E_a, E_b = electrons; V_{ab} = energy of photons.

ing radiation[9] (Fig. 9–1). Laser is a special form of electromagnetic energy that is within the visible or infrared regions of the electromagnetic spectrum (Fig. 9–2).

In a laser, when electrons are stimulated by an external power source at a rapid rate, resultant photons are aligned in a reflecting chamber. When they hit a semipermeable silver resonating mirror, photons are reflected back to a reflecting mirror. The back-and-forth reflection of photons between two mirrors through the laser medium further amplifies that light (Fig. 9–3). This process continues as more and more photons are stimulated, until the chamber cannot contain the energy level. Photons are then ejected through the semipermeable mirror and out a fiber-optic cable. The fiber optic is a threadlike filament composed of glass that guides the stimulated photons by directing them to the surface to be treated. As photons pass through the cylindric stylus, some of the excited atoms in the reflecting chamber begin to revert back to their ground state. This previously mentioned process of spontaneous emissions creates a lower intensity of emitted photons to the tissue. Another type of laser uses a diode in the applicator tip rather than a fiber optic.

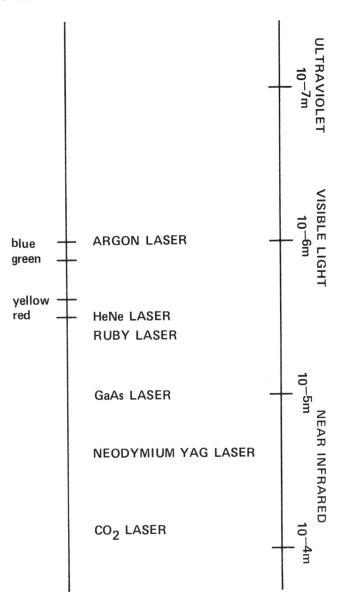

FIGURE 9–2. The visible light and infrared portions of the electromagnetic spectrum (EMS). Some different types of lasers are placed in their approximate location on the EMS.

Basic Components of Laser

There are three properties of the laser that distinguish it from incandescent and fluorescent light sources: coherence, monochromaticity, and a collimated beam.

The property of coherence denotes several things. All of the photons of light emitted from individual gas molecules are of the same wavelength. The individual light waves are locked in step with another. Having the same phase, waves are said to be temporally coherent. Also, they are all traveling in the same direction; this is called *spatial coherence* (Fig. 9–4).

When light is spatially coherent, it can be focused to a very small spot by a lens.

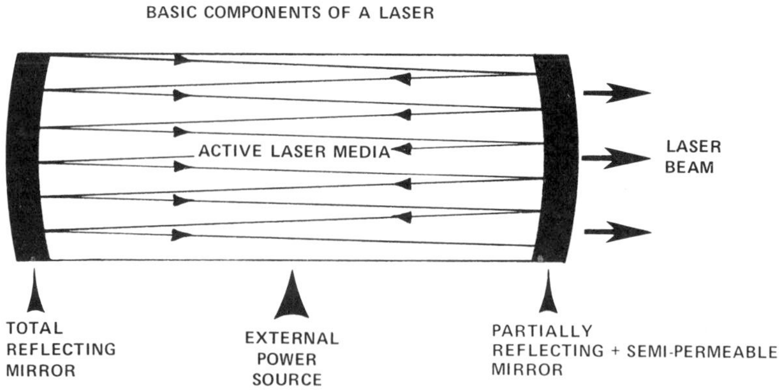

BASIC COMPONENTS OF A LASER
ACTIVE LASER MEDIA
LASER BEAM
TOTAL REFLECTING MIRROR
EXTERNAL POWER SOURCE
PARTIALLY REFLECTING + SEMI-PERMEABLE MIRROR

FIGURE 9–3. Basic components of laser.

Since light from a laser is similarly coherent, possible damage to the eyes can occur if that light is focused by the lens of the eye onto a small retinal spot.[11]

Monochromaticity refers to the specificity of light in a single, defined wavelength, which gives it added purity not found in most light sources. If this specificity is in the visible spectrum, it is of a single color. For example, HeNe produces a red light. A laser is one of the few light sources that produces a specific wavelength. The shorter the wavelength, the greater the purity of the light. HeNe has a 632.8-nm wavelength. Gallium arsenide (GaAs) has a wavelength of 910 nm.

The laser beam is well collimated. There is minimal divergence or moving apart of the photons.

Power is the rate at which energy is being produced and is measured in watts (joules/sec) or as a smaller unit, such as the milliwatt (mW) or 10^{-3} watts (W). If the laser produces one pulse per second, its average power, the amount of energy transferred in 1 second, would be 0.001 joule per 1 sec = 0.001 W or 1 mW. When the

λ
LASER
Spatial Coherence
LASER BEAM DIRECTION
Temporal Coherence

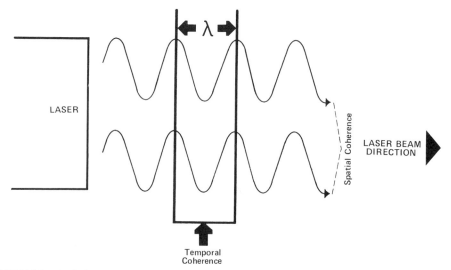

FIGURE 9–4. Coherence—Laser energy is highly coherent in temporal and spatial planes.

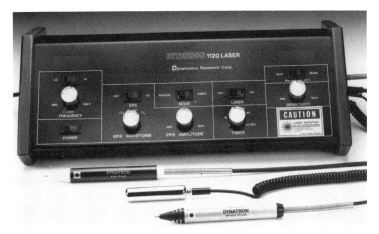

FIGURE 9–5. Dynatron 0.9 mw HeNe laser. (Courtesy of Dynatronics, Salt Lake City, UT.)

average power of a laser is below that which causes tissue heating, it is called a low-power or "cold" laser.[12] It also may be referred to as a low-energy or soft laser.

Dosage is equal to the total energy delivered. Therefore, it is equal to the average power multiplied by the time of treatment. When using an HeNe laser, such as the Dynatron 1120 (Fig. 9–5), in a chopped or pulsed mode, average power is approximately 0.45 mW.

Power density describes the concentration of power in a particular area. It is determined by power divided by area. A 1-mW laser source distributed over a 1-cm² area, therefore, has a power density of 1 milliwatt per square centimeter (1 mW/cm²).

When the laser is focused on the epidermis, the amount of energy absorbed is proportional to the absorption quality of the tissue. Human epidermis absorbs approximately 99 percent of the laser radiation.[12] Laser energy absorption is greater with darker or pigmented tissues. As tissues are not homogenous, the quality of each structure produces a varying absorption of laser energy. The physiologic variability of the effect on the tissue also depends upon wavelength, energy, and exposure time. This will be elaborated on throughout the chapter.

Classification of Laser

Laser can be classified as high-power or low-power (cold). At present, the most common image of laser radiation and its biologic effects is associated with damaging changes to cells and tissues through its thermal effects. This concept probably originated and was exaggerated by science fiction literature and movies. With the advent of the surgical laser, controlled heating and cutting have become more realistically associated with the device.

The different intensities of lasers are represented by different wavelengths. Tissue responses produced by a high-intensity laser are directly linked to intensity and include five effects: (1) elevation of tissue temperature; (2) dehydration of tissue; (3) coagulation of protein; (4) thermolysis; and, (5) evaporation.

The magnitude of thermal reactions produced by high-intensity lasers depends on: (1) the absorption, reflection, and transmission of the tissues at the laser wavelength; (2)

TABLE 9–1. Some Medical Uses of High-Intensity Laser

Laser	Spectrum	Most Frequent Use
CO_2	Invisible	Epithelial dysplasias
		Surgery: tumor destruction
Argon (skin)	Blue–green	Superficial vascular lesion such as removal of tattoos
Argon (eye)	Blue–green	Diabetic retinopathy
YAG	Invisible	Surgical incision

the power density of the laser beam; (3) the speed of incision or time of exposure; (4) the volume and the velocity of blood flow of local blood vessels; and (5) the degree of tension at the area of incision when cutting is used. Table 9–1 indicates some of the medical uses of high-intensity lasers.

Lasers with powers less than 60 mW (a low-power laser) will cause minimal to no thermal response. Total optic illumination in most cases is limited to less than 1 mW at a total peak power or to less than 0.5 mW in a pulsed mode. At this low milliwattage, the laser beam does not even warm the tissues.

Effects of low-power laser are direct effects of irradiation rather than secondary effects of tissue heating. Low-energy laser systems have been used experimentally and have been suggested clinically to stimulate wound and fracture healing and to obtain analgesic effects. The low-energy systems used include HeNe and GaAs.

HELIUM–NEON (HeNe) LASER

Helium–neon laser is produced by a tube containing atoms of these two gases (Fig. 9–5). The helium gas is elevated from the ground state to one of two excited states by electrical excitation. These states are a direct result of either stimulated or spontaneous emission. The atoms of the gas are in a vacuum chamber and are stimulated with a special light called a flash gun. The excited levels of the helium atom very closely approximate ground-state levels of the neon atom. When an excited approximate ground-state levels of the neon atom. When an excited helium atom collides with a ground-state neon atom, the energy produced is transferred to the latter, and the helium reverts to the ground state.

The wavelength of helium–neon laser is 632.8 nm (within the red band of visible light). It is directed toward the tissue in a pulsed or continuous mode by a fiber optic.[5] The helium–neon depth of penetration is up to 0.8 mm directly and from 10 to 15 mm indirectly. Direct penetration refers to the characteristic properties of laser that have not been altered. In indirect penetration, the light is transmitted into the deeper tissues through hyperscopic absorption properties of the surrounding tissue. Once this occurs, the coherent and collimated properties of laser are altered. Therefore, the difference between the two depths is due to the dispersion of light in tissue.

GALLIUM–ARSENIDE (GaAs) LASER

The first "semiconductor" laser, used in 1962, was the gallium–arsenide laser. This laser is housed in a diode (Fig. 9–6). A diode is an electrical component that allows electric current to pass in one direction through the device, offering high electrical resistance in the reverse direction. Using GaAs, upon which has been deposited a thin coating of zinc, a junction diode may be formed. This design allows the current to flow

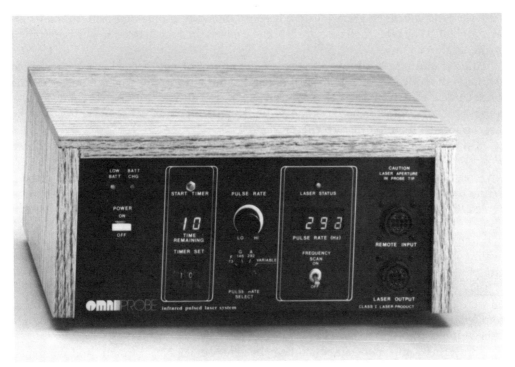

FIGURE 9–6. Omniprobe 0.9 mw GaAs infrared laser. (Courtesy of Physio Technology, Inc., Topeka, KS.)

more readily in the direction from the zinc to the GaAs. The laser reaction occurs in this junction region. The energy is delivered in the pulsed mode.

One further difference between the two low-powered lasers is that the indirect depth of tissue penetration of the GaAs output is 5 cm, compared with that of the HeNe laser, which is 10 to 15 mm. GaAs, at a wavelength of 910 nm, is within the infrared or invisible spectrum.

BIOPHYSICAL EFFECTS OF LASER

The investigation into the biologic and physical effects of cold laser radiation is still in its early stages. Some of the *preliminary proposed* physiologic effects attributed to low-power laser energy include an acceleration in collagen synthesis, an increase in vascularization of healing tissue, a decrease in micro-organisms, and pain reduction. Much of the work reported to date is empirical observation, which can serve as a foundation for the design of well-controlled laboratory and clinical studies on the bioeffects of laser irradiation.

Tissue Healing

In laboratory studies with animal models, exposure to low-power laser was reported to accelerate phagocytosis, facilitate collagen synthesis, and increase wound closure and contracture. Mester and colleagues[16] studied the effect of ruby laser on

Staphylococcus aureus, a gram-positive bacteria. Blood was obtained from human subjects and rats. The rate of phagocytosis of the bacteria was accelerated by the application of the laser.

Mester and Jaszsagi-Nagy[17] examined the effects of nonthermal laser on collagen synthesis in induced wounds in rats. Bilateral symmetric wounds were induced in the hindquarters of Wistar rats. One wound of each pair was irradiated. Analysis was completed 72 hours after surgery. The authors reported greater collagen synthesis in the laser-irradiated wounds than in the untreated site.

Cummings[18] studied the effect of HeNe laser irradiation on induced hindlimb wounds in rats. Rats were divided into three groups: daily laser treatment, every-other-day treatment, and sham laser. The rats that received laser achieved wound closure before those that received sham laser. The rats that received every-other-day treatment healed the most rapidly. The result of this study suggests that there might be an optimal dosage.

Kana and associates[19] examined the effect of HeNe and argon laser on wound healing in rats. An acceleration of wound healing was noted in the 4 per cm^2 per day groups, as compared to the higher-power laser group or controls.

Dyson and Young[20] studied the effects of varying frequencies of laser stimulation on wound contracture in mice. Treatment with 700-Hz laser increased the rate of wound contracture, total cell count, and the number of fibroblasts, as compared to 1200-Hz laser and a control group.

Braverman and associates[21] studied the effect of HeNe, infrared, and combined HeNe and infrared laser irradiation on wound healing in rabbits. All three experimental groups' wounds demonstrated greater tensile strength than the wounds of nonirradiated control rabbits.

Pain Modulation

Walker[22] investigated the effect of HeNe-laser irradiation on serum serotonin levels in patients with chronic pain. An increase in serotonin metabolism was noted in laser-treated patients. Serotonin has been implicated as an endorphin precursor.

Ponnudurai and coworkers[23,24] have studied the effect of low-power laser on pain threshold in rats in two studies. In the first, 1-mW HeNe laser was applied to the rats' tails at either 4, 60, or 200 Hz for 15 seconds. The 4-Hz frequency resulted inn a 50 percent increase in pain threshold, as measured by the rat-tail-flick test. In the second study, 1-mW HeNe laser applied at a frequency of 4 Hz to the base of the tail produced an increased pain tolerance to rat-tail-flick and hot-plate tests. Pretreatment with low-dose naloxone, an opiate antagonist (2 mg/kg), did not reverse the effects. High-dose naloxone (20 mg/kg) reversed the laser's analgesic effect, as measured by the hot-plate technique, but not by the tail-flick test.

Greathouse and colleagues[13] studied the effect of 1-mW GaAs laser on latency of superficial radial nerve in human subjects. No change in latency was noted when laser-treated subjects were compared with sham-irradiated controls. Conversely, Snyder-Mackler and coworkers,[25] using the identical protocol, found an increase in distal latency of the superficial radial nerve in HeNe-laser-irradiated subjects as compared to sham-irradiated controls. Differences may be attributable to the different wavelengths of the lasers studied.

INDICATIONS AND CLINICAL APPLICATION OF LASER

The purported indications for the therapeutic use of cold, or low-intensity, laser are typically separated into categories of tissue healing and pain management (acute or chronic). This section will discuss proposed clinical applications for laser.

Tissue Healing

Animal studies and anecdotal reports strongly suggest that low-power laser may accelerate healing rates of chronic open wounds and other soft-tissue injuries. Gogia and coworkers[26] reported positive results in two cases of patients who received HeNe laser and whirlpool to treat chronic open wounds. The wounds almost totally healed with this treatment.

Trelles and Mayayo[27] studied the effect of 2.4 joules of HeNe laser every other day for 24 days on experimentally-induced fractures in mice. Laser was applied through the skin. Histologic analysis revealed increased vascularization, more rapid formation of osseous tissue, and presence of a dense trabecular net in the treated animals as compared to controls.

Basically two different techniques for treating open wounds with laser have been reported in the literature: gridding the wound and surrounding the wound. To grid a wound, the clinician should imagine a grid or screen over the wound with 1 to 1½ cm² open squares. Irradiation of each square should take place for 20 seconds with the HeNe laser and 10 seconds with the use of the GaAs type (Seitz and Kleinkort, unpublished data). If indicated for cleansing and debridement, the whirlpool or saline cleansing should be introduced before laser application. One daily application of whirlpool is suggested. If there is eschar present, or if the wound is unusually large, the therapist may choose to surround the healthy tissue on the periphery of the wound. Stimulation is then applied every 2 cm² for 30 seconds using the HeNe laser and for 20 seconds using the GaAs. If the wound is closing from the outside, sterile saline or hydrogen peroxide can be poured into the wound. This fluid is then stimulated for 1 to 2 minutes with the laser. For wound healing, stimulation every other day at a frequency of 80 Hz, or continuously using the gridding or surrounding techniques is suggested by manufacturers of laser devices.

CASE STUDY

Case 1: Tissue Healing

The patient is a 55-year-old diabetic woman with a persistent, 10-cm diameter open wound over her right lateral malleolus. The wound has been treated with debridement and conventional wound management for 6 months. She has been referred for a trial of HeNe laser therapy.

Evaluation reveals a clean, dry wound with no evidence of re-epithelialization. No granulation tissue is apparent. The patient is anesthetic from the midcalf to the toes bilaterally. Her foot, calf, and anterior leg muscles are generally fair to fair+. She ambulates with a walker, partial weight bearing (PWB) on the right. Reflexes are absent at the knees and ankles bilaterally. There is no evidence of other skin breakdown.

The wound is covered with a transparent paper and is traced. Laser treatment will be delivered using a circumferential technique: 20 seconds of continuous HeNe laser per cm² of wound edge. Treatment will be given daily with weekly tracings being made to monitor closure. Other treatment will include debridement, as necessary, and cleaning and dressing the wound.

Pain Management

In acute pain management, the manufacturers' recommended application techniques employed in the studies cited below are straightforward. After the area of pain is localized, the laser is applied for 20 seconds with the GaAs laser or 30 seconds with the HeNe unit. The GaAs laser is usually set at a frequency of 73 Hz, and the HeNe is usually used in the continuous setting. The use of trigger points, or other such body points, in conjunction with the painful site can be included when treating the acute patient.

Laser use has been suggested to reduce pain in the acute and chronic states. Many different protocols are used, including direct stimulation over the site of dysfunction or stimulation of associated acupuncture, trigger, or motor points. Some of the more commonly treated dysfunctions will be discussed in this section.

In most circumstances, the patient should require no more than 8 to 12 treatments. If pain reduction has occurred after 4 or 5 sessions, the use of laser is discontinued. This is prudent clinical decision making, as with other physical agents.

BACK AND NECK DYSFUNCTION

There is some indication that neck and back pain may be affected by low-power laser. Snyder-Mackler and Bork[28] undertook a double-blind study to determine the effect of cold laser on musculoskeletal trigger points. They defined a trigger point as a site that elicits referred pain on deep palpation and demonstrates lowered skin resistance in comparison to surrounding tissue. Thirty patients with musculoskeletal pain were included in the study. Trigger points were treated for three successive treatments. Snyder-Mackler and Bork[28] noted that the patients who received the cold laser treatment demonstrated a significant increase in skin resistance when compared with the control. The difference was $p < 0.05$. They concluded that the results indicated that increases in skin resistance associated with the resolution of trigger points may be elicited by using cold laser therapy.

Snyder-Mackler and coworkers,[29] in a partial replication of the previous study, found identical results in a second group of patients. They also found that laser significantly decreased pain, as recorded on a visual analogue scale, when compared to placebo laser.

Kreczi and Klinger[30] used a randomized single-blind crossover design to study the effects of HeNe laser on patients with radiating back and neck pain. Mean pain levels, as measured by visual analogue scales, were significantly lower after laser treatment. In the crossover portion of the study, laser gave a better result than placebo in all variables measured.

Arthritis

Clinical results with laser application to inflammatory joint conditions suggest that laser may be beneficial to these conditions. Treatment of osteoarthritis and rheumatoid arthritis is most practical when only one or two joints require radiation. The only exceptions to this observation are in the hand, the foot, and the cervical, and lumbar areas. The treatment of a joint, as described in the articles below, is to approach it on all sides. The only time that circumferential exposure appears to be unproductive is when treating multiple joints in the foot or hand. In these cases, irradiation, both medially and laterally, are sufficient. The times remain the same as previously mentioned.

Goldman and associates[31] undertook a study using 30 people with classic or definite rheumatoid arthritis. They were classified by American Rheumatism Association criteria, 26 having classic, and 4 having definite, rheumatoid arthritis. There were 25 women and 5 men who ranged in age from 22 to 73 years. Twenty-one patients noted improvement of both their metacarpal phalangeal joints and proximal interphalangeal joints of both hands during laser therapy. Twenty-seven patients noted improvement of their proximal interphalangeal joints, and 26 noted improvement of their metacarpal phalangeal joints during therapy. The improvement was in both hand function and hand activity. The changes usually were bilateral, although more improvement in grip strength and tip pinch, and less erythema and pain, were noted on the side treated with laser perhaps explained in part by a placebo effect. Activity levels related to duration of morning sickness and motion restricted by joint heat, erythema, tenderness, pain, and swelling.

Bliddal and colleagues[32] reported the effect of low-power laser on 17 patients with rheumatoid arthritis. One hand was irradiated with HeNe laser at 6 j/cm^2. The contralateral hand was treated with sham laser. When the hands were compared, there was a slight decrease in pain in the laser-irradiated hand, but there was no change in joint motion and morning stiffness.

Snyder-Mackler and colleagues, in work in preparation, examined the effect of HeNe-laser irradiation on grip strength, range of motion, pain, stiffness, and activity level in a double-blind study of 152 patients with rheumatoid arthritis. The proximal interphalangeal (PIP) and metacarpophalangeal (MCP) joints of the patients' dominant hands were irradiated with HeNe laser or placebo. A significant increase in grip strength and decrease in pain variables was noted in the laser-treated patients.

Basford and coworkers[33] studied the effects of HeNe laser on range of motion, pain, joint tenderness, grip and pinch strength, activity level, and medication use in a blinded study of 81 patients with osteoarthritis of the thumb. The laser-treated group had a tendency for less tenderness of the treated MCP and interphalangeal (IP) joints, and an increase in three-finger-chuck-pinch strength in the treated hand as compared to the control hand. There was no statistical difference, however, between the groups in any of the variables tested.

Soft Tissue

The effects of low-power laser on soft tissue are equivocal. Investigators have used various strategies for assessing this effect. Lundeberg and associates[34] studied the effects of HeNe-laser irradiation to upper extremity acupuncture site on pain from lateral epicondylitis. No significant effect on pain was noted. Snyder-Mackler and colleagues, in work in preparation, studied the effects of HeNe laser irradiation on tennis elbow in an ABAB single-case design (Chapter 10) in a subject with chronic lateral epicondylitis.

No effect on pain and grip strength was noted, although significantly less medication was used during the treatment periods.

Siebert and coworkers[35] studied the effects of HeNe and GaAs laser on tendinitis. Patients were randomly assigned to a treatment or a placebo group (total = 64) and were treated for 10 consecutive days with low-power laser. Although all patients had a significant reduction in pain and symptomatology during the course of the study, no difference was found between the two groups.

CASE STUDY

Case 2: Pain

The patient is a 41-year-old woman with left lateral epicondylitis of 4 months' duration. She reports no history of specific trauma to the area.

Examination reveals a 9 cm² area of tenderness just distal to the left lateral epicondyle. There is some edema noted. She has pain with resisted isometric wrist extension and passive wrist flexion. There is a positive tennis-elbow test. Elbow and wrist range of motion and strength are within normal limits. There are no sensory changes. Her symptoms are consistent with pain and inflammation of the left-wrist extensor mass.

Plans for this patient, in addition to counterforce bracing and rest, include the use of low-power laser. HeNe laser will be delivered for 20 seconds to each cm² of painful area 3 times per week. Efficacy will be documented using a graphic rating scale and a log of medication usage.

DOCUMENTATION OF TREATMENT WITH LASER

Dosage is preferably described in joules/cm². Laser power is given in watts, and the irradiating surface area is also usually provided. Joules can be determined by multiplying the number of watts by the treatment time in seconds. The rehabilitation professional should document the exact location treated, the total treatment time, the mode used (continuous or pulsed frequency), and the type of laser.

PRECAUTIONS AND CONTRAINDICATIONS FOR LASER

Research and safety criteria are necessary for any new therapeutic agent. Investigations on the safety and effectiveness of laser continue in Europe, Russia, and the United States.

Lasers less than 1 mW are classified by the Food and Drug Administration (FDA) as a class III medical device. The low-power laser, at the time of this writing, is still considered an investigational device, and the user should have an investigational-device exemption (IDE) under the abbreviated requirements of section 812.2(b)a of the FDA regulations before therapeutic intervention with laser. The FDA is concerned not only with safety, but also with therapeutic efficacy. The FDA's Center for Devices and Radiological Health now regulates the manufacture and safe of laser products in the

United States (US Department of Health, Education and Welfare, 1979). This regulation requires the manufacturer to classify the laser product.

Several other organizations have followed suit with safety standards that are comparable. The basic concepts of the classification schemes of the American National Safety Institute (ANSI), the American Conference of Governmental Industrial Hygienists (ACGIH), the World Health Organization (WHO), the International Electrotechnical Commissions (IEC), and the FDA are as follows:

Class I laser products are essentially safe and are typically enclosed systems that do not emit hazardous levels.

Class II laser products are limited to visible lasers that are safe for momentary viewing but should not be stared into continuously unless the exposure limits (ELs) and the dazzle of the brilliant visible light source would normally preclude staring into the course.[36]

Low-power lasers are class II or I laser devices. They are considered an insignificant risk to humans unless held close to the cornea of the eye.

The safety of these devices can further be evaluated by ANSI Standard 2-136.0. A review of the maximal permissible emission value of the lasers less than 1 mW shows a good margin of safety.[26]

The most prominent safety standard for laser was first produced in 1973 and has since been revised: ANSI Standard 2976, *Safe Use of Lasers*. A new edition of the ANSI standard was approved in 1980.

There are some contraindications for use of laser to which the clinician should adhere: Refrain from using laser in the pregnant woman; laser should not be used over the unclosed fontanels of children; the use of laser near cancerous lesions should be avoided; and laser should not be radiated directly into the cornea.

Ophthalmologic research has shown that, in rabbits, laser levels of 25 mW may produce retinal lesions in the continuous-wave HeNe laser mode. These lesions were obtained after 2.5 seconds, with a rise of temperature at the lesion site of 7.8°C. No lesions were present, however, with the use of 2- or 5-mW lasers.[37]

Lappin[38] has measured ocular damage threshold for the HeNe laser in the rhesus monkey. Exposure time of radiation was 2 msec to 10 seconds, with peak power of 50 mW. Mean values of the visible-damage threshold for power versus time were determined for each eye in the macula and in the extramacula. Approximately 500 exposures were made to determine mean-damage-threshold levels in 70 eyes for the macular, and an extramacula area between the optic disc and the macula. The macula was found to have a lower damage threshold than the extramacular area, the ratio of thresholds decreasing as exposure time increased. The macular–extramacular threshold ratio varied from about 2:1 at 5 msec to 1.3:1 at 1 second.

Ham and associates[39] studied the retinal-burn thresholds for the HeNe laser in the rhesus monkey. They concluded that the threshold power for irreversible burn damage in the monkey is about 7 mW at the cornea for the worst case of accidental exposure to HeNe lasers. For this exposure, the whole beam entered the eye and was focused on a minimal spot size. Available data indicate that the human retina is less susceptible to thermal damage than that of the monkey or the rabbit. Until more reliable data are available, the total power of the HeNe laser entering the human eye should be limited to 1 mW or less. This recommendation is based solely upon the chance of irreversible thermal damage to the retina.

ULTRAVIOLET

Ultraviolet (UV) light has been used in physical therapy for decades. Although its uses have varied over the years, it has been used primarily in the treatment of dermatologic problems, most notably psoriasis. Although UV has largely been dropped from the treatment regimens of many physical therapy clinics, it is still used in some clinics. The objectives of this section are: (1) To present the types of UV lamps in use; (2) to describe how dosimetry is determined; (3) to present adverse effects; and, (4) to describe common pathologies for which UV light is used.

UV, as used therapeutically, is not technically a thermal agent. Treatment times are too short for substantial thermal effects to occur. Therapeutic UV lamps in issue in the United States are broad spectrum UVB (250–320 nm) and UVA (320–400 nm). Recently, narrow-band UVB (311–312 nm) has been used). UV can be delivered by a single-bulb lamp (fog) or, most commonly, in a multibulb cabinet. Newer equipment often has both UVA and UVB capabilities in the same cabinet. The purpose of therapeutic UV is usually to cause an erythemal response. This response usually occurs within 2 to 4 hours after treatment and usually peaks within 12 hours. Other effects that can accompany the erythema (but have longer latencies) are production of vitamin D, changes in skin pigmentation, and exfoliation of skin.

Physical Principles of Ultraviolet

There are two laws of optic physics that are relevant to the UV application — the inverse square law and the law of cosines. The inverse square law ($E = I/D^2$, where E is the illumination intensity, I is the lamp intensity, and D is the distance from the source) states that the intensity of illumination varies with the square of the distance between the source and the treatment surface. This means that cutting the distance between the lamp and the patient by 50 percent will increase the dosage by 400 percent. The law of cosines states that the energy of illumination varies proportionally to the cosine of the degrees of deviation from the perpendicular. This means that as the area being irradiated becomes more oblique, the dose decreases.

Dosimetry for Ultraviolet

Erythemal doses are graded sub, minimal-, first-, second; and third-degree erythema doses. The unit used to describe the dose is a unit of time (usually seconds to minutes). These doses are dependent upon age, skin color, and many other individual factors and, thus, cannot be generalized from patient to patient. This necessitates testing each patient before treatment. Testing is usually performed on the anterior aspect of the forearm, but probably should be performed in the area that is to be treated. A piece of UV-opaque material is windowed, as shown in Figure 9–7. Each of the four windows are cut to 1 to 2 cm^2 in area. The entire area in the UV field is draped except for the small testing area. The lamp is warmed up and placed so that the light is perpendicular to the test area. Traditionally, distances of 60 to 80 cm have been used for standard UVB dose testing. Times given here are for this distance. (Note that lamps may differ and manufacturers' recommendations for testing should be followed.) The first window is uncovered for 120 seconds, then the second is uncovered and both are irradiated for 60 seconds, the third is added for 30 seconds, and the final aperture is uncovered, and all

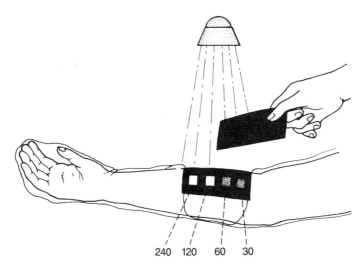

240   120   60   30

FIGURE 9–7. Determination of M.E.D. using a four-windowed shield. (Adapted from Stillwell, GK: Therapeutic Electricity and Ultraviolet Radiation, ed 3. Williams and Wilkins, Baltimore, MD, 1983.)

four are exposed for an additional 30 seconds. Thus, the total exposure for the four windows is 240, 120, 60, and 30 seconds, respectively. Dosimetry cannot be immediately determined because of the latency period. Ideally, the skin should be examined 8 hours after exposure to inspect for the area where mild reddening of the skin has occurred. If the patient cannot be seen by medical personnel, self-reporting is acceptable with the reliable patient.

A suberythemal dose is a treatment time insufficient for perceptible reddening of the skin to occur. A minimal erythemal dose (MED) is the time required for mild reddening of the skin, which appears within 8 hours of treatment and disappears within 24 hours. Pigmentation changes occur only with repeated exposure, and exfoliation rarely, if ever, occurs at MED. First-degree erythema also appears after approximately 6 hours. This erythema is more pronounced, is similar to a mild sunburn, and lasts for several days. There may be associated discomfort, which is proportional to the surface area irradiated. This level of treatment may eventually be followed by slight exfoliation. A second-degree erythema occurs after a latency period of 2 hours or less and resembles a severe sunburn. The skin is angrily red, hot, tender, and may be accompanied by edema. This dose is always accompanied by significant exfoliation and prolonged pigmentation changes. A third-degree erythema is a second-degree burn where blistering occurs. Once the MED has been determined, all other doses may be calculated using the conversion formula in Table 9–2.

Amount of exposure to maintain a specific erythemal dose increases over time,

TABLE 9–2. Ultraviolet: Conversion of Known Dose to Desired Dose

Erythema degree	MED	1st	2nd	3rd
Factor	1	2.5	5	10
Equation				

$$\text{Desired dose} = \frac{\text{Known dose (sec)}}{\text{Factor (dose desired)}} \times \text{Factor (known dose)}$$

much as tolerance to sunlight increases. It is necessary, therefore, to increase the time or to decrease the distance from the source in order to maintain therapeutic efficacy. The time required to maintain each level of erythema varies. MED usually is increased by 35 percent per treatment per day. First-degree requires an increase of 50 percent; second and third degree increases are from 75 percent to 100 percent per treatment. This progression is usually continued until exposure time reaches 5 minutes, at which time the distance is decreased to decrease the treatment time. The inverse square law is used to estimate an appropriate treatment time at the new distance. The equation for conversions is: $T = T_1 \times D^2)/D_1^2$, where T is the new time, D is the new distance, T_1 is the old time and D_1 is the old distance.

Therapeutic Applications of Ultraviolet

PSORIASIS

UV usually is used in one of two ways to treat this proliferative dermatosis: the Goeckerman regimen or psoralens UVA (PUVA). The Goeckerman regimen, developed at the Mayo Clinic, involves the use of a petroleum-based coal-tar mixture, which is used as a photosensitizing agent, followed by exposure to UVB. PUVA involves taking of oral psoralens (photosensitizing agents) plus UVA. Although both of these treatments are effective for control of psoriasis, PUVA has been shown to be considerably more effective. Unfortunately, PUVA therapy also results in an increased incidence of skin cancer.

Dosimetry

Dose is usually begun at the first-degree erythemal level. For the Goeckerman regimen, coal tar is applied and removed and an MED test is performed, as previously described. Treatment is delivered once or twice per day until the plaques clear. UVA has a longer latency until appearance of erythema. PUVA therapy usually results in a longer lasting erythema that is more intense than with the Goeckerman regimen. Therefore, initial dosage is usually determined by the referring dermatologist, who takes into consideration the patient's skin type and medication level. Ideally, the erythema should peak 48 hours after treatment as a first-degree dose. Because of the long latency of response, PUVA therapy is given at most every other day.

CYSTIC ACNE

Ultraviolet is now used rarely for this disorder, because improved pharmacologic means are available for controlling cystic acne. The goal of UV treatment with this patient population was to dry out the skin and promote skin exfoliation.

Dosimetry

Dosage at the second-degree erythemal level was used, as significant exfoliation of skin was the desired response. Dosimetry was determined by the method described above.

Adverse Effects and Treatment Precautions for Ultraviolet

Adverse effects of treatment include burns and redness of the skin acutely and premature aging and skin cancer chronically. Careful application of this physical agent should not result in burns. The patient should be informed of all risks and benefits of this type of therapy. Unfortunately, psoriasis often can not be adequately controlled by pharmacologic therapy alone. In spite of its attendant risks, therefore, UV therapy is sometimes required.

The therapist and patient must take precautions during treatment. Polarized goggles should be worn at all times. Exposure times should be carefully monitored. Erythemal responses should be graded carefully. Treatment times should be carefully increased from visit to visit, so as to maintain therapeutic levels of treatment without causing burns. Areas of skin that are rarely exposed to light (breasts and genitalia) should be exposed to only ⅓ to ½ the dose for the rest of the body.

Caution must be taken when the patient is taking medications, that is, certain antibiotics or diuretics that photosensitize.

Documentation of Treatment with Ultraviolet

Exposure in seconds, distance of the light source from the patient, and angle of incidence all figure into dosage and should be reported. Draping procedures should be documented for each treatment. The specific lamp used for treatment should be noted by its serial number. MED may vary from lamp to lamp due to varying outputs.

SUMMARY

The use of light in physical therapy has a long history. This chapter has described current practice using one of the older agents, ultraviolet, and one of the more recent, low-power laser. There is evidence that both agents can be used to effectively treat a number of conditions. Caution should be used in their application, and careful attention to details of indications for use, application time, and location should improve efficacy. The work supporting the efficacy of low-power laser in rehabilitation is preliminary and its use in the United States is restricted. The need for further well-controlled studies to support or refute its efficacy is apparent and required before it may be used to treat patients.

REFERENCES

1. Kleinkort, JA and Foley, RA: Laser acupuncture: Its use in physical therapy. American Journal of Acupuncture 12:51, 1984.
2. Watkins, AL: A Manual of Electrotheray. Lea & Febiger, Philadelphia, 1968, pp 12–15, 24–26, 197–199.
3. Bloom, AL: Gas Lasers. John Wiley & Sons, New York, 1971, pp 1–24.
4. Calder, N: Einstein's Universe. Greenwich House, New York, 1982, pp 29–30.
5. Goldman, L: Biomedical Aspects of the Laser. Springer-Verlag, New York, 1967, pp 1–7.
6. Lengyell, BA: Lasers-Generation of Lightly Stimulated Emission. John Wiley & Sons, New York, 1962, pp 1–15, 22–23, 83–99.
7. Kroetlinger, M: On the use of laser in acupuncture. International Journal of Acupuncture and Electrotherapy Research 5:297, 1980.
8. Kovacs, L: Experimental investigation of photostimulation effect of low energy HeNe laser radiation. In Laser in Basic Biomedical Research, IV. Plenum, New York, 1977.
9. Litwin, MS and Glew, DH: The biological effects of laser radiation. JAMA 187:842, 1964.
10. Caspers, K: Laser stimulation therapy. Physikalishe Medizin and Rehabilitation 18:426, 1977.
11. Dynatronics: Dynatron 1120 Operators Manual. Dynatronics, Salt Lake City, UT, 1983.
12. Basford, JR: Low-energy laser therapy: Controversies and new research findings. Lasers in Surgery and Medicine, 9;101, 1989.
13. Greathouse, DG, Currier, DP, and Gilmore, RL: Effects of clinical infrared laser on superficial radial nerve conduction. Phys Ther 65:1184, 1985.

14. Lehmann, JF and DeLateur, B: Therapeutic heat. In Lehmann, JF and Basmajian, JV (eds): Therapeutic Heat and Cold, ed 3. Baltimore, Williams & Wilkins, 1982, pp 404–562.
15. Fork, RL: Laser stimulation of nerve cells in aplysia. Science 171:907, 1971.
16. Mester, E, Mester, AF, and Mester, A: The biomedical effects of laser application. Lasers Surg Med 5:31, 1985.
17. Mester, E and Jaszsagi-Nagy, E: The effects of laser radiation on wound healing and collagen synthesis. Studia Biophysica 35(3):227, 1973.
18. Cummings, JP: The effect of low energy (He-Ne) laser irradiation on healing dermal wounds in an animal model. Phys Ther 65:737, 1985.
19. Kana, JS, et al: Effect of low-power density laser radiation on healing of open skin wounds in rats. Arch Surg 116:293, 1981.
20. Dyson, M and Young, S: Effects of laser therapy on wound contraction and cellularity in mice. Lasers Surg Med 1:125, 1986.
21. Braverman, B, et al: Effect of helium-neon and infrared laser irradiation on wound healing in rabbits. Lasers Surg Med 9:50, 1989.
22. Walker, J: Relief from chronic pain by low power laser irradiation. Neurosci Lett 43:339, 1983.
23. Ponnudurai, RN, et al: Laser photobiostimulation-induced hypoalgesia in rats is not naloxone reversible. Acupunct Electrother Res 13:109, 1988.
24. Ponnadurai, RN, Zbuzek, VK, and Wu, W-H: Hypoalgesic effect of laser photobiostimulation by rat tail flick test. Acupunct Electrother Res 12:93, 1987.
25. Snyder-Mackler, L and Bork, CE: Effect of helium-neon laser irradiation on peripheral sensory nerve latency. Phys Ther 68:223, 1989.
26. Gogia, PP, Hurt, BS, and Zirn, TT: Wound management with whirlpool and infrared cold laser treatment: A clinical report. Phys Ther 68(8):1239, 1988.
27. Trelles, MA and Mayayo, E: Bone fracture consolidates faster with low-power laser. Lasers Surg Med 7:36, 1987.
28. Snyder-Mackler, L, et al: Effect of helium-neon laser on musculoskeletal trigger points. Phys Ther 66(7):1087, 1986.
29. Snyder-Mackler, L, et al: Effects of helium-neon laser irradiation on skin resistance and pain in patients with trigger points in the neck or back. Phys Ther 69:336, 1989.
30. Kreczi, T and Klinger, D: A comparison of laser acupuncture versus placebo in radicular and pseudoradicular pain syndromes as recorded by subjective responses of patients. Acupunct Electrother Res: 11:207, 1986.
31. Goldman, JA, et al: Laser therapy of rheumatoid arthritis. Lasers Surg Med 1:1, 1980.
32. Bliddal H, et al: Soft-laser therapy of rheumatoid arthritis. Scand J Rheumatol 16:225, 1987.
33. Basford, JR, et al: Low-energy helium neon laser treatment of thumb osteoarthritis. Arch Phys Med Rehabil 68:794, 1987.
34. Lundeberg, T, Haker, E, and Thomas, M: Effects of laser versus placebo in tennis elbow. Scand J Rehabil Med 19:135, 1987.
35. Siebert, W, et al: What is the efficacy of "soft" and "mid" lasers in therapy of tendinopathies? A double-blind study. Arch Orthop Trauma Surg 106:358, 1987.
36. Goldman, L: Basic reactions in tissue. In Goldman, L (ed): The Biomedical Laser: Technology and Clinical Applications. Springer-Verlag, New York 1981, pp 6–9.
37. Kohtiao, A, et al: Temperature rise and photocoagulation of rabbit retinas exposed the CW laser. Am J Ophthalmol 62:3, 1966.
38. Lappin, PW: Ocular damage thresholds for the helium-neon laser. Arch Environ Health 20:2, 1970.
39. Ham, WT, et al: Retinal burn threshold for the helium-neon laser in the rhesus monkey. Arch Ophthalmol 84:6, 1970.

SELECTED READINGS (UV)

1. Beckett, RH: Modern Actinotherapy. London, 1955.
2. Goeckerman, WH: The treatment of psoriasis. Northwest Med 24:229, 1925.
3. Sams, WM: Phototherapy of psoriasis. In TB Fitzpatrick (ed). Sunlight and Man. Tokyo University Press, Tokyo, 1974, pp 793–796.
4. Stillwell, GK: Therapeutic Electricity and Ultraviolet Radiation (ed). Williams & Wilkins, Baltimore, 1983.
5. Stern, RS, et al: Photochemistry for psoriasis. NE to Med 300:809, 1979.
6. Sunlamp products: Performance standards, Federal/Register 44:65352-65358, 1979.

SECTION III

Clinical Decision Making

CHAPTER 10

Clinical Evaluation of Thermal Agents

Mary P. Watkins, M.S.,P.T.

Evaluation of the effectiveness and efficiency of therapeutic intervention is an essential function of every health-care professional. Participation of each individual in this process can vary from critical reading of the medical and scientific literature to conducting sophisticated research projects. In order to participate at all, health-care professionals must have an understanding of the existing problems and questions about current practice and have the ability to incorporate into practice those therapeutic advances that have been demonstrated to be effective by sound critical analysis. Acquisition of such understanding and ability depends upon a working knowledge of the aims, uses, and limitations of clinical investigation.

This book presents a comprehensive review of the physical and physiologic mechanisms that serve as the basis for the characteristics of energy delivered and the potential applications of thermal agents. From the physical sciences, for example, we have gained knowledge of heat-transfer mechanisms. From the biologic sciences, we have gained information about the responses of cells, tissues, and organs to thermal agents. In vitro laboratory studies include the influence of temperature changes on the viscoelastic properties of collagen and changes in ion fluxes across cell membranes when temperature is altered. In vivo animal studies have examined such changes as blood flow, muscle-spindle activity, synaptic transmission, and induction and resolution of inflammation and edema. These kinds of information are useful for establishing a rationale for employing thermal agents in the treatment of patients. Throughout this book, current instrumentation and techniques are also described, which demonstrate clinical application of heat, cold, laser, ultraviolet, and PEMF. In many instances, however, the therapeutic effects of these modalities are based on anecdotal reports or on empiric evidence of success in ameliorating patient problems.

Further clinical research is needed to accomplish our professional goal of providing high-quality patient care in an economically sound manner. Although findings based on normal subjects may help in understanding physiologic responses to therapeutic applications, they do not answer the important questions regarding clinical efficacy. Formal clinical studies that document the effects of treatment procedures applied to real clinical problems will help clinicians to: (1) Determine the appropriateness of current techniques; (2) develop new methods tested by scientific inquiry; and, (3) discard methods that do not stand up to such scrutiny.

The purpose of this chapter is to examine selected elements of the research process applicable to the clinical evaluation of thermal agents and other physical agents such as laser. General principles, samples of methodology, and instrumentation are presented to highlight the uses and limitations of the clinical-research process. Examples of research questions concerning the application of thermal agents will be used.

GENERAL PRINCIPLES OF CLINICAL RESEARCH

Planning and Preparation

The basic process of conceiving, planning, and preparing to conduct research can be described in several well-defined steps. These preliminary steps are:

1. Definition of the research question.
2. Collection of the relevant information.
3. Statement of the hypothesis or the specific aims of the research activity.
4. Selection and development of the method of study.
5. Preparation of the written research proposal.

This process applies to all types of research design and involves careful planning, including the recognition of problems that potentially can invalidate the outcome of a study. Several general guidelines can be defined to ensure well-planned and well-executed clinical research projects.[1,2]

The Research Question

The research question or problem must be specific and delimited, identifying the research variables precisely. The first potential failure in the research process is posing a question that is diffuse or broad, containing confounding elements that make it impossible to derive a useful answer. For example, "What is the effect of cold on edema?" The two key elements of this research question can be identified as: (1) the independent variable, cold, which the investigator will control, manipulate, or apply; and (2) the dependent variable, edema, which will be observed or measured to determine the effect of applying the modality. The question, however, is unmanageable. Many confounding elements, or extraneous variables, have not been taken into account. What kind of cold is being questioned? How often will it be applied? In what setting? On what kind of patient? What specific outcome is relevant—range of motion, limb circumference, limb volume, or functional abilities? These kinds of questions must be addressed and resolved during the process of defining the research question.

Collection of the Relevant Information

Background information must be carefully accumulated and analyzed. Clinical observation and experience are valuable sources of background information; indeed, the question at hand is often derived from some clinical event. Although clinically derived knowledge is important, it is never thorough enough to substitute for a critical review of the current medical and scientific literature.

As the investigator defines the problem to be studied and formulates the specific elements of the research project, several pertinent pieces of information should be incorporated, or at least considered. The approach to the literature review begins with preparing a list of topics, including details about the independent variable, the dependent variable(s), and the pathologic condition or patient population to be studied. This list will be transposed into appropriate "key words," which will then be used by the investigator to retrieve reference citations from the bibliographic indexes in medical or university libraries.[2]

Regarding the illustrative question of cold and edema, the literature search would include both laboratory and clinical studies. From animal studies, the investigator will learn the mechanisms of edema formation and, as discussed in Chapter 4, that the intensity and duration of cold application may influence the tissue response, possibly adversely. This knowledge should lead to careful consideration of the method of cold application to be used. From clinical studies, there is evidence that the application of cold may control swelling. In at least one study, however, compression wraps were also part of the treatment. This problem suggests a more definitive series of questions than did the first, vaguely stated question. In general, the investigator needs to know if his or her question has been studied, how it has been studied, what has not been studied, and what constitutes the scientific rationale for the proposed study. This information is necessary to solidify the importance of the current problem and to develop an appropriate approach to the research question.

At this point, the investigator should be able to pose an important, clinically relevant, sensible research question. Taking the initially stated global question, for example, a more refined question may be asked: "Is cold, or cold plus intermittent compression, more effective in reducing edema following ankle sprains in college athletes?" Then the question can be transposed into a working or research hypothesis.

Hypothesis or Specific Aims

Most research questions can and should be transposed into hypotheses. Certainly, if the study compares two treatment methods, a prediction of the outcome can be made based on the available background information. The hypothesis must be stated to clearly identify the independent and dependent variables and proposes a relationship between the two. This statement can be made in two ways: nondirectional or directional.

A statement of difference declares that the application of the independent variable will result in a change in the dependent variable. If the investigator predicts a change, but not the direction of that change, the statement is referred to as a *nondirectional hypothesis*. For example, "There will be a difference in the amount of residual ankle edema when sprains are treated with cold alone, compared with cold plus intermittent compression." A *directional hypothesis* predicts not only a difference but also the direction of that difference: "The application of cold plus intermittent compression will be more effective in reducing edema following ankle sprains than the application of cold alone."

Occasionally, a research hypothesis may be that "treatment 'X' will be as effective as treatment 'Y'." This statement should not be confused with the *null hypothesis*. The null hypothesis is a statistical statement of "no difference" that is used in the application of statistical procedures to determine significance of the research data.

In studies of a descriptive or correlational nature, when the purpose is to describe a particular phenomenon, a predictive hypothesis may not be appropriate. In this case, a clear statement of the specific aims of the study should be made.

Method

In order to answer the question or test the hypothesis, a method of study must be carefully selected and specifically described. The purpose of this major task is to make certain that: (1) All extraneous variables (factors other than the independent variable that could affect the outcome) are controlled for or eliminated; and, (2) the kind and use of the measurement tools are appropriate.

An explicit written description of the method must be prepared and must include the following details (1) the specific conditions of the study must be stated, such as the age, sex, and health status of subjects and the setting in which the study is to be conducted; (2) the testing instruments and their application are specifically defined to answer: what test, when used, how used, and by whom?; (3) the procedure for applying the independent variable is defined in order to outline, using our example, such details as: What type of cold?, How frequently administered?, How will the subject be positioned?, and What kind of supervision or monitoring?; and, (4) statistical procedures or other techniques that will be used to analyze the data are outlined. Through this protocol, operational definitions will be stated: The meaning of cold and the meaning of edema should become clear.

At this point in preparing to conduct a research study, the investigator must analyze the proposed method to ensure that the design is correct and meets certain criteria. This process may require consultation with other investigators and clinicians, as well as a pretrial pilot study. Three important criteria should be met: reliability, validity, and objectivity.[3]

Reliability is synonymous with dependability, stability, consistency, predictability, and accuracy. If the same set of objects are measured again and again with the same or comparable instruments under the same conditions, will the results be the same? There are statistical techniques to estimate the degree of reliability of a testing situation.[4,5] (These techniques, in many cases, simply serve to confirm the investigator's good common sense.)

Validity refers to the soundness, logic, and appropriateness of the study design.[6] The *internal validity* of a study depends upon the extent to which the method controls extraneous factors that interfere with the true relationship between the stated independent and dependent variables. Is the investigator measuring what he or she thinks is being measured? What factors, in addition to the application of cold alone or cold and compression, are important: weight bearing, elevation of the limb, anti-inflammatory medication? *External validity* refers to the extent to which the results can be generalized to other subjects, settings, or conditions. How representative are the findings to the "outside" world? Will cold-gel packs have the same effect as the application of chipped ice? Will the response of an athlete, anxious to return to competition, be the same as the response of a sedentary executive?

Objectivity means the extent to which the testing situation and the measurement tools control for the biggest kind of extraneous variable: the biases, subjective impressions, and feelings of the investigators and subjects.

The Research Proposal

At this point, the investigator prepares a written research proposal. This document reflects all of the preceding steps: identification of the research question, definition of the need and importance of the proposed study, relevant background from the literature review, and description of the specific protocol (method) to be followed. It, along with a written informed-consent form, will be reviewed by an appropriate institutional review board, which must approve the project.[1,7] The written protocol becomes the guide that must be strictly followed during every phase of the study.

Dissemination of Results

When data collection is complete and the results are analyzed according to plan, the investigator has one more responsibility — to share results with professional colleagues. The results of clinical studies may also be useful to the engineers and manufacturers responsible for the design, construction, and safety of therapeutic devices.

The information in the final report must be accurate and detailed enough so that the reader or listener can identify the question asked, assess the appropriateness of the method, replicate the study, and evaluate the strength and veracity of the conclusions.

The primary goal of any research is to improve or increase the body of knowledge in the relevant clinical or scientific arena. This can best be done by gathering and disseminating sound, reliable, accurate information.

TYPES OF CLINICAL RESEARCH

Some types of research are more rigorous than others, but all carefully planned and executed projects that follow the principles previously outlined will make a contribution to the existing body of knowledge. An understanding of the purposes and limitations of various research approaches will permit appropriate interpretation and analysis of information in the proper perspective. The research designs discussed here are those that seem most applicable to the clinical evaluation of thermal agents. Real and hypothetic examples will be cited.

The Single-Case Study

Many will argue that the report of a single case does not fulfill the criteria for research. On the other hand, the description of a single case can provide useful information, particularly if questions exist about the applicability of a known method of treatment in an unusual circumstance, or to elucidate a new approach to an old clinical problem. An innovative case report may be a stimulus for the author and others to investigate a topic in greater depth.

A report by Wing[8] illustrates that a well-planned, well-documented single case will contain several elements of the research process. The question asked was, "What is the effect of phonophoretically driven hydrocortisone on the range of motion (ROM) of the temporomandibular joint (TMJ) and pain level in a patient with TMJ dysfunction?" Supportive rationale was provided in the introductory paragraph. The methods for assessment of ROM and pain were presented and were conducted before and after treatment. The specific treatment protocol was described. The conclusion was stated clearly and appropriately: Phonophoresis with hydrocortisone "was influential in reducing pain and increasing ROM in this case." This statement, as written, acknowledges the most distinct disadvantage of the single-case study, which is the inability to generalize the result to a broader population. There is an inherent lack of control over extraneous variables, such as the effect of the passage of time, the patient's attitude toward treatment or, in this case, his desire to eat more heartily.

Single-Group Study

The same problems of lack of control and inability to generalize results exist in the single-group pretest, post-test design, whereby a number of subjects are tested before and after the application of a specific treatment regimen. Quillen and Rouillier[9] presented such a single-group study. The purpose of their project was to evaluate the effect of rapid pulsed-pneumatic compression, in conjunction with cold, on acute grade I sprains. Their conclusion, based primarily on edema reduction as measured by volumetric displacement, was that this form of compression was effective. A comparison of the pretreatment and post-treatment volumetric measurements was presented to support their conclusion. There can be more confidence in the effectiveness of treatment when the same or similar results are obtained in a group of individuals, in contrast to the single case.

The important questions, however, remain unanswered. Is the change in measurement caused by the treatment alone, or do other factors (i.e., time, bed rest, medication, or daily activities) contribute to the outcome? Is this group of patients different in some way from other patients with a similar clinical problem.

Campbell and Stanley[6] categorize these kinds of studies as "pre-experimental." The implication is that more rigor and control are needed to increase the value of the findings.

Comparative-Research Designs

Several approaches to comparative research can be used to study clinical questions. A common factor among them is that at least two carefully defined circumstances are compared. The choice of the approach to a specific research problem is based on: (1) the nature and content of the question to be studied and (2) a number of pragmatic details, such as the availability of subjects, the support of patients, their families, and other health-care providers whose intervention may have an effect on the study, and whether or not withholding treatment from some subjects is ethically sound.

GROUP STUDIES

Two traditional methods for comparison are the two-group pretest, post-test design and the two-group post-test-only design.[6] Both require a rigorous control of patient selection and group assignment. Both will test the effect of a treatment scheme imposed on one group, but not on the second. The difference between these two designs is that to use a pretest determination, there must be a common pre-existing condition that can be measured and remeasured after the experimental period. For example, the question, "Is cold or cold plus intermittent compression more effective in reducing edema following ankle sprains?" presupposes that edema is present and measurable before administrating the two treatment regimens. Measured pretreatment edema becomes one criterion for patient selection, and a change in that edema becomes a determination of effectiveness. In contrast, the post-test-only design applies when the condition to be measured (the dependent variable) does not exist before treatment. If the question were, "Does the application of cold packs prevent edema following arthroscopic meniscectomy?", the preoperative condition would not necessarily include edema and, therefore, a pretreatment measurement would be irrelevant and noncontributory to answering the research question.

Both of these traditional experimental designs customarily require the most rigorous control of subject selection and assignment to treatment or control groups. The designs, for example, by classic definition require that subjects for study be drawn randomly from some defined, existing population. This requirement assumes that such a population is available to the investigator at the time a study sample is to be selected. In the case of studying the effect of cold on edema in college athletes, the investigator could hope that a huge number of athletes will suffer ankle sprains at 4 PM on a particular Wednesday. Of course, such an event is unrealistic. Furthermore, if that should happen and if the study sample could be randomly drawn from that number, would the investigator have adequate manpower, equipment, and facilities to conduct the evaluations and treatments outlined in the research protocol in a timely manner? This is highly unlikely and suggests one of the serious practical problems in performing traditional experimental research in the real clinical world.

Traditional designs can and are employed in the clinical setting despite such problems, although compromises are usually made. The study sample is often derived by the method of sequential assignment, rather than by random selection. In a two-group comparative study requiring 15 patients per group, for example, 30 slips of paper (15 with the number 1, and 15 with the number 2, written on them) can be placed in a hat and drawn out one by one. The order of the drawn numbers becomes the method of assigning the eligible patients as they appear to either group 1 or group 2.

A second kind of adaptation or compromise can be made when the investigator believes that certain characteristics of subjects must be controlled by the process of group assignment. A common variable in clinical studies is the age of the subjects. In this case, an investigator who believes that healing time or functional recovery, or any element of the dependent variable, may be affected by age may choose to match the subjects according to this criterion and may assign subjects to groups in pairs, according to age.

TIME-SERIES DESIGNS

Research questions about treatment effectiveness and efficiency focus on the patient and on the management of the patient's problem in the clinic. In the clinical setting, practical issues such as time, numbers of patients with specific disorders, space and, at times, ethical considerations make it difficult to conduct two- or multi-group studies with random samples. Procedures for conducting research have been described that may apply when the clinic is the "laboratory," the clinician is the "investigator," and the patient referred for treatment is the "subject." Of particular relevance in this clinical setting is that the time-series designs presented here can be applied to a single subject, as well as to groups of subjects. As the phrase "time series" implies, these methods of evaluation are based on serial assessment of the dependent variable over time. Depending upon the question, this may mean repeated measures over a period of hours, days, or weeks. The most important factor is that decisions about the measured variable are based not on a single assessment, but on a series of assessments.[10-13]

The simplest time-series model is the simple baseline design (A–B), in which A is a period of baseline measurement, and B is a period of measurement while treatment is being administered. In this, and in all time series designs, the baseline period continues until the measured values are stable over repeated measures.[10,13] Figure 10–1 (top) represents a hypothetic example of the use of the A–B design to investigate the effect of ultrasound on range of motion of the shoulder in a patient with frozen shoulder. The

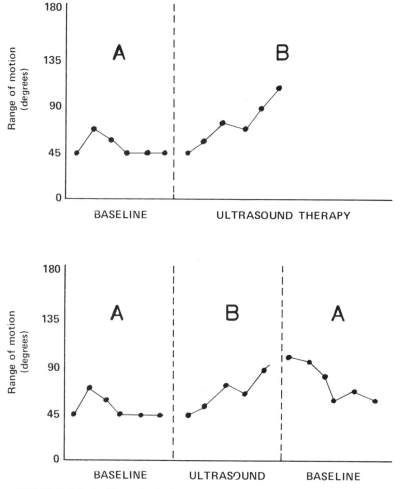

FIGURE 10–1. Hypothetical record representing the time series designs.

results of this study would be less than convincing, because there is no way to be sure that some confounding variable is not responsible for the effect during phase B.

The investigator may have more confidence in the effect of treatment during phase B, if the treatment can be withdrawn for a period of time while baseline measurements are made again. If, during the second baseline period, the treatment effect is reversed toward the original baseline, and all other activities or aspects of management of the patient are unchanged, the evidence is strengthened that the treatment administered during phase B was responsible for the change in measurement values. The A–B–A, or even an A–B–A–B, time design can be used to evaluate treatment of conditions in which a return to baseline values might be expected, such as in the chronic inflammatory states of rheumatoid joints or limitations of motion secondary to long-term changes in joint structure (Fig. 10–1, bottom). These designs will not work when return to baseline is not expected. For example, when a patient is treated following a temporary period of immobilization and resumes normal activity, a return of limited motion or weakness should not happen. In this case, the A–B–A design is inappropriate.

A variation of time-series research is the *multiple-baseline design*, in which more than one measurement is obtained and evaluated. Two or more baseline measures can be derived in several ways: (1) within a single subject, studying multiple joints, limbs, or muscle groups; (2) across subjects, whereby the same method is applied to several subjects over a staggered time course; or, (3) across setting, whereby a single subject is studied in different treatment settings introduced sequentially.[2,12]

SEQUENTIAL MEDICAL TRIALS

The sequential-medical-trials model is a comparative experimental system in which the results of each pair of observations, as they are obtained, determine if the experiment must continue in order to reach a definitive answer or if the experiment is to be terminated.[2,14,16] This system is based on alternative treatments randomly administered to individuals or to paired subjects. Subjects are admitted to the study until a decision is made about which of two treatments is superior. That decision is determined by the sequential plan, chosen in advance, based on the selected probability of obtaining a statistically significant result.

Formulas and calculations for these determinations have been presented by Bross[14] and Armitage.[15] Using the Bross model at a significance level of 0.05, for example, a grid is constructed. This grid, with a hypothetic set of data, is illustrated in Figure 10–2. When a preference for one treatment over the other is made for each pair of observations, an X is placed in the direction (vertical or horizontal) of that preference. As soon as the path of Xs crosses one of the bold lines, indicating a decision in favor of one of the two treatments (or in favor of neither, if the central portion lines are crossed), the study is terminated. In order for the Xs to progress, a clear decision within each pair must be made — preference for one or the other treatment must be achieved in each pair. If there is no preference (that is, if neither achieves, or if both achieve, the selected goal for success), then no X is recorded for that pair. This represents a potential fault with the design in that data are lost from the total evaluation of the comparison, unless the investigator reports this occurrence separately.

The essential requirements for employing the sequential-medical-trials model include those that apply to all research designs: The alternative treatments and the measurement procedure must be specifically defined, and the criteria for subjects to be included in the study must be established in advance. Two other important require-

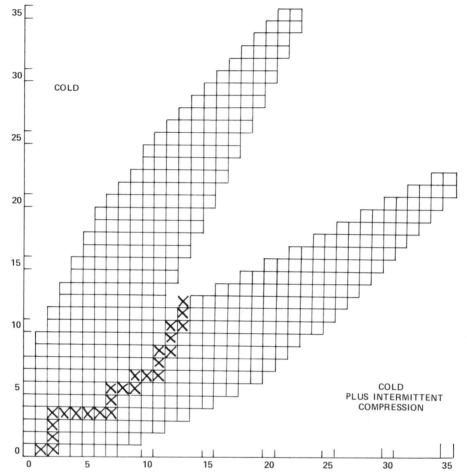

FIGURE 10–2. Sequential medical trials grid with significance level of p ≤ 0.05. Data are hypothetical, comparing cold alone and cold plus intermittent compression in the treatment of ankle sprains.

ments must be fulfilled. First, observations are made in pairs, one for each treatment. If the comparison is between two treatments in the same subject (within-subject comparison), the order of presentation or administration of each of the treatments is random. Second, because the decision to place the Xs is based on a preference (i.e., treatment A or B or neither is better), the criterion or definition of "better" must be specified. For example, if the dependent variable is passive range of motion, what value will indicate "better": an increase of 15 degrees over the initial value; some percentage of the initial value; or a value relative to a normal value, perhaps of the uninvolved extremity?

Using the sample question, "Is cold, or cold plus intermittent compression, more effective in reducing edema following ankle sprains in college athletes?", this research model can be illustrated. The investigator will define "ankle sprain, perhaps limiting the sample to grade-2 sprains, and will determine the exact methods of applying the two treatments. The management of all subjects should be the same in all respects, except for the application of intermittent compression in one group. The number of treatments and treatment days should be specified. The daily activities of the subjects during the experimental period should be specified to control for such variables as weight bearing on the involved ankle. The criterion measure should be defined, perhaps a 50 percent reduction in foot and ankle edema measured volumetrically on the fourth day postinjury.

Hypothetically, 50 athletes suffered grade-2 sprains during an academic year. The effect of the two treatments was determined on each of 25 pairs and recorded on the grid (Fig. 10–2). With these 25 pairs, the central bold line was crossed, thereby indicating that neither method was "better." In 13 pairs, cold plus intermittent compression resulted in a 50-percent reduction in edema on the fourth day and, in 12 pairs, cold alone resulted in achieving that criterion. Furthermore, the opposite member of each pair had not achieved the criterion measure. It can be noted, however, that, with the results obtained from the 20th pair, cold alone would not be found to be "better." At that point, however, it was not known if cold plus compression would be determined to be superior or, as happened, if neither could be considered significantly better.

The efficiency of a sequential medical trial is a major advantage for the clinical investigator. Patients who meet the defined criteria are admitted to the study as they appear. This process is easily adapted to the clinical setting, where the ongoing clinical service cannot be disrupted in a major way, and where it is unlikely that a large number of patients are available at any one time to be randomly assigned to treatment groups. The recording of results on each pair is immediate. This process means three things: (1) data analysis is simple; (2) the study is terminated as soon as a preference is determined; and, (3) when there is a clear demonstration of superiority, the impact on clinical decision making can be immediate.

The major argument against sequential trials is that an answer may be obtained after a small number of observations, or it may require a relatively large number of observations—as many as 58 pairs to reach either favorable choice, using the Bross model.[2] Numbers are of concern in interpretating the roles of chance and traditional statistical significance.[17]

This design is certainly more rigorous than the single-case study or the single-group design. It is economical and practical as a research approach in the setting of a busy clinical practice. As an example, Light and coworkers[18] have employed this model to compare two methods of stretching in patients with chronic knee-flexion contractures.

The approaches to research presented here are not all-inclusive, but rather were selected to exemplify the kind of options and some of the constraints that must be considered in order to answer any question about the value of a therapeutic regimen.

INSTRUMENTATION FOR CLINICAL EVALUATION

Clinical evaluation of thermal agents depends upon the use of measurement techniques that will provide accurate documentation of therapeutic effectiveness. Selecting appropriate measuring tools must be based on: (1) the therapeutic aims of treatment; (2) the reliability, validity, and objectivity of the measurement procedures; and, (3) the value of the evaluation to the advancement of knowledge and practice of the clinician. Throughout this book, a number of clinical signs and symptoms have been discussed repeatedly: pain, edema, limitation of motion, and interference with normal muscular function. Each problem means something special to the patient and should be of major concern to the clinician. Appropriate evaluation procedures, therefore, should accurately document changes in the clinical conditions.

Many clinical characteristics are measurable in quantitative terms, for example: temperature, limb volume, muscle force, range of motion, and recovery time. Some values are qualitative in nature, for example: pain assessment and manual muscle-test grades. The importance of this distinction is that the approach to statistical analysis of data depends on an understanding of the measurement values.[2]

The following discussion will be limited to a review of the instrumentation that is currently available to the clinician or that is economically feasible to acquire and useful for measurement of the clinical problems enumerated above.

Pain Assessment

The presence of pain for many patients is a most debilitating problem. Pain relief, therefore, becomes a priority in clinical management. For this reason alone, the evaluation of pain is important. In addition, the comprehensiveness of the evaluation may also provide information about the causes of pain.

The complexities of the pain experience include, not only the sensation itself, but also the impact of the patient's past experience, emotional state, and cultural attitudes on the interpretation of the quality and magnitude of the symptom. Herein lies one of the difficulties, for both the patient and the clinical investigator, in determining pain levels and changes in the pain state.

Many methods of approaching documentation of the pain experience have been described and evaluated for applicability, reliability, and validity.[19] The need for pain-assessment methods has been recognized, as the development of clinics to specifically treat patients with chronic pain has grown over the past 2 decades.[20]

McGILL PAIN QUESTIONNAIRE

In 1975, Melzack introduced the McGill pain questionnaire (MPQ).[21] This assessment tool is considered comprehensive in that it records information about sensory, affective, and evaluative dimensions of the patient's pain experience. One section of the MPQ consists of work descriptors, divided into three major categories and 20 subcategories. The sensory category (see Fig. 2–8, columns 1–10) is subdivided into groupings that describe spatial ("shooting"), temporal ("flickering"), pressure ("stabbing"), thermal ("burning") and sharp–dull aspects of pain. The affective category (columns 11–15) includes words such as "exhausting," "vicious," and "terrifying." The evaluative words (column 16) relate to the patient's view of the total pain experience. Columns 17 to 20 consist of miscellaneous words, which represent a mixture of the three major categories. The patient is asked to select one word from each subcategory that applies to his pain and to skip a section if no word applies.

The scores obtained from this section of the questionnaire are the number of words chosen (NWC) and the pain-rating index (PRI). The PRI is derived by ranking each word per subcategory by its position in the list and summing the ranked values.

The questionnaire also includes an index of present pain intensity (PPI), which is derived from an ascending, ranked list of words: 0 = no pain to 5 = excruciating.

An abbreviated form of the MPQ has been described, which consists of 15 descriptive words (11 representing sensory qualities, and 5 representing affective qualities).[22] Each word is scored on an intensity scale from 0 = no pain to 3 = severe pain. The short form appears to be sensitive to changes in pain state and can be administered in 2 to 5 minutes, as compared to the 5 to 10 minutes required to complete the standard MPQ.

RATING SCALES

Several kinds of pain-rating scales have been described. *Verbal rating scales (VRS)* consist of word descriptors presented in ascending order, such as: "mild," "discomforting," "distressing," "horrible," and "excruciating." This example is incorporated in the McGill pain questionnaire. This descriptive scale implies a rank ordering, but should not imply equal intervals between ratings and may lack adequate sensitivity to small changes.[23]

A standard *visual analog scale (VAS)* consists of a 10-centimeter line labelled at the extreme ends: "No pain" at one end, and "pain as bad as it can be" at the other.[24] The VAS asks the patient to report pain intensity. The extreme case may state "as bad as it can be," which would indicate an affective quality of the assessment. In either case — "no pain" or "as bad as it can be" — the VAS measures only a unidimensional aspect of the pain experience. Using this scale, the patient is asked to make a mark along the line, which represents the level of pain. The distance from the "no pain" end of the scale to the patient's mark is the pain score.[25] When patients are assessed repeatedly using the VAS, they are usually presented with the line on a fresh piece of paper and do not see their previous markings, as suggested by Jacobsen.[26] Scott and Huskisson,[27] however, reported increasing errors in pain estimates, as time increased between assessments, when patients did not see their previous records.

Another pain-rating method is the *numerical rating scale (NRS)*, on which numbers 0 to 10 (or some greater range) are aligned, and the patient is asked to circle the number that applies to his or her pain intensity. Downie and coworkers[28] found good correlation between VRS, NRS, and VAS in patients with various rheumatic disorders. They concluded that the NRS is a good compromise between the VRS, which provides only a few choices, and the VAS, where the freedom to mark anywhere along the line may be confusing to patients.

Other behavioral measures may be useful in clinical investigation to define or interpret the impact of pain.[19] For example, "up-time" versus "down-time" may be documented by asking the patient how long each day he or she spends lying down or sleeping. Records of medication intake also may indicate changes in pain levels.

When pain scales or questionnaires are used to generate research data, every possible precaution must be taken. For example, some patients have difficulty with the vocabulary used in the MPQ. If the test is too demanding, patients may not complete the test, as designed.[23] Melzack[21] discussed this potential problem regarding the reliability of the MPQ. He suggested that instructions be read aloud and that the researcher or an assistant may need to help patients comprehend the words presented. Jensen and colleagues[25] have suggested that supervision may result in fewer errors in using other rating scales, as well. Of course, the ability of the researcher or assistant to interact with a patient without bias is another potential source of variability.

PRESSURE ALGOMETER

In 1986, Fischer[29,30] described the use of a pressure gauge attached to a rubber disc (1 cm²) for measuring pressure threshold and pressure tolerance (Fig. 10–3). This instrument has been used to document trigger-point sensitivity and responses to therapeutic intervention when pain, especially myofascial pain, is an important problem.[31,32] The advantage of this instrument is that it provides objective, quantitative data.

The disc is placed on the skin, and increasing pressure is applied at a 90-degree angle by the examiner. *Pressure threshold* is defined as the minimal pressure that induces discomfort, as reported by the subject. The gauge reading in kilograms or newtons, at

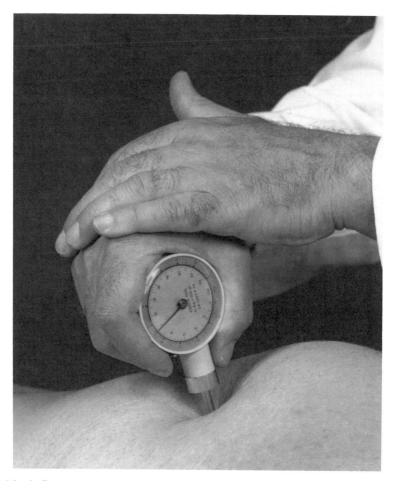

FIGURE 10–3. Pressure Algometer. (Courtesy of Pain Diagnostics and Thermography Corp, Great Neck, New York)

the time the subject so indicates, is the pressure-threshold value. *Pressure tolerance* is defined as the maximal pressure the subject can tolerate. The gauge reading at the time the subject says "stop" is the pressure-tolerance value.

Fischer[33] studied 50 normal adult volunteers to document pain-threshold values over nine muscles of the shoulder, trunk, and hip. The results indicated that values were higher for men than women, that there were few differences in values between sides of the body, and that values differed from muscle to muscle. In a three-part study, Reeves and coworkers[34] documented intra- and inter-rater reliability, using patients with myofascial pain as subjects. Their results showed good correlation between trials (generally, $r = .70$ or above) and that there was a significant difference in algometer values taken over trigger points, as compared to nearby non-trigger point locations.

Two clinical studies using the pressure algometer have been reported. Jimenez and Lane[35] documented increases in both pain threshold and pain-tolerance values, following a 21-day multidisciplinary treatment program, in patients with chronic pain. Jaeger and Reeves[36] studied the effect of a spray-and-stretch procedure on symptoms of myofascial pain in patients with chronic head and neck pain. They documented a significant increase in threshold values following treatment. During this study, patients also were asked to rate their pain intensity using a VAS. Although there was a significant decrease in VAS scores following treatment, there was a poor correlation between the VAS scores and algometer readings. This finding suggests that, at least in patients with chronic pain problems, the algometer data may be limited. Apparently, it does not reflect the complexity of the pain experience in chronic conditions.

OTHER CONSIDERATIONS

When pain assessment measures are used to evaluate the effects of thermal agents (or any other physical-therapy procedure), the investigator must take into account other aspects of the patient's management. Of particular importance is the administration of analgesics and anti-inflammatory drugs, which will undoubtedly influence the pain state. Cooperation between the patient, physician, and physical-therapy investigator is mandatory during a clinical trial. Clinical judgment will determine the reasonable course to follow in this case. Occasionally, stopping or withholding medication may be possible. If not, as is likely, medication administration may be regulated to ensure that no new medication is introduced and that the dosage schedule remains constant during the trial. At the very least, a record of drug intake should be maintained, as it will be if the patient is hospitalized. Control of compliance[37,38] by an outpatient is more difficult to regulate, but every attempt should be made to document the extent of this important extraneous variable.

The presence and magnitude of pain often accompanies or results in other physiologic changes. Concurrent muscle spasm or muscle guarding may interfere with range of motion. Pain may be the limiting factor in the patient's performance of daily activities. The converse may also occur if, for example, the patient has no pain at rest but, because of muscle tightness, has pain on motion. Many times, therefore, other measures of clinical effectiveness may be, and should be, obtained concurrent with the assessment of pain.

Range of Motion

Techniques of goniometry are well known to physical therapists. When these techniques are used accurately, they provide quantitative data about limitation in joint range of motion (ROM).

For research purposes, a specific protocol must be selected and defined, to include such details as the type of goniometer, placement landmarks, patient position, and patient participation. The last consideration may seriously affect the validity of testing. The choice is whether to measure passive, active–assisted, or active ROM. The results may be quite different, depending upon muscle guarding, spasm, segmentalreflex interactions or the patient's ability to follow instructions.

Common methods have been described[39,40] and are used as guides throughout the United States. Reliability of these methods has been evaluated.[41,42] Accurate goniometry requires skill and consistent performance of the examiner. These attributes may be assessed by determining intra-rater reliability on repeated trials. Each investigator is obliged to determine his own reliability before initiating a study, using as a sample the same kind of patient and clinical problem that will be studied.[43] Knowledge of intra-rater variability for specific measurements should be used to establish criteria for a change in patient status. Based on Boone's[42] data, for example, a change of greater than

5 degrees in the upper extremity, and 6 degrees in the lower extremity, must occur to state an improvement or a decline in ROM. Because of the documented differences between testers, it seems appropriate to use only one examiner in a given study.

Volumetric and Girth Measurements

Edema is a common problem in several of the clinical conditions for which thermal agents are employed and may be a major cause of pain, limitation of motion, and decreased functional ability. Reduction of swelling, therefore, becomes another important therapeutic goal. Two relatively inexpensive and efficient methods for obtaining quantitative data about limb edema are volumetric measurement and girth measurement.

Volume of an entire limb or a distal-limb segment can be estimated using a water displacement system,[44,45] in which the part to be evaluated is submerged in a water tank with an outflow spout from which the water displaced by the limb is collected in a graduated cylinder. The indicator of limb volume is the quantity of displaced water, measured in milliliters. The accuracy of this method depends upon: (1) the initial level of water in the tank relative to the outflow spout; (2) the position of the limb in the tank, particularly depth of submersion; and, (3) the state of relaxation of the patient's limb. Tanks made of clear material such as Plexiglas (Volumeters Unlimited, 524 Double View Drive, P.O. Box 145, Idyllwild, CA) are probably best to permit the examiner to observe the position of the limb within the tank (Fig. 10–4).

Smyth and associates[46] investigated the reproducibility of volumetric measurement in both normal subjects and patients with acute joint inflammation. The variability in repeated measures, taken several times in succession, was less than 1 percent for hands and a maximum of 0.6 percent for feet in normal subjects. When measurements were taken at 8:30 AM and 3:30 PM, changes (both increases and decreases) were noted. The greatest change was a 1.7 percent decrease in the left hands of female subjects. Throughout 5 days of repeated measures, the maximal coefficient of variation was 2.3 percent for hand measurements and 1.5 percent for foot measurements. Two case

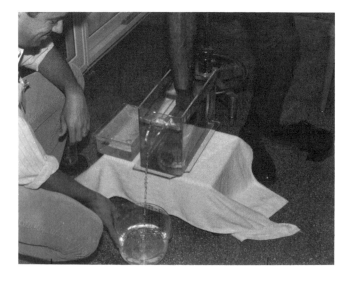

FIGURE 10–4. Foot and ankle volume is being measured using a volumeter.

studies were presented, both employing anti-inflammatory medications. In both cases, volumetric measures documented a marked decrease in volume in response to treatment: an 11 percent decrease in the hand measurement of the patient with rheumatoid arthritis, and a 7.4 percent decrease in the foot measurement of the patient with gout.

This method of volumetric measurement is appropriate when the swelling is distally located (i.e., hand and wrist or foot and ankle), or when swelling involves a large area from distal to proximal. If swelling is limited to a more proximal site (i.e., knee, thigh, or upper arm), this measurement method may not be sensitive enough to detect a change in such a delimited location, because the entire limb must be immersed. In that case, girth (or circumferential) limb measurements may be more appropriate. The only equipment required is a measuring tape; one made of flexible steel or fiberglass is probably preferred to one of cloth or plastic, which may change in length over time by stretching. Because examiner skill is required in placing and reading the tape, intra-rater reliability should be evaluated before using this procedure. Limb posture and relaxation of the part to be measured may be confounding variables. Careful instructions to the patient, therefore, are necessary.

Evaluation of Muscle Performance

Muscle strength may not be of primary concern during the acute stage of injury or illness; however, restoration of normal muscle performance is usually found on any list of long-term therapeutic goals. The direct effects of cold on muscle strength have been discussed in Chapter 4. In addition, skeletal-muscle performance may be altered secondary to the demonstrated effects of thermal agents on nerve-conduction velocity, muscle-spindle activity, and synaptic transmission. For these reasons, muscle strength may be an important dependent variable in evaluating the long-term effects of applying thermal agents.

If so, the investigator must make a series of decisions in selecting the appropriate test instrument. The first problems to solve are the *operational definitions* of strength and the selection of criteria for determining whether strength is improving or declining. None of the currently used terms (such as force, tension, work, and power) are synonymous, although all can be used to describe a quality of being "strong" or "weak." Criteria for improvement or decline should be based on knowledge of the reliability or reproducibility of the selected test procedure. The second important consideration must be both the local and systemic *conditions* of the patients who will be studied. For example, testing procedures that require patients to generate high levels of force may be impractical and inappropriate in the presence of acute inflammation or serious debilitation secondary to prolonged bed rest. A third factor relates to the nature of the *research question.* If it is one in which the muscle testing should be correlated with functional activity, a determination of the functional requirements of the muscles to be tested will have to be made. Then, the investigator can select a test condition, such as isometric or dynamic, at low or high speed, that most closely relates to those functional requirements.

There is an imposing array of testing instruments for the measurement of muscle strength. Only four of the choices will be mentioned, to illustrate the available spectrum: the manual muscle test, the cable tensiometer, the hand-held dynamometer, and the isokinetic dynamometer. These instruments represent the diversity of information that can be obtained under the category of "strength" testing.

The manual muscle test[47] was developed by Lovett and Merrill in 1912 and, since that time, it has periodically fallen in and out of favor without careful analysis of the attendant reasons. One of the criticisms has been that it is not an "objective test." The objectivity of this test very definitely depends on the skill and precision of the examiner and on the adherence to strict rules for grading. Under sensible, controlled conditions, the reliability of the manual muscle test was assessed by Lilienfeld and coworkers[48] and, based on their study results, this test was effectively employed during the polio era. This study has been criticized, however, because muscle scores were weighted by a muscle-bulk factor, which makes it impossible to relate the data to current practices of muscle testing.[49] A more recent study of inter-rater reliability was presented by Silver and associates.[50] This study demonstrated 97 percent agreement within plus or minus a half grade between three examiners, testing patients with chronic renal disease. This study affirms that standardized procedures and practice are important.

The qualitative ranking of muscle strength by manual muscle testing can be used to determine change, particularly in muscles that cannot move through the complete arc of motion against an externally applied resistance. In fact, there may be no other measure in common usage to assess muscle strength in this circumstance. The arguments against the manual muscle test become more appropriate when the variable of the examiner's manual resistance is introduced, as in the range of grades above "fair" (50%). Not only is the examiner's resistance part of the determination, but the grade of "normal" (100%) may be interpreted to mean full recovery and normal function, which is not necessarily so. Watkins and colleagues,[51] for example, documented deficits in isokinetic torque production in the socalled uninvolved thigh musculature of patients with hemiparesis whose manual-muscle-test grades for quadriceps and hamstrings muscles were graded "normal."

When the muscles under study are able to develop higher levels of force, the quantitative measures of that force can, and should, be employed.

The cable tensiometer measures *isometric* tension.[1] The recorded values are pounds of kilograms of force. A calibrated length of cable is placed within a fixed cable or chain system, which is attached to the subject's limb and against which the muscle or muscle group exerts force. The force, translated through the calibrated cable, is recorded using a tensiometer attached to that cable. The advantage of this instrument is that, with the versatility of hardware attachments, the subject and tensiometer can be aligned to test a muscle at several points within the arc of motion.

A hand-held dynamometer is a device that measures the force exerted between the examiner's hand and the part being tested.[52,53] It is designed to test maximal voluntary isometric contraction. How accurate a reflection of maximal performance the dyna-mometer is may depend on whether a "make-test" or "break-test" protocol is used. In a make-test, the examiner holds the dynamometer in a fixed position and instructs the subjects to exert maximal force against the instrument. In a break-test, the subject holds the limb in a fixed position and the examiner exerts force through the instrument until the part gives way. Bohannon[54] found a significant difference in elbow-flexor forces between methods, using a sample of 27 healthy women.

Good to excellent reliability of measures using a hand-held dynamometer have been documented in tests of normal children, children with Duchenne's muscular dystrophy, and patients with peripheral neuromuscular disorders.[53,55] This instrument should be considered when patients have weakness, but manual-muscle-test grades are above "fair," and when testing small muscle groups or children.[53] The magnitude of force that can be measured is limited by the range of the instrument (e.g., the Sparks' limit is 0 to 60 lbs, or 27.2 kg) and the strength of the examiner, who must resist the patient's contraction.[52]

The capability of testing *dynamic* muscular performance requiring motion through an arc of motion is no longer limited to weightlifting and values such as the ten-repetition maximum of DeLorme and Watkins,[56] although this method may continue to be used if it suits the needs and criteria of a particular research question.

The concept of isokinetic exercise and the introduction of isokinetic dynamometers[57] interfaced with recording devices (such as the Cybex II, Lumex Corporation, Cybex Division, Ronkonkoma, NY) have expanded the choices of instrumentation for clinical measurement of strength. With isokinetic-exercise devices, which are based on the force–velocity principle, speed of motion can be preselected, and the instrument will prevent acceleration beyond that preset speed. Several measures of muscular performance, such as peak torque and joint angle at peak torque, can be obtained from the torque curves generated by the patient's attempt to accelerate. The Cybex II is designed to assess isometric or concentric contractions, whereas other devices (such as the KINCOM, Chattecx Corporation, Chattanooga, TN) permit assessment of eccentric contraction, as well. Assessment of performance over a range of speeds that may more closely simulate functional requirements is a potential advantage of these systems.[59] Further study, however, of both the reliability and validity is warranted, as related to functional performance.

Assessment of muscular performance can make an important contribution to the evaluation of long-term effects of thermal agents. There is, however, one final caution: All of these procedures designed to measure muscle strength depend on the *voluntary* participation and cooperation of the patients. Apprehension, inattention, lack of motivation, and the inability to follow instructions are factors that may interfere with the validity of these measures.

Functional Tests

In the course of therapeutic intervention, the question of the effectiveness and efficiency of treatment procedures eventually becomes: "How well does the patient function in carrying out the physical activities relevant to the patient's lifestyle?" In considering the efficacy of thermal agents and any comparison of specific modalities, the question may be: "How quickly does the patient return to his or her optimal level of function?" In this case, the measure is "recovery time." "Function," "recovery," and "time to recovery" then can become dependent variables in clinical studies. Again, the first necessary step is to define operationally those terms in a manner relevant to the specific research question.

The performance of functional tasks can be documented qualitatively or quantitatively. The system of noting whether a patient can perform a given activity independently, with an assistive device, or not at all can be translated into a qualitative rating scale for research purposes.

A number of quantitative measures are available or could be created. These are timed tests of functional performance in which the dependent variable is the time (usually in seconds) it takes to accomplish a defined task. An objective and standardized test of hand function by Jebsen[60] is an example of such a measure of upper-extremity function, including such items as writing a short sentence and stacking checkers. The time required to walk a fixed distance or climb a set of standard stairs[61] are other examples of timed tests.

Temporal and spatial characteristics of gait may also be quantitatively and reliably measured.[62,63] The basic implements of the method described by Boenig[62] are a mat or paper strip secured to the floor, inked tapes on the shoes of the subject, and a stop watch. Using this method, the data obtained include step length, stride length, step width, foot angle, and cadence. Using more sophisticated instrumentation, such as the computerized gait described by Wall and associates,[63] additional data can be collected, namely, stance time, double-support time, and velocity of walking.

All of the preceding examples of clinical instrumentation can be employed by physical-therapy clinicians for both the assessments of individual patients who are referred for treatment and, with careful planning and organization, the evaluation of therapeutic effectiveness or efficiency of thermal agents.

Related Evaluative Procedures

The practitioner and clinical investigator should be aware of other instruments relevant to the evaluation of thermal agents. Some have been cited elsewhere in this book. These measurements do not directly document *clinical* progress or outcomes. The information they provide, however, may be correlated with signs and symptoms that limit function. These techniques may be useful to draw attention to and further elucidate the underlying mechanisms of pathology or to document the nature and extent of a patient's problem. Because of the distance between these techniques and the functional status of patients, only one, thermography, will be defined, and others will be noted for the reader's information.

THERMOGRAPHY

Clinical thermography is a method of detecting and recording infrared radiation specifically from the body surface. One of the available systems is liquid-crystal-contact thermography, which uses selected cholesteric esters embedded in elastomeric sheets. The configuration of crystals allows calibration of color responses to specific temperature ranges.[64] These sheets are placed in contact with the area to be assessed. As the colors are displayed through a clear plastic frame, they are photographed to record the colored thermogram (Fig. 10–5).

Thermography is based on the principles that infrared rays are radiated from any object having a temperature above absolute zero,[65] and that superficial blood flow contributes to surface temperature.[66] Variations of detected emissions over a given area may represent autonomic or metabolic reactions to pathologic conditions.

The reported applications of this instrumentation include detection of spinal-root compression,[64] observation of pain,[67] evaluation of low back pain,[68] and evaluation of myofascial-pain syndromes.[32] The accuracy of thermography will be influenced by several factors including room temperature, ambient infrared radiation, materials (such as oils and powder) on the skin surface, and pressure.[69] Obviously, thermography could not be used to evaluate the immediate effects of a thermal agent, because the surface temperature would simply reflect the temperature of the applied agent. It may be more useful during initial assessment to delineate the specific area to be treated.

Effects of thermal agents on blood flow and blood volume have been discussed in

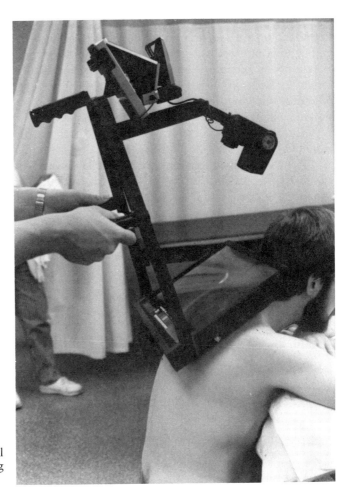

FIGURE 10–5. The cervical area is being examined using liquid crystal thermography.

Chapters 4 through 8. Techniques to ascertain assessment of these functions include the Doppler ultrasound flow meter,[70,71] plethysmography,[71,72] and ^{133}Xe washout studies.[72] Electromyography and nerve-conduction-velocity studies[73] have been cited elsewhere (see Chapters 4, 5, and 7) and may continue to provide insight regarding neuromuscular responses to thermal agents.

SUMMARY

This chapter has identified the need and selected methods for conducting clinical studies to evaluate the effectiveness and efficiency of applying thermal agents for ameliorating conditions of pain, swelling, limited motion, and functional limitations. Such evaluation cannot be done by informal opinions of practitioners whose private experiences are not tested in a well-organized manner. It must be done through sound, systematic research, most properly conducted in the clinical setting where the physical therapist and associates become the investigators, and the patients referred for treatment become the subjects of study.

The success of this kind of clinical research depends on multiple collaborations. Coordination and cooperation among physical therapists, physicians, other allied health professionals and, most certainly, the patients are important to ensure adequate control of extraneous variables. Consultation with a biostatistician during the process of establishing the appropriate research design will facilitate proper application of data-analysis procedures. In the case of thermal agent evaluation, the accuracy of energies delivered should be determined by the appropriate biomedical or electrical engineer. In summary, it is foolhardy to expect that clinical research can or should be done by a single individual.

The data derived from this kind of collaborative clinical investigation will contribute to the professional body of knowledge about therapeutic intervention and will enhance the process of clinical decision making to the benefit of both the practitioner and the patient.

REFERENCES

1. Currier, DP: Elements of Research in Physical Therapy, ed 2. Williams & Wilkins, Baltimore, 1984.
2. Payton, O: The Validation of Clinical Practice, ed 2. FA Davis, Philadelphia, 1988.
3. Rothstein, JM (ed): Measurement in Physical Therapy. Churchill-Livingstone, New York, 1985, pp 5–42.
4. Colton, T: Statistics in Medicine. Little, Brown, Boston, 1974, p 39.
5. Fleiss, JL and Shrout, PE: The effects of measurement errors on some multivariate procedures. AJPH 67:1188, 1977.
6. Campbell, DT and Stanley, JC: Experimental and Quasi-Experimental Designs for Research. Rand McNally College Publishing, Chicago, 1963.
7. Code of Federal Regulations 45 CFR 46: Protection of human subjects (HHS). US Government Printing Office, Washington, 1983.
8. Wing, M: Phonophoresis with hydrocortisone in the treatment of temporomandibular joint dysfunction. Phys Ther 62:32, 1982.
9. Quillen, WS, et al: Initial management of acute ankle sprains with rapid pulsed pneumatic compression with cold. Journal of Orthopaedic and Sports Physical Therapy 4:39, 1982.
10. Ottenbacher, KJ: Evaluating Clinical Change Strategies for Occupational and Physical Therapists. Williams & Wilkins, Baltimore, 1986.
11. Barlow, DH and Hersen, M: Single-case experimental designs. Arch Gen Psychiatry 29:319, 1973.
12. Martin, JE and Epstein, LH: Evaluating treatment effectiveness in cerebral palsy. Phys Ther 56:285, 1976.
13. Wolery, M and Harris, SR: Interpreting results of single-subject research designs. Phys Ther 62:445, 1982.
14. Bross, I: Sequential medical plans. Biometrics 8:189, 1953.
15. Armitage, P: Sequential Methods in Medical Research. John Wiley & Sons, New York, 1971.
16. Gonella, C: Designs for clinical research. Phys Ther 53:1276, 1973.
17. Oldham, PD: Measurement in Medicine. JB Lippincott, Philadelphia, 1968.
18. Light, KE, et al: Low-load prolonged stretch vs. high-load brief stretch in treating knee contractures. Phys Ther 64:330, 1984.
19. Williams, RC: Toward a set of reliable and valid measures for chronic pain assessment and outcome research. Pain 35:239, 1988.
20. Schaefer, CA: The pain clinic approach. In Michel, TH (ed): International Perspectives in Physical Therapy, I: Pain. Churchill-Livingstone, New York, 1985, pp 233–258.
21. Melzack, R: The McGill pain questionnaire: Major properties and scoring method. Pain 1:277, 1975.
22. Melzack, R: The short-form McGill pain questionnaire. Pain 30:191, 1987.
23. Chapman, CR, et al: Pain measurement: An overview. Pain 22:1, 1985.
24. Huskisson, EC: Measurement of pain. Lancet 2:1127, 1974.
25. Jensen, MP, et al: The measurement of clinical pain intensity: A comparison of methods. Pain 27:117, 1986.
26. Jacobsen, M: The use of rating scales in clinical research. Br J Psychiat 111:545, 1965.
27. Scott, J, et al: Accuracy of subjective measurements made with or without previous scores: An important source of error in serial measurement of subjective states. Ann Rheum Dis 38:558, 1979.
28. Downie, WW, et al: Studies with pain rating scales. Ann Rheum Dis 37:378, 1978.
29. Fischer, AA: Pressure threshold meter: Its use for quantification of tender spots. Arch Phys Med Rehabil 67:836, 1986.
30. Fischer, AA: Pressure tolerance over muscles and bones in normal subjects. Arch Phys Med Rehabil 67:406, 1986.

31. Fischer, AA: Documentation of myofascial trigger points. Arch Phys Med Rehabil 69:386, 1988.
32. Simons, DG: Myofascial pain syndromes: Where are we? Where are we going? Arch Phys Med Rehabil 69:207, 1988.
33. Fischer, AA: Pressure algometry over normal muscles: Standard values, validity and reproducibility of pressure threshold. Pain 30:115, 1987.
34. Reeves, JL, et al: Reliability of the pressure algometer as a measure of myofascial trigger point sensitivity. Pain 24:313, 1986.
35. Jimenz, AC, et al: Serial determinations of pressure threshold in chronic pain patients. Arch Phys Med Rehabil (abstract). 66:545, 1985
36. Jaeger, B, et al: Quantification of changes in myofascial trigger point sensitivity with the pressure algometer following passive stretch. Pain 27:203, 1986.
37. Carpenter, J: Medical recommendations followed or ignored: Factors influencing compliance in arthritis. Arch Phys Med Rehabil 57:241, 1976.
38. Vincent, P: Factors influencing patient non-compliance. Nurs Res 20:509, 1971.
39. Moore, ML: The measurement of joint motion. Part II: The technic of goniometry. Phys Ther Rev 29:256, 1949.
40. Joint Motion: Method of Measuring and Recording. American Academy of Orthopaedic Surgery, Chicago, 1963.
41. Hellebrandt, FA, et al: The measurement of joint motion. Part III: Reliability of goniometry. Phys Ther Rev 29:302, 1949.
42. Boone, DC, et al: Reliability of goniometric measurement. Phys Ther 58:1355, 1978.
43. Miller, PJ: Assessment of joint motion. In Rothstein J (ed): Measurement in Physical Therapy. Churchill-Livingstone, 1985, pp 103–136.
44. Engler, HS and Sweat, RD: Volumetric arm measurements: Technique and results. Am Surg 28:465, 1952.
45. Devore, GL, et al: Volume measuring of the severely injured hand. AJOT 22:16, 1968.
46. Smyth, CJ: A method for measuring swelling of hands and feet. Acta Rheum Scand 9:293, 1963.
47. Daniels, L and Worthingham, C: Muscle Testing: Techniques of Manual Examination. WB Saunders, Philadelphia, 1980.
48. Lilienfeld, AM, Jacobs, M, and Willis, M: Study of reproducibility of muscle testing and certain other aspects of muscle scoring. Phys Ther Rev 34:279, 1954.
49. Lamb, RL: Manual muscle testing. In Rothstein J (ed): Measurement in Physical Therapy. Churchill-Livingstone, 1985, pp 47–55.
50. Silver, M, et al: Further standardization of manual muscle testing for clinical study. Phys Ther 50:1456, 1970.
51. Watkins, MP, Harris, BA, and Kozlowski, BK: Isokinetic testing in patients with hemiparesis: A pilot study. 64:184, 1984.
52. Edwards, RHT, et al: Hand-held dynamometer for evaluating voluntary-muscle functions. Lancet 2:757, 1974.
53. Stuberg, WA, et al: Reliability of quantitative muscle testing in healthy children and in children with Duchenne muscular dystrophy. Phys Ther 68:977, 1988.
54. Bohannon, RW: Make tests and break tests of elbow flexor muscle strength. Phys Ther 68:193, 1988.
55. Wiles, CM, et al: The measurement of muscle strength in patients with peripheral neuromuscular disorders. J Neurol Neurosurg and Psychiat 46:1006, 1983.
56. DeLorme, TL and Watkins, AL: Progressive Resistance Exercise: Technic and Medical Application. Appleton-Century-Crofts, New York, 1951, p 23.
57. Thistle, HG, et al: Isokinetic contraction: A new concept of resistive exercise. Arch Phys Med Rehabil 48:279, 1967.
58. Farrell, M, et al: Analysis of the reliability and validity of the kinetic communicator exercise device. Med Sci Sport and Exercise 18:44, 1986.
59. Watkins, MP and Harris, BA: Evaluation of isokinetic muscle performance. Clinics in Sports Medicine 2:37, 1983.
60. Jebsen, RH: An objective and standardized test of hand function. Arch Phys Med Rehabil 50:311, 1969.
61. Vignos, PJ, Spencer, GE, and Archibald, KC: Management of progressive muscular dystrophy of childhood. JAMA 184:103, 1963.
62. Boenig, D: Evaluation of a clinical method of gait analysis. Phys Ther 57:795, 1977.
63. Wall, JC, Dhanendran, M, and Klenerman, L: A method of measuring the temporal/distance factors of gait. Biomed Eng 11:409, 1976.
64. Pochaczevsky, R, et al: Thermographic study of extremity dermatomes in the diagnosis of spinal root compression syndromes. In Gautheric, M and Albert, E (eds): Biomedical Thermography. Alan R Liss, New York, 1982, p 339.
65. Atsumi, K (ed): Medical Thermography. University of Tokyo Press, Tokyo, 1973, p 11.
66. Love, TJ: Thermography as an indicator of blood perfusion. Proc NY Acad Sci 335:429, 1980.
67. Hobbins, WB: Thermography and pain. In Gautheric, M and Albert, E (eds): Biomedical Thermography. Alan R Liss, New York, 1982, p 361.
68. Rubal, BJ, Traycoff, RB, and Ewing, KL: Liquid crystal thermography: A new tool for evaluating low back pain. Phys Ther 62:1593, 1982.

69. Fujimasa, I, Sakurai, Y, and Atsumi, K: Some physical and physiological aspects of thermography. In Atsumi, K (ed): Medical Thermography. University of Tokyo Press, Tokyo, 1973, p 31.
70. Guyton, AC: Textbook of Medical Physiology, ed 6. WB Saunders, Philadelphia, 1981, p 209.
71. Hirsh, J: Noninvasive tests for thromboembolic disease. Hosp Pract (Sept) 1982, p 77.
72. Lasen, NA, Henriksen, O, and Sejrsen, P: Indicator methods for measurement of organ and tissue blood flow, Section 2. In Shepherd, JT and Abboud, FM (eds): Handbook of Physiology. The Cardiovascular System. American Physiological Society, Bethesda, 1983, p 40.
73. Goodgold, J and Eberstein, A: Electrodiagnosis of Neuromuscular Diseases, ed 2. Williams & Wilkins, Baltimore, 1978.

CHAPTER 11

The Application of Cold and Heat in the Treatment of Athletic Injuries

Wayne Smith, M.Ed., P.T., A.T.C.

Kraus[1] has described athletic injuries as "those injuries produced by circumstances inherent in respective athletic performances." These injuries can vary from minor strains and sprains to fractures. The goal in treatment of an injured athlete with musculoskeletal dysfunction is to restore the greatest possible degree of function in the shortest period of time. Physical agents, such as cold and heat, can be instrumental in reducing an athlete's recovery time.[2-7] The objectives of this chapter are: (1) To review the literature on thermal agents as applied to injured athletes; and, (2) to suggest guidelines to follow in treating athletic injuries.

COLD

Cold has become an increasingly versatile agent among sports-medicine practitioners. It is not only useful in first aid to control hemorrhage and edema, but also to relieve pain and muscle spasm. The use of cold enhances ease of passive and active exercises of muscles and joints and reduces the morbidity immediately following acute injury.[4,8-11]

Edema

One of the earliest attempts to establish guidelines for application of cold in sports medicine advocated the use of cold (8°C) whirlpool baths to control hemorrhage and edema.[12] Bennett[12] believed that this temperature would allow vasoconstriction but avoid the vasodilation response reported by Lewis.[13] Although there was no formal research undertaken, Bennett's[12] article did serve as an impetus for future clinical practice. Therapists and trainers assumed that the properties of cold were effective in treating acute injuries because of their physiologic effects.[14-16]

However, it was only after Hocutt and associates[17] compared cold with heat that any clinical documentation was formulated. Their study assessed patients recovering from ankle sprains. Participants were categorized according to the severity of injury, and according to the use of cryotherapy versus the use of heat therapy (each 15 minutes, 1–3 times daily, for a minimum of 3 days). Therapy commenced either less than 1 hour, from 1 to 36 hours, or more than 36 hours, after traumatic injury. Patients who were treated on the first day of injury with cold (i.e., whirlpool baths or ice packs) returned to pre-injury activities on an average of 8 days sooner than did their counterparts, who were treated with heat (i.e., warm soaks or heating pads).[17] The significance of the study was threefold: (1) It was the first controlled study of its kind reported in the literature; (2) it attempted to establish parameters with regard to temperature and duration of cold application; and (3) it was found that early cryotherapy allowed patients to return to full activities sooner than late cryotherapy or early heat treatments. The findings of Hocutt and associates[17] have been supported by other investigations. Cote and coworkers[18] compared the effects of cold, heat, and contrast baths in minimizing edema in acute ankle sprains and concluded that cold therapy was the more appropriate of the three treatment regimens if the objective was to minimize swelling.

COLD AND COMPRESSION

Cold has been reported to be effective when combined with other modalities in treating athletic injuries.[17-20] The addition of compression to cold application appears to enhance the effectiveness of treating sprains.[2,19-22] A basic cause of swelling is a change in capillary-filtration pressure. Edema will occur when factors controlling the equilibrium between intra- and extravascular fluids are disturbed. The use of a mechanical intermittent-compression device appears to help maintain the homeostasis, with respect to osmotic pressures and hydrostatic pressures in the capillary beds, by encouraging lymphatic and venous return. Several clinical studies have sought to evaluate the efficacy of combining cold and intermittent compression in treating ankle sprains. Starkey,[21] using high school athletes, compared the simultaneous use of cold, elevation, and intermittent inflatable compression with that of cold, elevation, and compression wrapping. According to Starkey,[21] 30 minutes of intermittent compression at a 15-second cycle, along with cold and elevation, proved to be more effective in edema reduction than were cold, elevation, and compression wrapping. In addition, time lost from practice was reduced with the former regimen by approximately 2 days.[21] Similar results were reported by Quillen and Rouillier,[22] who combined cold and elevation with a rapid pneumatic-pulse compression (70 to 90 mm Hg), along with a cold wrap placed around the injured joint, followed by removal of the cold and a continuation of compression for an additional 15 minutes. Volumetric displacement measurements of the foot and ankle confirmed the significant reduction in edema. More recent research confirms earlier studies of the effectiveness of cold and compression. Sloan and associates[23] comparative treatment of cold versus cold and compression in the treatment of artificially induced acute inflammatory edema, found that the most effective treatment was a combination of both modalities.

CASE STUDY

Case Study 1

Case number one illustrates the use of cold and compression.

A 16-year-old male high school athlete sustained an inversion sprain to his right ankle. He reported to the training room and was seen by the school trainer, complaining of pain on weight-bearing. Physical examination of the right ankle revealed no gross deformities, limited range of motion (ROM), palpable tenderness distal to the right lateral malleolus, and moderate swelling of the anterolateral aspect of the right foot and ankle complex. Initial treatment consisted of a combination of 30 minutes of cold, intermittent compression (50 mm Hg), and elevation. The patient was given crutches and a compression wrap and instructed in a home program of 20 minutes of ice and elevation for a period of 24 hours. On the second day postinjury, he reported to the trainer, who noted a marked reduction of edema; then a prescribed regimen of cryokinetics was instituted; cold whirlpools (9°C for 15 minutes), followed by ROM exercises and weight-bearing as tolerated. On the fourth day postinjury, swelling and pain appeared stabilized, and the patient progressed to a program of 15 minutes of alternating cold application and light resistive exercises. The athlete resumed full activities by the ninth day postinjury.

COLD AND HIGH VOLTAGE PULSED CURRENT

High voltage pulsed current, along with ice to reduce effusion, has become a popular therapy mode (Fig. 11–1). Although research is pending regarding the efficacy of the use of this modality with cold, several preliminary reports have suggested that this combination appears to be effective in the management of musculoskeletal trauma, including sprains.[17,18,23] Lambonie and Harris[20] have reported good results in reducing edema using cold, compression, and high voltage pulsed current at 30 pulses per second and negative polarity for 30-minute periods. Smith[24] reported similar results in post-

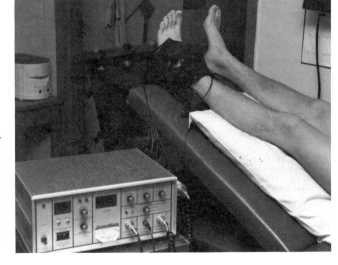

FIGURE 11–1. The use of cold in combination with high-voltage pulsed current for the acute management of an ankle sprain. Note: The lower extremity is elevated, and the stimulating electrodes are on the medial and lateral ankle under the cold pack.

fracture using cold packs, elevation, and high voltage pulsed current at 60 pulses per second (pps), negative polarity, and reciprocal stimulations for 10 seconds per pad. A more well-controlled study published by Michlovitz, Smith, and Watkins,[25] however, comparing ice versus ice and high voltage pulsed current (negative polarity) at 28 and 80 pps for the treatment of acute ankle sprains, found no significant difference in the treatment's effect on foot and ankle volume or ROM in dorsiflexion. More studies, using different stimulus characteristics and larger patient samples, therefore, are warranted.

Muscle and Tendon Injury

Conditions that involve injury at the musculotendinous junction, or at the tendon itself, can pose a difficult problem for the trainer. The joint must be kept mobile to avoid morbid complications during healing without producing further damage. In an attempt to initiate early motion in these painful conditions, cold has been demonstrated to be effective in relieving pain and allowing passive and active exercising.[10,17,22,23] Grant[8] and Hayden[9] both reported that ice massage of 5 to 7 minutes duration achieved sufficient anesthesia to permit ROM and mobilization exercises. Waylonis,[26] who later repeated Grant's[8] study under controlled conditions, measured some of the physiologic changes in ice massage — pain stimuli, blood flow, and skin temperature. Waylonis[26] reported that although numbness occurred at 5 minutes of application, those who received a 10-minutes application had a greater reduction of temperatures to the deeper tissues.

Prentice[27] used electromyography (EMG) to evaluate the effectiveness of heat and cold, along with some form of stretching for inducing skeletal-muscle soreness. The study involved a fourway comparison among heat and contract–relax stretching, cold and static stretching, heat and static stretching, and a control group. The findings indicated that those who received a combination of 20 minutes of ice pack followed by static stretching exhibited less EMG activity than did the 3 other groups. The implications for using cold and stretching in such conditions as muscle spasm, therefore, may have some validity, as shown by experimental research.

Yackzan and associates[28] investigated the efficacy of 15 minutes of ice massage in reducing delayed muscle soreness to determine the optimal time within a stated protocol. Three groups receiving cold were tested: those receiving ice immediately after exercise, those receiving it 24 hours after exercise, and those receiving it 48 hours after exercise were studied. Pain and range of motion were assessed after the patient's undergoing eccentric-based exercises to the elbow flexors. This investigation reported no consistent patterns of significant differences in various comparisons between the treated, versus the untreated, arms and of the treated arms that were iced at different times. The result of this study failed to demonstrate that cold alone was effective in preventing the occurrence of or in alleviating pain in delayed muscle soreness. Therefore, cold in combination with stretching exercises may be the preferred technique.

Cryokinetics

In the preceding paragraphs, reference was made to the use of cold and exercise. Cryokinetics (cold and exercise) is an important component of an athlete's rehabilitation program. The key to successful rehabilitation is the use of cold along with graded exercises. Ice is used to numb the affected area; 10 to 12 minutes of application are

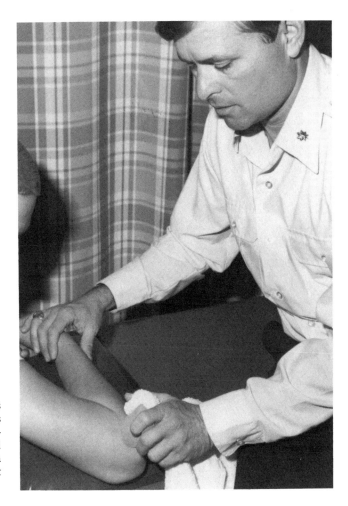

FIGURE 11–2. Cryokinetics in the management of tennis elbow. Ice massage is being applied to the area of the lateral epicondyle to be followed by a slow, gentle stretch of the wrist extensor muscles.

usually necessary to achieve the required analgesia (Fig. 11–2). Unlike the potential dangers involved when pain-alleviating pharmaceutical agents are injected to enable the patient to perform exercises, the use of cryokinetics has a built-in safety valve. Although the clinical application of cold produces a degree of analgesia, judicious application is generally not enough to completely anesthetize the involved tissue. If an athlete is experiencing pain during analgesia of the injured part when exercising, it indicates to the practitioner that the patient is exercising too vigorously. In order to avoid pain during exercise, the patient's activity level should be decreased.

Cryokinetics is easily performed under proper instruction and supervision. Initially, cold is used to numb the injured part by applying ice massage, ice packs, immersion baths, or towels soaked in ice water (Fig. 11–3). If the therapist or trainer chooses to use an immersion bath, a technique sometimes employed for injuries of the distal joints, the duration of treatment should not exceed 15 minutes, and the clinician should ensure that the patient has an intact peripheral circulation. An extremity's prolonged exposure to cold has been reported to result in nerve palsies.[29]

Because use of cold can be a valuable tool in the early management of rehabilitation of the injured athlete, it is important that the therapist or trainer knows the specific

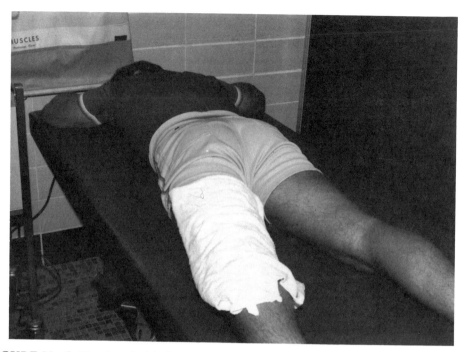

FIGURE 11–3. Towel soaked in ice water is applied along the length of the hamstrings. This will be followed by a hamstring stretch in a long sit or supine position.

effects cold has on the body, when to use this agent, where to apply it, and how it can help in the rehabilitation process. Tables 11–1, 11–2, and 11–3 provide the reader with the basic guidelines for the application of thermal agents in three common sports-related injuries. These should serve as guidelines only and not as cookbook formulas.

HEAT

The effects of heat on circulation, metabolism, and neural activity must be taken into account when beginning a new phase of rehabilitation. Heat improves capillary flow and increases the fluid quantity of tissues by speeding the blood flow and dilating the vessels in the heated areas. As a result, metabolism of heated parts is increased, hastening chemical changes and diminishing congestion brought about by the inflammatory process. Heat may reduce muscle spasm by increasing the threshold of sensory endings or altering gamma motoneuron activity (see Chapter 5); hence, it is a pain-relieving modality. To help the therapist decide when it is safe to apply heat to the injured athlete, certain criteria should be met. There should have been no increase in swelling of the affected part within the prior 24 hours, and there should be minimal point tenderness, with no severe aching of the body part. If heat is applied too soon after an injury, inflammation and extravasation of blood from vessels and synovial fluid may be exacerbated.

TABLE 11-1. Therapeutic Guidelines for the Application of Cold
and Heat in the Management of Ankle Sprains

Conditions	Management Phase	Basic Management	Combination Treatment	Objectives of Treatment
Inversion Ankle sprain (grade 2-3)	Phase 1: Immediate 0-72 hr	Cold Ice pack 15-30 min Whirlpool 12-20 min (13° to 21°C) Ice towels 15-30 min	Compression Constant Intermittent HVPC stimulation	Reduce swelling and pain
	Phase 2: Subacute 72-96 hours	Cold Cryokinetics 7-10 min ice massage Whirlpool (13°-21°C) Heat (edema controlled) Whirlpool 15-20 min (35.5°-38°C) Hot pack × 15-20 min Ultrasound (dosage dependent) continuous Phonophoresis	Passive/active exercising Same as above Mobilization	Improve mobility; Increase blood flow Same as above Selective heating of joint structures Tissue repair; Induce medication to injury site
	Phase 3	Heat Whirlpool 12-20 min (37°-39°C) Ultrasound (dosage dependent)	Isokinetic cycle Preprogram jogging Friction massage to fibular collateral ligament	Strengthening Improve blood flow Reduction of adhesions or scarring

Techniques of Heat Application

The method of heat application is usually predicated on convenience of application, availability of method, and the depth of absorption. In most training rooms, heat is usually administered by either hydrocollator packs, hydrotherapy, or ultrasound. Hydrotherapy is the most frequently used modality in treating postacute sprains, strains, and contusions. When choosing a therapeutic temperature, the therapist must take into account the disadvantages of, and the precautions necessary when using, whirlpools. Studies have shown that topically applied wet heat to raise superficial tissue tempera-

TABLE 11–2. Therapeutic Guidelines for the Application of Cold
and Heat in the Management of Thigh Contusions (Charley Horse)

Conditions	Management Phase	Basic Management	Combination Treatment	Objectives of Treatment
Thigh Contusion (Charley Horse, grade 2–3)	Immediate 0–48 hr	Cold Ice pack 15–30 min Cool whirlpool 10 min (13°–21°C)	Elevation crutches Compression wrap Rest HVPC stimulation	Control hemorrhaging Reduce muscle spasms and pain
	Subacute 48 (variable) hr	Cryokinetics 10 min ice massage to injury site Ice pack 15–20 min	Isometric exercise; passive ROM to tolerance Electrical stimulation; exercise	Improve blood flow; mobility; strengthening Muscle re-education; reduce stasis
	Phase 3 Injury site stabilized or chronic	Heat Whirlpool (38°–39°C) Ultrasound (dosage-dependent)	Isokinetic cycle; Pre-program Passive stretching	Strengthening injury site; improve blood flow Heat deeper tissues; clot reabsorption

tures is best produced when temperatures between 37°C and 43°C are obtained.[31] Therefore, water should be within these temperature ranges, using variances that take into account the amount of edema and patient sensitivity. Researchers have found that whirlpool baths at temperatures between 40.5°C and 41.6°C produce up to 140 ml of increased volume in extremities.[32] Consequently, whirlpool baths at high temperatures are contraindicated in cases when edema is a potential problem.

The practice of full-body immersion for treating extremities at high temperature should be avoided. Two serious problems can result from this technique. As blood vessels throughout the body dilate, blood is drawn away from the parts not submerged. The change in blood pressure can result in the person fainting. Also, there is danger of the athlete suffering from heat exposure, since the body's surface is surrounded by water that is warmer than normal body temperature. Heat may not be able to dissipate from the body through evaporation or radiation. Special care should be taken by the trainer to avoid full-body immersion of an athlete who has just completed vigorous exercising. A proper cool-down is first necessary to dissipate the internal body heat that has resulted from exercise.

The clinical application and guidelines for administration of ultrasound and hot packs have already been discussed in previous chapters. The literature involving control studies using these modalities among the athletic population is sparse. The significance of what is reported, however, can be applied to the population. Ultrasound is commonly used by therapists and trainers as an adjunct in the management of soft-tissue injuries.[4,6]

The technique of delivering anti-inflammatory drugs by ultrasound (phonophoresis) (Figs. 11–4 and 11–5) is becoming increasingly popular among practitioners.

TABLE 11–3. Therapeutic Guidelines for the Application of Cold
and Heat in the Management of Achilles Tendonitis

Conditions	Management Phase	Basic Management	Combination Treatment	Objectives of Treatment
Achilles tendinitis	Swelling and redness present	Cold Ice pack 15–30 min Cool whirlpool 10 min (13°–21°C)	Crutches 1/4 inch heel lift HVPC 15–30 min	Reduce swelling; pain reduction
	Gradual onset: Crepitation; pain Present	Cryokinetics 5–10 min ice massage	Nonweight bearing Heel cord stretching; temporary orthotic 1/4 in heel lift	Increase blood flow Mobility Biomechanical control
	Phase 3 Pain intermittent Edema not present	Ultrasound (dosage dependent) Heat Whirlpool 10–15 min (37°–79°C)	Phonophoresis, active exercising, and flexibility program; consider permanent orthotic control	Induce medication Increase blood flow Biomechanical control if necessary
	Chronic (>3 wk) Intermittent pain with excessive activities	Ultrasound (continuous) before friction massage or Ice massage, ice pack, or whirlpool	Friction massage to Achilles tendon	Heat tissues Reduce adhesions Reduce irritation after massage

Kleinkort and Wood[33] have reported its effectiveness using hydrocortisone administered by ultrasound in treating certain types of tendinitis of the elbow and the Achilles tendon.

Smith and coworkers,[34] comparing phonophoresis with other modes of treatment —ice and iontophoresis—in treating shinsplint syndrome, found it to be an effective treatment mode for pain control, but not significantly superior to the other treatment regimens.

When using this procedure in treating joint and tendon dysfunction, one must take into account the stage of inflammation. After considering the physiologic effects of continuous wave ultrasound in elevating tissue temperature and increasing the possibility of edema, phonophoresis may have its greatest value in treating subacute and chronic conditions rather than acute conditions. Depth of penetration, which may be up to 6 centimeters, and anatomic positioning are also factors to keep in mind when using phonophoretic treatments. Intensities between 1.0 and 1.5 W/cm^2 for a 5-minute

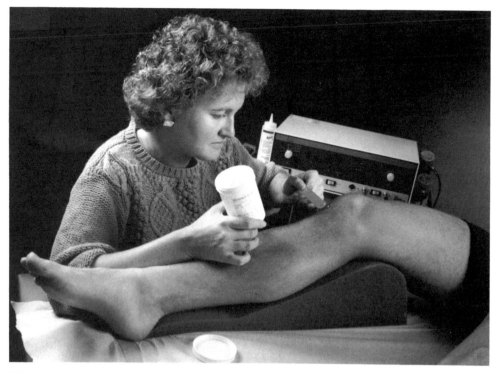

FIGURE 11–4. Preparing for a phonophoresis treatment. Massaging a 10 percent solution of hydrocortisone ointment into the skin overlying the patellar tendon. This will be followed by ultrasound.

duration appear to have commonly been used. Conditions such as subdeltoid bursitis may be difficult to treat using phonophoresis, due perhaps to the excessive amount of tissue the drug must pass through to reach the inflamed area.

Plantar fasciitis, a common occurrence in runners, appears to respond to the therapeutic application of ultrasound. Clark and Stenner[35] studied the effects of ultrasound among patients who were diagnosed for plantar fasciitis. Of the 10 patients treated, 8 reported they felt improvement after nine applications of 15 to 20 minutes of 1.5 W/cm^2 continuous ultrasound. Kleinkort and Wood,[33] on the other hand, reported poor results after six phonophoretic treatments. They postulated that thickened epidermis may have hampered delivery of the hydrocortisone to significant levels. The success of the Clark and Stenner[35] study may have been attributed to the thermal effect of ultrasound, that is, blood flow and tissue metabolism.

Ultrasound is often used to facilitate the healing of soft-tissue structures during the post-traumatic period or postsurgical period. Frieden and associates[36] studied the therapeutic effects of ultrasound following partial rupture of Achilles tendon in male rats. Through the use of electron microscopic analysis, ultrastructural changes within the treatment group were consonant with those changes that would occur in a more advanced stage of healing.

However, the intensity applied by the therapist must be a consideration. Histologic studies using ultrasound on traumatized tissues (hematomas) indicate that intensities of 1.5 W/cm^2 or greater were needed to effect the healing process.[37] Heat can be of value to the patient when it is used to warm connective tissue that has been scarred following

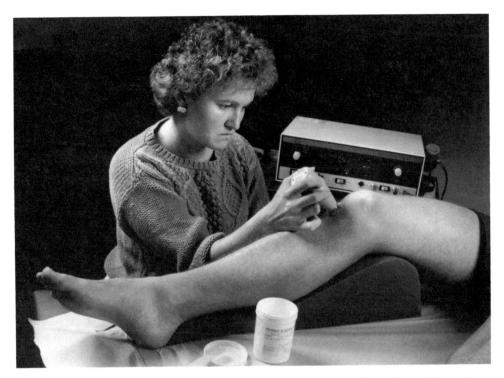

FIGURE 11–5. Phonophoresis (driving in medication by ultrasound) to the patellar tendon in the management of tendinitis.

injury or surgery. Strains involving the tearing of either muscle or connective tissue are a common occurrence among athletes. The cellular response by the body is to produce fibroblasts which, in turn, leads to the production of collagen. Injury and subsequent immobilization can affect movement of tissues, causing joint stiffness. Studies have shown that, under heated conditions, the viscous properties of collagenous tissue can become altered, allowing residual elongation of this tissue when combined with a superimposed load. Sapega and coworkers[38] have suggested that prolonged low-intensity stretching at elevated temperatures and maintaining that stretch while the tissues cool can be effective in gaining range of motion. Lengthening of connective tissue is maximized, while the deterioration of tensile strength by heating prior to stretching is minimized.

CASE STUDY

Case Study 2

A treatment plan that used cold and heat is illustrated in case study 2.

A 23-year-old female distance runner developed left Achilles peritendinitis while participating in a 6-mile run. She was initially treated with ice and high voltage pulsed current and given a ¼-inch heel lift for a period of 72 hours, at which time swelling and pain subsided. She continued to have intermittent discomfort, however, 5 days postinjury. Physical examination revealed tightness in the gastrocnemius-soleus muscle complex with mild crepitation within the Achilles tendon. Rehabilitation of the gastrocnemius-soleus muscle tendon unit consisted of flexibility exercises and 6 minutes of 1.5 W/cm² continuous ultrasound to the Achilles tendon, followed by 5 minutes of friction massage to alleviate scar tissue. The patient was able to resume activities 3 weeks after onset of the initial injury.

SUMMARY

The implications for using heat and cold among athletes have been reviewed. Cold appears to be effective in reducing swelling and managing the inflammatory process. It is also an effective pain-controlling modality when combined with exercise. Heat is still a universal treatment for pain after the acute stage of injury. It has many beneficial physiologic effects that the practitioner must take into account when beginning a new phase of rehabilitation.

REFERENCES

1. Kraus, H: Evaluation and treatment of muscle function in athletic injury. Am J Surg 98:353, 1959.
2. Esterson, P, Knortz, K, and Wallace, L: Immediate care of ankle injuries. Journal of Orthopaedic and Sports Physical Therapy 1:46, 1979.
3. Knight, K: Ice for immediate care of injuries. Physician Sports Medicine 10:137, 1982.
4. Knight, K: Cryotherapy Theory, Technique and Physiology, ed 1. Chattanooga Corporation, Chattanooga, TN, 1985.
5. Millar, A: Strains of the posterior calf musculature (tennis leg). Am J Sports Med 7:172, 1979.
6. Moore, RJ: Uses of cold therapy in the rehabilitation of athletes: Recent advances. Presented at 19th AMA National Conference on the Medical Aspects of Sports, San Francisco, June 18, 1977.
7. Novich, M: Physical therapy in treatment of athletic injuries. Tex State J Med 61:672, 1965.
8. Wise, D: Physiotherapeutic treatment of athletic injuries to muscle-tendon complex of the leg. Can Med Assoc J 8:117, 1977.
9. Grant, AE: Massage with ice (cryokinetics) in the treatment of painful conditions of the musculoskeletal system. Arch Phys Med Rehabil 45:233, 1964.
10. Hayden, CA: Cryokinetics in early treatment program. Am J Phys Ther 44:990, 1964.
11. Knight, K: Cryostretch for muscle spasm. Physician and Sports Medicine 4:129, 1980.
12. Bennett, D: Water at 67° to 69° to control hemorrhage and swelling encountered in athletic injuries. Journal of National Athletic Trainers Association 1:12, 1961.
13. Lewis, T: Observation upon the reaction of the vessels of the human skin to cold. Heart 15:177, 1930.
14. Moore, RJ, Nicolette, RL, and Behnke, R: The therapeutic use of cold (cryotherapy) in the care of athletic injuries. Journal of National Athletic Trainers Association 6:12, 1967.
15. Aquired, J, et al: A re-examination of Lewis' cold-induced vasodilation in the finger and the ankle. Athletic Training 15:248, 1980.
16. Knight, K and Laodere, RB: Comparison of blood flow in the ankle of uninjured subjects during therapeutic application of heat, cold and exercise. Medicine and Science in Sport and Exercise 12:217, 1980.
17. Hocutt, JE, et al: Cryotherapy in ankle sprains. Am J Sports Med 10:316, 1982.
18. Cote, W, Prentice, W, and Hooker, D: Comparison of three treatment procedures for minimizing ankle sprain swelling. Phy Ther 68:1072, 1988.
19. Brown, S: Ankle edema and galvanic muscle stimulation. Physician and Sports Medicine 9:137, 1981.
20. Lamboni, P and Harris, B: The use of ice, airsplints, and high voltage galvanic stimulation in effusion reduction. Athletic Training 18:23, 1983.
21. Starkey, J: Treatment of ankle sprain by simultaneous use of intermittent compression and ice pack. Am J Sport Med 4:142, 1976.
22. Quillen, WS and Rouillier, LH: Initial management of acute ankle sprains with rapid pulsed pneumatic compression and cold. Journal of Orthopaedic and Sports Physical Therapy 4:39, 1982.
23. Sloan, J, Giddings, P, and Hain, R: Effects of cold and compression on edema. Physician and Sports Medicine 8:116, 1988.
24. Smith, W: High galvanic therapy in the symptomatic management of acute tibial fracture. Athletic Training 16:59, 1981.

25. Michlovitz, S, Smith, W, and Watkins, M: Ice and high voltage pulsed stimulation, a treatment of acute lateral ankle sprain. Journal of Orthopaedics and Sports Physical Therapy 9:301, 1988.
26. Waylonis, GW: The physiological effects of ice massage. Arch Phys Med Rehabil 48:37, 1967.
27. Prentice, WE: An electromyographic analysis of the effectiveness of heat or cold and stretching for inducing relaxation of injured muscle. Journal of Orthopaedic and Sports Physical Therapy 3:133, 1982.
28. Yackzan, L, Adams, C, and Francis, K: The effects of ice massage on delayed muscle soreness. Am J Sports Med 12:159, 1984.
29. Drez, D, Faust, DC, and Evans, JP: Cryotherapy and nerve palsy. Am J Sports Med 2:256, 1981.
30. Stopka, C: Hydrotherapy: Invaluable and now inexpensive. Athletic Trainer 22:219, 1987.
31. Abramson, D, et al: Comparison of wet and dry heat in raising temperature of tissues. Arch Phys Med Rehabil 12:654, 1967.
32. Magness, J, Garrett, T, and Erickson, D: Swelling of the upper extremity during whirlpool baths. Arch Phys Med Rehabil 5:297, 1970.
33. Kleinkort, J and Wood, F: Phonophoresis with one percent versus ten percent hydrocortisone. Phys Ther 55:1321, 1975.
34. Smith, W, Winn, F, and Parrette, R: Comparative study using four modalities as shin splint treatments. Journal of Orthopaedic and Sports Physical Therapy 8:77, 1986.
35. Clark, GR and Stenner, L: Use of therapeutic ultrasound. Physiotherapy 62:185, 1976.
36. Frieden, S, et al: A pilot study: The therapeutic effects of ultrasound following partial rupture of Achilles tendons. Journal of Orthopaedics and Sports Physical Therapy 10:39, 1988.
37. Stratton, SA, Heckman, R, and Francis, RS: Therapeutic ultrasound: Its effects on the integrity of a non-penetrating wound. Journal of Orthopedic and Sports Physical Therapy 5:278, 1984.
38. Sapega, A, et al: Biophysical factors in range of motion exercise. Physician and Sports Medicine 9:57, 1981.

CHAPTER 12

The Use of Heat and Cold in the Management of Rheumatic Diseases

Susan L. Michlovitz, M.S., P.T.

A well-planned therapy program is an integral part of the comprehensive management of the patient with rheumatic disease. The overall objective of physical therapy is to improve or maintain the patient's level of function.

The physical therapy evaluation serves as a foundation from which a treatment program can be designed. In developing treatment goals, it is important to assess pain (at rest and on activity), range of motion (ROM), muscle strength, posture, gait, and functional status (such as stair climbing, activities of daily living, occupational demands). The component parts of a treatment plan are developed from short- and long-term goals and can include techniques for pain relief, exercises for increasing/maintaining ROM and muscle strength, and cardiovascular conditioning. Assistive and adaptive devices may be required to improve gait and functional activities. An important aspect of treatment, patient education, should include joint protection and energy-conservation techniques.

Physical agents, including electrical stimulation, heat, and cold can be used as an adjunct to provide pain relief before exercise or positioning, decrease muscle-guarding spasm, improve ROM, or facilitate muscle re-education. In most cases, it is important to emphasize that the use of a physical agent is only an adjunct in the total treatment plan and may only help reach short-term goal. Most important to consider is that the patient with arthritis has a chronic disease often associated with exacerbations and remissions and unrelenting pain.

The purposes of this chapter are to: (1) Discuss the role of thermal agents in the total treatment strategy; (2) review previous work that has used heat or cold agents as an adjunct in the management of arthritis; and, (3) suggest guidelines for application of these agents and evaluation of treatment outcome.

GENERAL CONSIDERATIONS

All of the thermal agents have been incorporated at some point in the various treatment regimens for arthritis management. The decision of which agent to use in which situation is not always clear. Certain basic questions come to the forefront. Should a superficial or a deep-heating agent be applied? Is heat or cold the more effective in treating the arthritis patient? Will cold increase stiffness in persons with arthritis? Will deep heat accelerate the destruction of joint structures in the patient with inflammatory arthritis? As will become evident in the forthcoming review and discussion, some of these questions have been partially or fully answered. Others still require further investigation.

The choice of when to apply a thermal agent and which to use is dependent on a number of factors, including some of the following:

1. *Inflammatory versus noninflammatory polyarthritis.* As an example, if the goal of medical treatment of rheumatoid arthritis is to reduce joint inflammation and temperature, it may be best to choose a physical agent that will alter only skin and subcutaneous tissue temperature (such as hot packs or cold packs). These will provide pain relief and relaxation through reflex mechanisms and counterirritation, rather than a deep-heating agent (such as continuous wave ultrasound or diathermy), which has the potential to increase joint temperature and inflammation. In the case of osteoarthritis, when muscle-guarding spasm or joint contracture is present, heating can usually be more aggressive.

2. *Acute versus chronic inflammation.* When a joint is actually inflamed (hot and swollen), heat application may exacerbate symptoms. During this time, cold application or electrical stimulation can be effective in reducing pain and inflammation. Cold also can be effective during the chronic stages of rheumatoid arthritis to provide pain relief before exercise (see subsequent section on rheumatoid arthritis).

3. *Loss of range of motion.* The origin of the limitation in motion must be delineated. If joint capsular shortening or musculotendinous contracture are limiting mobility, deep heat in combination with a slow, gentle stretch can be more effective than heat or stretch used in isolation. If the patient can tolerate cold application, simultaneous use of cold and low-load stretch may produce desired results. This technique should be used with caution, because cold analgesia before exercise may mask both pain and potential damage to soft tissue. If the joint space is reduced, then the techniques to increase ROM will be less successful.

4. *Position for treatment.* The patient should be discouraged from sitting while receiving a thermal agent to the trunk, hips, or knees. This is particularly important to stress with the patient who has inflammatory arthritis. This patient will have a tendency to develop flexion contractures, which will be facilitated with the patient in the seated position. Joints should be positioned so pain is not markedly increased. If one of the goals of treatment is to decrease pain, the therapy administered should not increase pain. A sharp, aggravating pain must be differentiated from a more subdued aching of short duration (less than 2 hours), which can be expected when performing exercise or positioning to maintain or increase ROM.

5. *Numbers of joints involved.* With multiple joint involvement, the use of some of the thermal agents may be impractical. For example, application of hot packs to more than four joints can be cumbersome. In this instance, hydrotherapy (especially Hubbard tanks and therapeutic pools) can assist in reducing the effects of gravity and

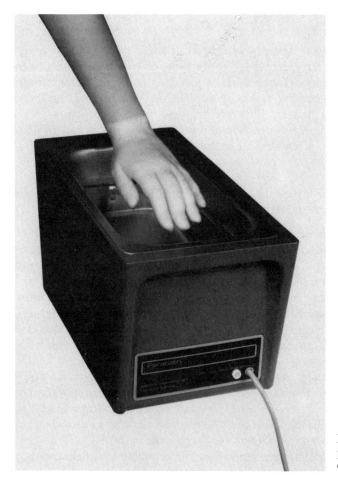

FIGURE 12-1. A home model paraffin unit. (Courtesy of Talcott Laboratories, Houston, PA.)

stress on painful joints, thus promoting ease of motion. In addition, psychologic aspects of pool therapy should not be overlooked.

6. *Clinic versus home care.* If a patient is placed on a home care program, some thermal agents are more practical to use than others. A table-top paraffin unit can be purchased or rented (Fig. 12-1); this is more practical and safe to use than the suggested "home mixtures" that are prepared in a double boiler or crock pot. Electric heating pads should be avoided because of the potential for falling asleep on the pad and producing a burn. If the heating pad has a control that only activates the unit when the person depresses a button then, with careful instruction, it may be safe for home use. There are presently hot packs that can be heated in a microwave oven before use. (Fig. 12-2) Cold packs can be made from ice chips and a plastic bag. Diathermy and ultrasound should be applied only by or under the *direct* supervision of a qualified professional, which precludes their unsupervised application at home by the patient or a family member.

7. *Precaution/Contraindication.* Some medical conditions and patient appliances preclude the choice of many of the thermal agents; thorough evaluation and good clinical judgment can screen for cases when a thermal agent can be potentially harmful. These conditions were discussed in earlier sections of this text, and some will be reiterated later in this chapter.

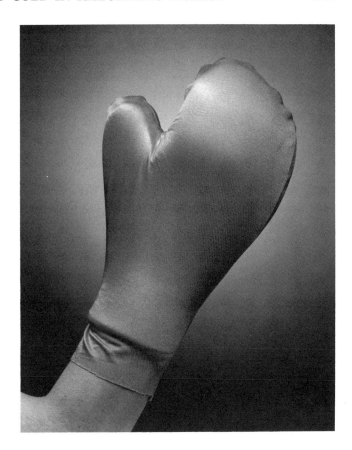

FIGURE 12-2. A heat mitt, which can be heated in a microwave oven. (Courtesy of Southwest Technologies, Inc. Kansas, MO.)

8. *Preconceived notions.* Many patients with arthritis have experienced periods of unrelenting pain and loss of function. They may have been given useful tips by well-meaning neighbors and friends. Many friends and neighbors have offered a myriad of topical salves and home remedies. It is not uncommon to hear a patient say, "Cold is bad for arthritis." Some people with arthritis favorably respond to heat, some to cold. Often the choice is empirically based. Therefore, patient education regarding the disease process and principles and goals of conservative management can be one of the keys to successful therapeutic intervention.

POLYARTICULAR ARTHRITIS: GUIDELINES FOR MANAGEMENT WITH THERMAL AGENTS

Foremost in the therapist's choice of thermal agent usage should be the goals of treatment of the arthritic patient. Short- and long-term goals can be determined after a completed evaluation of the patients' functional status, extent of joint involvement, and pain. Unlike some patients receiving treatment in a physical rehabilitation program (for example, postfracture or tendon repair), the patient with a rheumatic disease most likely will have chronic problems. Patients must be well educated about their disease, functional abilities, and limitations. These patients, more likely than not, will return for treatment more than once. Patients will be done a disservice if a hot or cold agent is

TABLE 12 – 1. Features of Inflammatory and Degenerative Arthritis

Findings	Degenerative Arthritis (Osteoarthritis)	Inflammatory Arthritis (Rheumatoid Arthritis)
Joints commonly involved		

Findings	Degenerative Arthritis (Osteoarthritis)	Inflammatory Arthritis (Rheumatoid Arthritis)
Joint swelling	Uncommon	Common
Morning stiffness	Minimal	Often greater than 1 hr
Joint changes	Osteophytes	Pannus (synovial membrane proliferation)
Sedimentation rate	Normal or minimally elevated	Elevated
Additional Findings	Heberden's and Bouchard's nodes	Rheumatoid nodules Baker's cysts Vasculitis Osteoporosis Peripheral sensory deficit

*Adapted from Katz.[1]

given without providing them with information and instructions about long-term management.

Successful therapeutic management of arthritis is difficult to achieve and assess. The more than 100 rheumatic diseases are not all managed in the same way. For the purpose of discussion in this chapter, two different categories of polyarticular arthritis will be considered—disorders associated with systemic disease and inflammation (for example, rheumatoid arthritis) and disorders primarily associated with joint degeneration (for example, osteoarthritis with some localized inflammation). Refer to Table 12–1 for an overview of disease characteristics. The application of thermal agents for each of the two categories will be reviewed separately.

Rheumatoid Arthritis

Rheumatoid arthritis (RA) is a systemic disorder of unknown etiology characterized by articular inflammation.[1,2] Often there is a natural course of exacerbations and remissions. The synovial lining cells hypertrophy, forming a vascularized granulation tissue (pannus). Digestants in the synovial fluid and pannus destroy periarticular tissue and articular surfaces. Pannus causes periarticular adhesions as well as weakening of capsular and ligamentous structures. The end result can be hypermobility or hypermobility and deformity. As a result of inflammation, joint temperature is elevated.[3] Treatment, including medication, splinting, and thermal agents, is aimed at reducing pain and inflammation, and exercise is also important for preserving ROM and muscle strength.

Other dysfunctions associated with RA include, but are not limited to, osteoporosis, bursitis, tendinitis, skin breakdown, rheumatoid nodules, and arteritis.

HEAT

The stage of the disease process, particularly with inflammatory arthritis, must be taken into account. A patient with rheumatoid arthritis who has an acutely inflamed joint may find his or her symptoms further exacerbated by heat application. During this time, the application of ice packs may aid in reducing pain and inflammation. If the disease process is in the subacute stage, superficial heat or cold may be equally effective in reducing discomfort and in ultimately improving function.

Superficial heating agents are probably the most commonly applied of the thermal agents for persons with RA. The patient will usually report temporary relief of or decrease in pain following such application. Patients can be instructed in the use of hot packs and paraffin for home use allowing carryover from the hospital or clinic setting.

The majority of studies that investigated superficial heat application measured the effects of an agent on the hands of patients with rheumatoid arthritis (Table 12–2). Harris and Millard[4] reported a slight increase in pain, tenderness, and swelling, and an increase in grip strength, following daily paraffin applied to patients with RA. The treatment was given at a temperature of 44°C for a duration of 6 weeks. The results of treatment were not considered to be statistically significant. When they applied paraffin daily for 3 weeks, no different was found between treated and untreated groups. Gallagher and associates[5] conducted a study in which the control group was given active range-of-motion (AROM) exercises, while the test group received both paraffin and AROM exercises daily for 10 days. There was no significant difference found between the control and test groups when strength, AROM, pain, stiffness, and functional dexterity were measured. The results of both experiments would suggest that paraffin is of little value in the final outcome when applied for a few weeks or less. Paraffin treatment continues to be one of the most widely recommended[1,6] and employed thermal agents in the management of rheumatoid arthritis. Although the long-term benefits may not be apparent, clinical experience suggests that heat before exercise will relax and psychologically prepare a patient in pain for exercise.

TABLE 12–2. Heat Application to the Hands of Patients with Rheumatoid Arthritis

Investigator	Thermal Agent and Treatment Protocol	Control	Conclusions
Finsterwald (unpublished)	Paraffin on one hand followed by exercise, 10 days, BID Fluidotherapy on other hand, 43.5°C with exercise while in heat unit, 10 days, BID	None	Preliminary results suggest patients with Fluidotherapy showed greater improvement
Gallagher, Eshlemann, and Schumacher[5]	Paraffin followed by AROM, daily for 10 days	AROM	No significant difference between the groups
Harris and Millard[4]	Paraffin daily for 3 wks; paraffin daily for 6 wks; both groups did exercises	No treatment	No differences among all groups at 3 wks, but group treated for 6 wks was slightly improved at the end of this time
Mainardi and associates[11]	Electric mitten at 40°C, 30 min BID for 2 yr	Opposite hand received no heat	No further changes on x-ray that could be attributed to heat application

The newest thermal agent, Fluidotherapy, is a useful adjunct in the conservative management of a person with arthritis. Exercise can be performed while the hand or foot is within the heated unit. Finsterwald and associates (unpublished data) have compiled information that compares paraffin with Fluidotherapy applied to the hands of persons with rheumatoid arthritis. Paraffin followed by an exercise regimen was used with one of the patient's hands, while the other hand was treated simultaneously with Fluidotherapy at 43.5°C and exercise. Preliminary results suggest that Fluidotherapy provided greater pain relief, increase in strength and ROM, and improvement in functional skills than did paraffin. In this study, no controls were used. It may be difficult to use control subjects in some clinical settings, such as one where a portion of a treatment regimen is denied to patients. Some research protocols are designed to compare and contrast different treatment techniques used in a particular rehabilitation setting with a single patient population.

There are far fewer studies in the literature on the results of deep-heat application to patients with inflammatory arthritis. Soren[7] treated patients with rheumatoid wrists and hips with ultrasound at 2.5 W/cm² for 8 to 10 treatments, 2 to 3 times a week, for a total of 10 to 15 sessions. The findings show that ultrasound produced no improvement in more than 60 percent of the 40 patients studied. Pain appeared to be reduced when ultrasound was given to rheumatoid nodules at an intensity of 1.0 to 2.5 W/cm² for 8 to 10 treatments.[8] No other improvements or changes were noted.

Controversy exists regarding the long-term effects of heat application to persons with inflammatory arthritis.[9] Persons with active rheumatoid arthritis can have elevated joint temperatures up to 37°C.[3] Normal intra-articular temperature is 3°C to 5°C lower. One could consider that further elevating joint temperature with a thermal agent during the period of acute or subacute inflammation may be additive and thus more detrimental to joint structures. Many of the treatments of RA aim to reduce joint temperature by reducing inflammation. Intra-articular corticosteroid administration and splinting of an inflamed joint are examples of two methods that have been used to reduce inflammation within a joint. Concern regarding elevation of joint temperature by a thermal agent in patients with active rheumatoid arthritis probably emerged as a result of studies conducted in the laboratory of Harris and McCroskery.[10] They demonstrated, in an in vitro study, that collagen cartilage lysis by rheumatoid synovial collagenase was four times greater when temperatures of the preparation were elevated to 36°C.

A 2-year study was conducted by Mainardi and associates[11] to investigate the long-term results of daily heat application to the hands of persons with rheumatoid arthritis. Heat was applied to one hand through an electric mitten at 40°C for 30 minutes 2 times a day for 2 years. The other hand of each person served as a control. X-ray examination revealed that no further evidence of joint destruction could be attributed to the heat-treated hands. Therefore, more clinical investigations on the long-term effects of heat therapy to rheumatoid joints seem to be warranted.

HYDROTHERAPY

Hydrotherapy is often recommended for patients with inflammatory and degenerative arthritis for decreasing pain, thus facilitating the ease with which exercises can be performed. An 8-week, biweekly course of hydrotherapy and exercises for patients with rheumatoid arthritis was evaluated by Dial and Windsor.[12] When the patients were evaluated at the end of the program, they demonstrated a significant improvement in ROM and a decrease in time required to perform functional tasks. By 1 month postprogram, the patients tended to return to preprogram status. The long-term benefits of the program appeared to be the psychosocial improvement expressed by the patients. This can be very important in assisting to improve the self-image of the patient with a chronic disability.

Contrast baths have long been used in arthritis and sports rehabilitation. Documentation of the short- and long-term effectiveness of this treatment is lacking. The studies that have appeared in the literature measured the changes in skin temperature produced by contrast baths in normals and in persons with rheumatoid arthritis.[13-15] The skin temperature changes in those with arthritis were less dramatic than were those with no pathology. Although this may provide some insight into the peripheral vascular status of some arthritic patients, any other clinical correlations do not seem to be apparent.

COLD

Cryotherapy has been gaining increased popularity in arthritis treatment during the last 2 decades. Ice packs were applied for 20 minutes 3 times a day for 1 month to the knees of patients with rheumatoid arthritis.[16] An increase in ROM and sleep duration and a decrease in pain (as measured by a visual analog pain scale) and in oral analgesic intake were reported. There were no changes in synovial fluid composition. In this study, one knee was treated with ice, while the other knee had no cold application, thus serving as a comparison. Pegg, Littler, and Littler[17] used 5-minute ice pack applications and exercise daily for 2 weeks in treating the knees and elbows of rheumatoid patients. Stiffness and pain were reduced in most patients, and ROM improved in 50 percent of the patients. When the same investigators changed treatment to immersing patients' hands in cold water (dipping in and out for 10 minutes), the treatment was less effective.

In a small sampling, Wright and Johns[18] and Backlund and Tiselius[19] found that immersion of the hands in a cold bath *increased* the stiffness of finger joints. Studies by Kirk and Kersley,[20] in which cold application to the knees *reduced* stiffness, do not support these findings. In the case of cold application to the knee, the temperature of the joint structures was probably not lowered, whereas cold application to the hand may have lowered the temperature of the joint capsule, thus increasing elastic stiffness. This may account for the differences reported by the investigators. Some patients with inflammatory arthritis will not tolerate cold application, particularly those with cryo-globulinemia and cold hypersensitivity syndromes.[21]

HEAT VERSUS COLD

Heat and cold both seem to be valuable adjuncts in the rehabilitation of persons with rheumatoid arthritis. Logically, the next subject to be addressed is the comparison of heat and cold. Two studies compared ice-pack with hot-pack application to the knees of RA patients. Kirk and Kersley[20] reported that 60 percent of their subjects preferred cold applications. Both groups improved in ROM without one being more statistically significant than the other. All patients were on a standard exercise program. Williams and associates[22] reported no statistically significant differences in pain or ROM when using heat and exercise or cold and exercise in the management of the rheumatoid arthritic shoulder.

Utsinger and associates[23] compared 1 week of ice packs (2 times a day) with 1 week of hot packs (3 times a day) applied to the same patients on alternating weeks. Fifty percent preferred hot packs to cold, and 18 percent had no preference for one over the other. All patients showed improvement in some of the measured variables (sleep duration, pain, timed functional tests). In those patients who preferred cold, naloxone was administered before a subsequent cold application. In most of these patients, after the administration of naloxone, cold was no longer effective in reducing pain. The investigators suggest that cold may be effective in reducing pain by facilitating activation of endorphins.

If the disease process is chronic with no active joint inflammation, and if the patient has soft-tissue tightness secondary to lack of active mobility or to immobilization, a more vigorous approach is suggested. Deep heat in conjunction with a slow, gentle stretch may be most beneficial.[24] Suggestions for patient positioning for stretching are elaborated on in an article by Kottke and associates.[25] Caution must be used in considering a stretch to an unstable joint (such as medial and lateral instability at the knee) or in a patient with osteoporosis. Before attempting stretching or splinting of hypomobile joints, x-ray findings should be reviewed to help the therapist determine if it would be realistic to expect an increase in ROM.

Thermal agents should be used very cautiously in patients with vasculitis or skin ulceration.

Osteoarthritis

Osteoarthritis is characterized by joint cartilage destruction with subsequent osteophyte spur formation at joint margins.[2] Associated synovitis can occur with advanced disease. Acute inflammatory flareups may be induced by trauma. Pain is present on passive motion and during weight-bearing. The course of this disorder appears to be exacerbated by abnormal stresses, such as those caused by obesity, placed on joints (see Table 12–1).

HEAT

In degenerative arthritis, pain and limited ROM, rather than joint inflammation, are the primary problems. Heating, then, may be more vigorous in treating this patient population. Often, the patient with a osteoarthritis will be obese. If this is the case, diathermy, particularly capacitance shortwave diathermy (SWD), may be contraindicated or may be used only with extreme caution.[26] Elderly patients with the disease, women more likely than men, may have osteoporosis. Again, caution should be used when having these patients perform a stretch to increase their ROM; active motion may be a more appropriate choice.

Hot packs are routinely used to relieve the symptoms of pain and muscle spasm in patients with inflammatory and degenerative rheumatic diseases. There is a dearth of literature supporting the effectiveness of such treatment. Hot-pack application was shown to reduce muscle spasm and provide analgesia in patients with neck and shoulder syndromes.[27]

Hamilton and Bywaters[28] compared superficial-heating agents with deep-heating agents in patients with inflammatory and degenerative joint diseases. All patients in the study received each of the four treatments reported, for a duration of 1 month. Although most of the patients showed improvement in stair-walking time, ROM, and strength, no single treatment was shown to be significantly better than any other. The treatments performed included SWD, infrared, paraffin, and cold SWD (as the control group). Each of these agents was incorporated into a complete rehabilitation program. It is interesting to note that patients who received a dose of thermal energy fared no better than did those receiving the control treatment.

If the therapist or physician determines that it may be more advantageous to heat deep structures to accomplish treatment goals (for example, to elevate the temperature of the knee joint capsule structures), then diathermy or continuous-wave ultrasound would be selected as the heating agent. More clinical investigations have been made about the effects of deep heat on osteoarthritis than the effects of deep heat on rheumatoid arthritis.

DePreux[28] administered ultrasound to patients' hips and reported a decrease in pain and an improvement in gait. Ultrasound was delivered at an intensity of 1.5 to 2.0 W/cm^2, 10 minutes per field, for a total of 10 to 20 sessions. Unfortunately, no control group was used against which to compare the efficacy of this treatment. When Aldes and Jadeson[30] administered ultrasound to the cervical and lumbar spines of 311 elderly patients, ROM was improved and pain was reduced in 70 percent of the patients. A sham ultrasound group was compared with the ultrasound-treated group, which received 8 to 12 treatments at an intensity of 1.3 to 11.9 watts for 3 to 10 minutes.

Intra-articular steroid injections, nonsteroidal anti-inflammatory drugs (NSAIDs), and thermal agents have all been used in the management of osteoarthritis of the knee. Wright[31] compared the effects of: (1) a placebo pill (one tablet, 2 times a day); (2) a placebo injection (intra-articular normal saline, a total of four injections over an 8-week period); and, (3) SWD 3 times a week for 6 weeks. Both the group receiving SWD and the group receiving a placebo injection improved waking time, had a decrease in pain, and required fewer oral analgesics. These two groups showed a greater improvement than did those who had taken the placebo pill.

Deep heat in conjunction with exercise has been used to increase ROM in patients with soft-tissue contractures secondary to arthritis. But a decrease in ROM at the knee was reported by Vanharanta[32] following SWD given to rabbits who had "experimentally induced" osteoarthritis. Immobilization of the knee was the model used to produce soft-tissue tightness in the rabbits' knees. SWD applied during an 11-week period was felt by the investigator to have been additive to the effects of immobilization. In this study, no exercise was used in conjunction with the heat treatments. Conversely, Gibson, Winter, and Grahame[32] reported an increase in knee flexion and a decrease in pain when SWD was used in combination with exercise in patients with osteoarthritis of the knee. The treatment was given 3 times a week for 2 weeks.

Many patients with degenerative arthritis often have the same functional limitation of motion (owing to soft-tissue tightness) as do patients with periarthritis, an inflammation of structures around the joint. Therefore, results of treatment of patients with periarthritis could be related to the results of physical management of patients with osteoarthritis. Lehmann and associates,[34] studying patients with periarthritis of the shoulder, reported a greater increase in ROM using ultrasound and exercise than using a combination of microwave diathermy (MWD) and exercise. Both ultrasound and MWD were given daily for 8 days. When Mueller and associates[35] compared sham ultrasound treatment to ultrasound at 2.0 W/cm^2 in a similar group of patients for the same duration of treatment as the study by Lehmann and associates,[34] no difference in function was found between the two groups. Again, these two studies are representative of the conflicting results found in the literature.

HEAT VERSUS COLD

A comparison among the effects of untuned SWD, SWD, and ice on the knees of patients with osteoarthritis, was made by Clark and associates.[36] Each treatment was given 3 times a day for 3 weeks. Most patients showed improvement on evaluation 3 months post-onset of treatment, but those receiving ice showed early progress in pain reduction. Results of this study suggest that cold may be valuable in decreasing pain, thus facilitating the ease with which exercise can be performed. A summary of studies that compare heat with cold can be found in Table 12–3.

FACTORS INFLUENCING THE OUTCOME OF TREATMENT

The results of treatment techniques for persons with rheumatic diseases are varied. A number of factors can obscure the outcome of a particular treatment or combination of therapeutic modalities. The *natural course of the disease*, often associated with spontaneous exacerbations and remissions, has been mentioned earlier in this chapter. Because of the *variable course* of inflammatory arthritis, including its exacerbations and remissions, it may be difficult to claim the effectiveness of one particular treatment modality.

The *stage of the disease* is also important to consider. Decreasing pain and improving functional level may be much more realistic in someone with early RA and minimal x-ray changes than in a patient with severe joint destruction and muscle atrophy.

Concurrent use of medications with physical therapy management or changes in medication can change the patient's response to treatment. For example, numerous NSAIDs are currently in use. Although many of these have similar actions, including reduction of inflammation and pain,[37] a patient may respond more favorably to one than to another. So, if there is a change in the NSAID or other medication taken by the patient during the course of physical therapy, the patient may improve owing to the new medication. If one is not aware of this change in medication, one may be tempted

TABLE 12–3. Summary of Clinical Studies that Compared Heat Versus Cold in Arthritis Management

Investigator	Subjects Treated	Heat Agent	Cold Agent	Control Group	Conclusions
Clarke and associates[36]	Osteoarthritic knees	SWD, t.i.w., 3 wk	Ice packs, t.i.w., 3 wk	Untuned SWD	Patients with cold made better early progress; no long-term (3 mo later) differences among 3 groups
Hamer and Kirk[38]	Frozen shoulders not due to primary joint disease	US at 0.5 W/cm² for 5–8 min; Codman's exercises	Iced towels for 15 min; Codman's exercises	None	Both decreased pain and in conjunction with exercise increased ROM; no significant advantage of one over the over
Kirk and Kersley[20]	Rheumatoid arthritic knees	Hot packs daily for 5 days; standard exercise	Ice packs daily for 5 days; standard exercise	Comparison of hot packs and cold packs alternated for 1 wk at a time	60% preferred cold; ROM improved with both treatments
Utsinger, Bonner, and Hogan[23]	Rheumatoid arthritic knees	Hot packs TID, 1 wk	Ice packs TID, 1 wk	Comparison of hot packs to cold packs on same patient	50% preferred HP; naloxone blocked efficacy of cold
Williams, Harvey and Tannenbaum[22]	Rheumatoid arthritic shoulders	Hot packs, t.i.w. 3 wk	Ice packs (crushed ice), t.i.w., 3 wk	None	Reduction in pain scores in both groups

to attribute the improvement to the physical therapy program. Conversely, a poor response to a change in medication may be erroneously interpreted as a poor response to a program of heat and exercise. It may be difficult to weigh the individual components of a total management program to evaluate the efficacy of each. Patients who are taking pain-relieving medications for their arthritis, or who are recovering from arthritis surgery, may be mildly obtunded as a side effect. Their abilities to participate in their therapy or to provide information about the treatment may be altered.

Pain management in arthritis is particularly difficult to effect and assess. Common methods of pain management used in arthritis therapy include heat, cold, electrotherapy, EMG biofeedback, relaxation and imagery, and medications. If the pain associated with rheumatic diseases were easy to manage, there would not be so many different treatment modes used. The pain associated with arthritis can be chronic. Therefore, psychosocial reactions to pain can compound the physiologic changes.

The variables of pain from patient to patient must be considered. All patients react differently to pain, owing to psychosocial and other factors. This observation may make it more difficult for the therapist or physician to evaluate a patient's pain. Many different methods have been used with patients with arthritis, and with other particular dysfunctions, to assess the effectiveness of a thermal agent (Table 12–4). In addition, an evaluation of patients' functional status and ROM may, or will, give you a better idea of their pain status than will use of only a subjective scale. Therefore, an idea of the pain

TABLE 12–4. Pain Assessment Pre- and Post-Thermal Agent

Investigator	Thermal Agent	Diagnosis	Pain Assessment
Clark and associates[36]	Ice or SWD	Osteoarthritis of knee	Maximal pain score of 17 could be gained by 0 = nil, 1 = slight, 2 = moderate, 3 = severe (pain at rest, with walking, overall pain with other activities); night pain, preventing onset of sleep = 1, occasionally awakening person from a sleep = 1, night pain every night = 2
Hamer and Kirk[38]	Ice or US	Frozen shoulder	Graded on a 5-point scale; 0 = painless, 2, 3 = spontaneous night pain disturbing sleep, 4, 5 = severe distressing night and day pain
Hogan, Lockard, Utsinger (reported by Kangilaski)[16]	Ice Packs	Rheumatoid arthritis (knees)	Visual analogue pain scales (VAPS); sleep duration
Mainardi and associates[11]	Electric mitten (heat)	Rheumatoid arthritis (hands)	Joint tenderness and swelling assessed by same observer: 0 = none, 1 = mild, 2 = moderate, 3 = severe
Williams, Harvey and Tannenbaum[22]	Hot packs or ice packs	Rheumatoid arthritis (shoulders)	McGill pain questionnaire (Parts I and IV)

level and a more objective evaluation of ROM and function can all be used in the total evaluation of treatment efficacy.

Many of the patients with rheumatic diseases that a therapist or physician will see have been through a *multitude of treatments* during the course of their disease. They may be discouraged by the numbers of types of treatments they have undergone. They also may have feelings of *frustration and depression* secondary to the chronic nature of their disorder.

In addition to the patients' having undergone a number of pain-reducing modalities and exercise techniques, the *technique of application* of the particular modalities may have varied. It is important for the therapist to be as thorough as possible when obtaining information about past treatments: How often was the treatment given? If hot packs were given, for example, over what body surface were they applied? Were the hot packs followed by exercise or positioning? Was relief obtained? For how long?

Some patients may come for one treatment, then may fail to keep subsequent appointments. Would you, as a therapist, assume they did not return because they improved? They may not return because they felt their symptoms were exacerbated by the therapy given.

EVALUATION OF TREATMENT RESULTS

Objective measurements are required when assessing the outcome of a rehabilitation program. Subjective impressions by the patient or therapist may be useful in identifying the patients' impression of the treatment but will not be helpful in documentation of the validity of a certain regimen. Three general areas should be assessed — pain, ROM and muscle strength, and functional skills.

An objective measurement of pain is difficult to perform. Some investigators[4,37] have relied on the subjective response of the patient to determine if pain has remained the same, has increased, or has decreased. Others[11] determine pain status by the impression of the evaluator. More useful information can be obtained from other measures such as a visual analog pain scale, McGill pain questionnaire, sleep duration, and expression of pain during different activities (i.e., pain at rest, pain with activity) (see Table 11–2).

The clinical tool available for evaluating range of motion is the goniometer. With the arthritis patient, however, the level of function and ability to perform activities of daily living may not be predictable from goniometric findings. The patient who has a chronic disease such as rheumatoid arthritis most likely will have adapted to that loss of motion by the use of substitute motions and adaptive devices. Muscle strength can be evaluated by a manual muscle test, isokinetic testing, and measurements of grip and pinch strength.

Functional skills can be evaluated by the use of timed functional tests.[5,22,36] Recording the time it takes a patient to walk a designated distance on a level surface or to climb stairs are measures that can be duplicated in subsequent test sessions.

Some of the objective measurements are difficult and unrealistic to perform in a clinical setting. Special techniques have been used in research facilities and clinical laboratories. A list of suggested clinical and laboratory tests can be found in Table 12–5.

Time of evaluation should be documented. Was the treatment applied and the evaluation performed at the same time each day? This would be of particular importance in the patient with rheumatoid arthritis, who would most likely have a decreased

TABLE 12–5. Assessment Techniques Used for Patients with Rheumatic Diseases

Clinical	Research Facility/Laboratory
Amount and frequency of analgesic intake	Gait analysis (using force plates, EMG, high-speed photography)
Duration of morning stiffness	Joint fluid analysis
Goniometric measurements	Sodium clearance
Gait analysis (stride length, step length, step width)	Joint stiffness
Isokinetic testing	
Joint circumference	
Hand grip strength	
Manual muscle test	
Sleep duration	
Timed functional tests	
Visual analog pain scales	
Walking time	

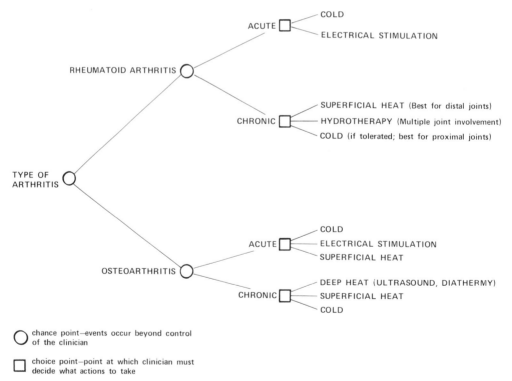

FIGURE 12–3. Clinical decision-making flow chart for application of thermal agents in arthritis. For all cases, the best choice also depends on whether the patient will be using the modality at home. If so, ease of application must be considered. (Courtesy of Bette Ann Harris, M.S., P.T., Boston, MA.)

performance early in the day owing to morning stiffness. The time, dosage, and name of medication intake should be recorded.

SUMMARY

Treating the patient who has a rheumatic disease can be both a rewarding and a challenging experience. Treatment regimens and goals must be tailored to the needs of the patient with a chronic dysfunction. Guidelines for the choice of thermal agent in the patient population with arthritis are outlined in Figure 12–3. The evaluation of short- and long-term efficacy of thermal agents applied to the patient with rheumatic disease seems to require further investigation. The intent of this chapter was to point out problems specific to patients with arthritis, to review studies that have been reported in the literature, and to suggest guidelines for integration of thermal agents into a total treatment program.

REFERENCES

 1. Katz, WA: Rheumatic Diseases: Diagnosis and Management. JB Lippincott, Philadelphia, 1977.
 2. Rodnan, GP and Schumacher, HR (eds): Primer on the Rheumatic Diseases, ed 8. Arthritis Foundation, Atlanta, 1983, p 12.
 3. Hollander, JL and Horvath, SM: Intra-articular temperature as a measure of joint reaction. J Clin Invest 28:469, 1949.
 4. Harris, R and Millard, JB: Paraffin-wax baths in the treatment of rheumatoid arthritis. Ann Rheum Dis 14:278, 1955.
 5. Gallagher, LA, Eshleman, JK, and Schumacher, HR: A controlled study of the effects of paraffin bath on the rheumatoid hand. Presented at Arthritis Health Professionals Meeting at the National Arthritis Foundation Meetings, Atlanta, 1980.
 6. Policoff, LD: Physical medicine and rehabilitation in the management of the arthritic patient. In Katz, WA: Rheumatic Diseases: Diagnosis and Management. JB Lippincott, Philadelphia, 1977.
 7. Soren, A: Evaluation of ultrasound treatment in musculoskeletal disorders. Physiotherapy 51:214, 1965.
 8. Clarke, GR and Stenner, L: Use of therapeutic ultrasound. Physiotherapy 62:185, 1976.
 9. Feibel, A and Fast, A: Deep heating of joints: A reconsideration. Arch Phys Med Rehabil 57:513, 1976.
10. Harris, ED and McCroskery, PA: The influence of temperature and fibril stability on degradation of cartilage collagen by rheumatoid synovial collagenase. N Engl J Med 290:1, 1974.
11. Mainardi, CL, et al: Rheumatoid arthritis: Failure of daily heat therapy to affect its progression. Arch Phys Med Rehabil 60:390, 1979.
12. Dial, CA and Windsor, RA: A pilot study of the impact of a water exercise program for rheumatoid arthritis. Presented at Arthritis Health Professionals Meetings, Arthritis Foundational Annual Conference, Atlanta, 1980.
13. Woodmansey, A, Collins, DH, and Ernst, MM: Vascular reactions to contrast both in health and in rheumatoid arthritis. Lancet 2:1350, 1938.
14. Martin, GM, et al: Cutaneous temperatures of the extremities of normal subjects and of patients with rheumatoid arthritis. Arch Phys Med 27:665, 1946.
15. Fricke, EJ and Gersten, JW: Effect of contrast baths on the vasomotor response of rheumatoid arthritis patients. Arch Phys Med 33:210, 1952.
16. Kangilaski, J: Baggie therapy: Simple relief for arthritic knees. JAMA 247:317, 1981.
17. Pegg, SMH, Littler, TR, and Littler, EN: A trial of ice therapy and exercise in chronic arthritis. Physiotherapy 55:51, 1969.
18. Wright, V and Johns, RJ: Physical factors concerned with the stiffness of normal and diseased joints. Bull Johns Hopkins Hosp 106:215, 1960.
19. Backlund, L and Tiselius, P: Objective measurement of joint stiffness in rheumatoid arthritis. Acta Rheum Scand 13:275, 1967.
20. Kirk, JA and Kersley, GD: Heat and cold in the physical treatment of rheumatoid arthritis of the knee: A controlled clinical trial. Ann Phys Med 9:270, 1968.
21. Ritzmann, SE and Levin, WC: Cryopathies: A review. Arch Intern Med 107:754, 1961.
22. Williams, J, Harvey, J, and Tannebaum, H: Use of superficial heat versus ice for the rheumatoid arthritic shoulder: A pilot study. Physiotherapy Canada 38:8, 1986.

23. Utsinger, PD, Bonner, F, and Hogan, N: Efficacy of cryotherapy and thermotherapy in the mangagement of rheumatoid arthritis pain: Evidence for endorphin effect (abstr). Arth Rheum 25:S113, 1982.
24. Warren, CG, Lehmann, JD, and Koblanski, JN: Heat and stretch procedures: An evaluation using rat tail tendon. Arch Phys Med Rehabil 52:465, 1971.
25. Kottke, FJ, Pauley, DL, and Ptak, RA: The rationale for prolonged stretching for correction of shortening connective tissues. Arch Phys Med Rehabil 47:345, 1966.
26. Lehmann, JD (ed): Therapeutic Heat and Cold. Williams & Wilkins, Baltimore, 1982.
27. Cordray, YN and Kruen, EM: Use of hydrocollator packs in the treatment of neck and shoulder pains. Arch Phys Med Rehabil 39:105, 1959.
28. Hamilton, DE and Bywaters, EGL: A controlled trial of various forms of physiotherapy in arthritis. Br Med J 1:542, 1959.
29. DePreux, T: Ultrasonic wave therapy in osteoarthritis of the hip joint. Br J Phys Med 15:14, 1952.
30. Aldes, JH and Jadeson, WJ: Ultrasonic therapy in the treatment of hypertrophic arthritis in elderly patients. Ann W Med Surg 6:525, 1952.
31. Wright, V: Treatment of osteoarthritis of the knees. Ann Rheum Dis 23:389, 1964.
32. Vanharanta, H: Effect of shortwave diathermy on mobility and radiologic stage of the knee in the development of experimental osteoarthritis. Am J Phys Med 61:59, 1982.
33. Gibson, T, Winter, PJ, and Grahame, R: Radiotherapy in the treatment of osteoarthritis of the knee. Rheumatol Rehabil 12:42, 1973.
34. Lehmann, JF, et al: Comparison of ultrasonic and microwave diathermy in the physical treatment of periarthritis of the shoulder. Arch Phys Med Rehabil 35:627, 1954.
35. Mueller, EE, et al: A placebo-controlled study of ultrasound treatment for periarthritis. Am J Phys Med 33:31, 1954.
36. Clarke, GR, et al: Evaluation of physiotherapy in the treatment of osteoarthrosis of the knee. Rheum Rehabil 13:190, 1974.
37. Melvin, JL: Rheumatic Disease: Occupational Therapy and Rehabilitation, ed 2. FA Davis, Philadelphia, 1982.
38. Hamer, J and Kirk, JA: Physiotherapy and the frozen shoulder: A comparative trial of ice and ultrasonic therapy. NZ Med J 83:191, 1976.

Glossary

Absorption: The taking up by the body of radiant heat, causing a rise in tissue temperature.

Acute pain: A short, sharp, cutting pain. Usually associated with acute inflammation or inflammation of serous membranes; also posterior spinal-root pains.

Adhesion: 1. A holding together or uniting of two surfaces or parts, as in wound healing. 2. A fibrous band holding parts together that are normally separated.

Aeration: 1. Act of airing. 2. Saturation or charging of a fluid with gases.

Afterdischarge: The discharge of impulses from a reflex center after stimulation of the receptor has ceased. Results in prolongation of response.

Alternating current: Abbr: A.C. An electric current that reverses direction at regular intervals.

Analgesia: Absence of normal sense of pain.

Anastomosis: 1. A natural communication between two vessels; may be direct or by means of connecting channels. 2. The surgical or pathologic connection of two tubular structures.

Anesthesia: Partial or complete loss of sensation, with or without loss of consciousness, as result of disease, injury, or administration of an anesthetic agent, usually by injection or inhalation.

Anoxia: Without oxygen. Term is often used incorrectly to indicate hypoxia.

Antidromic: Denoting nerve impulses traveling in the opposite direction from normal.

Arachidonic acid: A precursor of prostaglandin. It is metabolized in the body to produce a group of chemicals called eicosanoids. Included in these are prostaglandin, thromboxane, and leukotrienes. Synthesis of prostaglandin and thromboxane is directly inhibited by nonsteroidal anti-inflammatory agents such as salicylates, indomethacin, and ibuprofen.

Arteriovenous (A-V) anastomosis: Anastomosis between an artery and a vein by which the capillary bed is bypassed.

Atrophy: 1. A wasting; a decrease in size of an organ or tissue. 2. To undergo or cause atrophy. Etiol: May result from death and resorption of cells, diminished cellular proliferation, pressure, ischemia, malnutrition, decreased activity, or hormonal changes.

Attenuation: 1. The change (decrease) in a beam of radiation as it passes through matter. 2. In acoustics, the reduction in sound intensity of the initial sound source as compared with the sound intensity at a point away from the source.

Axonotmesis: Nerve injury that damages the nerve tissue without actually severing the nerve.

Axon reflex: A reflex that does not involve a complete reflex arc, hence is not a true reflex. The afferent and efferent limbs of the reflex are branches of a single nerve fiber, the axon (axon-like dendrite) of a sensory neuron. An example is vasodilation resulting from stimulation of skin.

Bactericidal agent: Destructive to, or destroying, bacteria.

Bradykinin: A plasma kinin. See: kinin.

Buoyancy: The upward pressure exerted by the fluid in which an object is immersed.

Bursa: A pad-like sac or cavity found in connecting tissue, usually in the vicinity of joints. It is lined with synovial membrane and contains a fluid, synovia, that acts to reduce friction between tendon and bone, tendon and ligament, or between other structures where friction is likely to occur.

Bursitis: Inflammation of a bursa, especially those located between bony prominences and muscle tendon, as the shoulder and knee.

Calibration: Determination of the accuracy of an instrument by comparing the information or measurement provided with that of a known standard or an instrument known to be accurate.

Capacitance: 1. State of being able to store electric charge. 2. Ratio of the charge transferred from one to the other of a pair of conductors to the potential difference between the conductors.

Capacitor: Electronic device for storing electric charges.

Cavitation: The vibrational effect on gas bubbles by an ultrasound beam.

Chemotaxis: Movement of cells in response to a chemical stimulus or message; for example, the movement of neutrophils to the site of injury or inflammation.

Chlorination: Treatment of water by addition of chlorine and its compounds for the killing of bacteria. For effective disinfection, a concentration of 0.5 to 1 part chlorine per million parts of water is necessary.

Chondroblast: A cell that forms cartilage.

Chronic pain: The persistance of pain beyond the usual or expected course of an acute disease, or after a reasonable amount of time for an injury to heal has elapsed.

Clonus: Spasmodic alternation of muscular contraction and relaxation.

Collagen: A fibrous insoluble protein found in the connective tissue, including skin, bone, ligaments, and cartilage. Collagen represents about 30 percent of the total body protein.

Collimation: The process of making parallel.

Complement: A series of enzymatic proteins in normal serum that, in the presence of a specific sensitizer, destroy bacteria and other cells. Complement components and complement regulators include at least two dozen substances. Once activated, the components are involved in a great number of immune defense mechanisms, including anaphylaxis, leukocyte chemotaxis, and phagocytosis.

Compliance: Cooperative performance in relation to prescribed therapy or medicines.

Condensation: Making more dense or compact.

Conductance: The conducting ability of a body or a circuit for electricity. The best conductor is one that offers the least resistance, such as gold, silver, and copper. When expressed as a numerical value, conductance is the reciprocal of resistance. The unit is the mho.

Conduction: 1. The process whereby a state of excitation affects successive portions of a tissue or cell, so that the disturbance is transmitted to remote points. Conduction occurs not only in fibers of the nervous system but also in muscle fibers. 2. The transfer of electrons, ions, heat, or sound waves through a conductor or conducting medium.

Conductor: Medium transmitting a force, a signal, or electricity. (Examples: aluminum and copper.)

Connective tissue: Tissue that supports and connects other tissues and tissue parts. The cells of connective tissue are comparatively few in number, the bulk of the tissue consisting of intercellular substance or matrix, the nature of which gives each type of connective tissue its particular properties. Connective tissues are highly vascular, with the exception of cartilage. Connective tissue proper includes the following types: mucous, fibrous (areolar, white fibrous, yellow fibrous, or elastic), reticular, and adipose. Dense connective tissue includes cartilage and bone (osseous tissue).

Consensual: Reflex stimulation of one part or side as a result of excitation of another part or opposite side.

Consensual response: Any reflex occurring on opposite side of body from point of stimulation.

Contraction: A shortening or tightening, as that of a muscle, or a reduction in size; a shrinking.

Contracture: 1. A condition of fixed high resistance to the passive stretch of a muscle, as may result from fibrosis of tissues surrounding a joint. 2. Permanent contraction of a muscle due to spasm or paralysis.

Contusion: An injury in which the skin is not broken; a bruise.

Convection: The transfer of heat by means of currents in liquids or gases.

Convergence: In reflex activity, the coming together of several axons or afferent fibers upon one or a few motor neurons; the condition whereby impulses from several sensory receptors converge upon the same motor center, resulting in a limited and specific response.

Cryoglobulinemia: Presence in the blood of an abnormal protein that forms gels at low temperatures. Found in association with pathologic conditions such as multiple myeloma, leukemia, and certain forms of pneumonia.

Cryotherapy: The therapeutic use of cold.

Debridement: The removal of foreign material and dead or damaged tissue, especially in a wound.

    d., enzymatic. Use of proteolytic enzymes to remove dead tissue from a wound. The enzyme does not attack viable tissues.

Decubitus ulcer: Ischemic necrosis and ulceration of tissue, especially over a bony prominence. Due to pressure from prolonged confinement in bed or from a cast or splint.

Diathermy: The therapeutic use of a high-frequency current to generate heat within some part of the body. The frequency is greater than the maximal frequency for neuromuscular response and ranges from several hundred thousand to millions of cycles per second.

Dielectric: An insulating substance offering great resistance to passage of electricity by conduction.

Diffraction: The change that occurs in light when it passes through crystals, prisms, or parallel bars in a grating, in which the rays are deflected and, thus, appear to be turned aside. This produces dark or colored bands or lines or other phenomena. Term is also applied to similar phenomena in sound and electricity.

Dipole: 1. Two equal and opposite charges separated by a distance. 2. In chemistry, one portion of the molecule has a certain charge, and the other portion has an equal and opposite charge.

Direct current: Abbr: DC or dc. An electric current flowing continuously in one direction.

Diuresis: Secretion and passage of large amounts of urine. This condition occurs in diabetes mellitus. It can be an early sign of chronic interstitial nephritis. May also be due to hysteria, result of fear and anxiety, ingestion of large quantities of liquids, diabetes insipidus, or the action of drugs that have the ability to cause diuresis.

Dorsal rhizotomy (posterior rhizotomy): Section of the dorsal root of the spinal nerve for relief of pain.

Edema: A local or generalized condition in which the body tissues contain an excessive amount of tissue fluid.

Effusion: Escape of fluid into a part.

Elasticity: The quality of returning to original size and shape after compression or stretching.

Elastin: An extracellular connective-tissue protein that is the principal component of elastic fibers.

Electrode: A medium intervening between an electric conductor and the object to which the current is to be applied. In electrotherapy, an electrode is an instrument with a point or a surface from which to discharge current to the body of a patient.

Electromotive force: Abbr: EMF. Energy that causes flow of electricity in a conductor. The energy is measured in volts.

Emigration: Passage of white blood corpuscles through the walls of capillaries and veins during inflammation.

Endogenous opiate-like substance: Chemical substance, polypeptides, produced in the brain, that act as opiates and produce analgesia by binding to opiate-receptor sites involved in pain perception. The threshold for pain is therefore increased. (Examples: endorphins, enkephalins.)

Eschar: A slough, especially one following a cauterization or burn.

Evaporation: 1. Change from liquid form to vapor. 2. Loss in volume due to conversion of a liquid into a vapor.

Extravasation: The escape of fluids into the surrounding tissue.

Extravascular: Outside a vessel.

Exudate: Accumulation of a fluid in a cavity, or matter that penetrates through vessel walls into adjoining tissue, or the production of pus or serum. In comparison with a transudate, there are more cells, protein, and solid material in an exudate.

Fibroblast: Any cell or corpuscle from which connective tissue is developed.

Firbrosis: Abnormal formation of fibrous tissue.

Gate control theory: The hypothesis that painful stimuli may be prevented from reaching higher levels of the central nervous system by stimulation of larger sensory nerves.

Granulation tissue: 1. Formation of granules or state or condition of being granular. 2. Fleshy projections formed on the surface of a gaping wound that is not healing by first intention or indirect union. Each granulation represents the outgrowth of new capillaries by budding from the existing capillaries and then joining up into capillary loops supported by cells that will later become fibrous scar tissue. Granulations bring rich blood supply to the healing surface.

Ground: In electronics, the negative or earth pole that has zero electrical potential.

Hemarthrosis: Bloody effusion into a cavity of a joint.

Hematoma: A swelling or mass of blood (usually clotted) confined to an organ, tissue, or space and caused by a break in a blood vessel.

Hemorrhage: Abnormal internal or external discharge of blood. May be venous, arterial, or capillary from blood vessels into tissues, into or from the body. Venous blood is dark red; flow is continuous. Arterial blood is bright red; flows in spurts. Capillary blood is of a reddish color; exudes from tissue.

Hertz: A unit of frequency equal to 1 cycle per second. Abbreviated Hz.

Histamine: A substance, produced from the amino acid histidine, that is normally present in the body. It exerts a pharmacologic action when released from injured cells. The red flush of a burn is due to the local production of histamine.

Homeostasis: State of equilibrium of the internal environment of the body that is maintained by dynamic processes of feedback and regulation.

Hyaluronic acid: An acid mucopolysaccharide found in the ground substance of connective tissue that acts as a binding and protective agent. Also found in synovial fluid and vitreous and aqueous humors.

Hydrotherapy: Scientific application of water in treatment of disease.

Hyperalgesia: Excessive sensitivity to pain. Opposite of hypalgesia.

Hyperemia: 1. Congestion. An unusual amount of blood in a part. 2. A form of macula; red areas on skin that disappear on pressure. 3. In physical therapy, increase in quantity of blood flowing through any part of the body, shown by redness of the skin caused by the application of heat.

Hyperreflexia: Increased action of the reflexes.

Hyperthermia: 1. Unusually high fever. 2. Treatment of disease by raising bodily temperature, accomplished by introduction of the malaria organism, injection of foreign proteins, or by physical means.

Hypertrophy: Increase in size of an organ or structure that does not involve tumor formation. Term is generally restricted to an increase in size or bulk not resulting from an increase in number of cells or tissue elements, as in the hypertrophy of muscle.

Hypotonic: 1. Pertains to defective muscular tone or tension. 2. A solution of lower osmotic pressure than another.

Immune response: The reaction of the body to substances that are foreign or are interpreted as being foreign.
  Nonspecific immune response: Does not involve antibody stimulation, but includes the inflammatory reaction, phagocytosis of micro-organisms, and complement activation.

Impedance: Resistance met by alternating currents in passing through a conductor; consists of resistance, reactance, inductance, or capacitance. The resistance due to the inductive and condenser characteristics of a circuit is called reactance.

Inductance: That property of an electric circuit by virtue of which a varying current induces an electromotive force in that circuit or a neighboring circuit. The unit of inductance, or self-inductance, is the henry.

Inflammation: Tissue reaction to injury. The succession of changes that occur in living tissue when it is injured. The inflamed area undergoes continuous change as the body repair processes start to heat and replace injured tissue. Inflammation is a conservative process modified by whatever produces the reaction, but it should not be confused with infection; the two are relatively different conditions, although one may arise from the other.

i., Acute: Inflammation in which the onset is rapid and the course relatively short.

i., Chronic: Inflammation that progresses slowly, is of long duration, and usually results in the formation of scar.

i., Subacute: A relatively mild inflammation that may become worse and then is severe or chronic.

Insulator: That which insulates. Specifically, a substance or body that interrupts the transmission of electricity to surrounding objects by conduction; anything that exerts great resistance to the passage of electric current by conduction. The electrical resistance of an insulator is expressed in ohms.

Intravascular: Within blood vessels.

Inverse-square law: Law stating that the intensity of radiation or light at any distance is inversely proportional to the square of the distance between the irradiated surface and a point surface. Thus a light with a certain intensity at a 4-foot distance will have only one fourth that intensity at 8 feet and would be 4 times as intense at a 2-foot distance.

Ischemia: Local and temporary deficiency of blood supply due to obstruction of the circulation to a part.

Joule's law: The principle that the rate of production of heat by a constant direct current is directly proportional to the resistance of the circuit and the square of the current.

Kallikrein: An enzyme normally present in blood plasma, urine, and body tissue in an inactive state. When activated, kallikrein is one of the most potent vasodilators. It forms kinin, q.v.

Keloid: Scar formation in the skin following trauma or surgical incision. Tissue response is out of proportion to the amount of scar tissue required for normal repair and healing. The result is a raised, firm, thickened red scar that may grow for a prolonged period of time. The increase in scar size is due to deposition of an abnormal amount of collagen into the tissue. Blacks are especially prone to developing keloids.

Kinin: A general term for a group of polypeptides that have considerable biologic activity. They are capable of influencing smooth muscle contraction, inducing hypotension, increasing the blood blow and permeability of capillaries, and inducing pain.

Kininogen: Substance that produces a kinin when acted upon by certain enzymes.

Labile cells: Cells that continue to proliferate throughout life, replacing cells that are continually being destroyed.

Laser: Acronym for light amplification by stimulated emission of radiation. The instrument converts various frequencies of light into one small and extremely intense unified beam of one wavelength radiation.

L. High power: Emits intense heat and power at close range. A tool used in surgery and in diagnosis.

L. Low power: The average power of a low-power laser is 50 mW or lower. Also known as "cold" laser.

Leukocyte: White blood corpuscle. There are two types: granulocytes (those possessing granules in their cytoplasm) and agranulocytes (those lacking granules). Granulocytes include juvenile neutrophils (3%–5%), segmented neutrophils (54%–62%), basophils (0%–0.75%), and eosinophils (1%–3%). Agranulocytes include lymphocytes, large and small (25%–33%), and monocytes (3%–7%).

Macrophage: Cells of the reticuloendothelial system having the ability to phagocytose particulate substances and to store vital dyes and other colloidal substances. They are found in loose connective tissues and various organs of the body. They include Kupffer cells of the liver, splenocytes of the spleen, dust cells of the lung, microglia of spinal cord and brain, and histiocytes of loose connective tissue.

Magnetic field: The space permeated by the magnetic lines of force surrounding a permanent magnet or coil of wire carrying electric current.

Margination: Adhesion of leukocytes of walls of blood vessels in first stages of inflammation.

Monochromatic: Having one color.

Monocyte: A large mononuclear leukocyte having more protoplasm than a lymphocyte.

Mottling: Condition that is marked by discolored areas.

Necrosis: Death of areas of tissue or bone surrounded by healthy parts.

Neovascularization: The endothelial response in small vessels of the connective tissue in wound healing that results in the formation of new capillary beds that invade the injured inflamed sites.

Nerve conduction velocity: The speed at which an impulse travels the length of a nerve.

Neurapraxia: Cessation in function of a peripheral nerve without degenerative changes occurring. Recovery is the usual outcome.

Neuraxis: The cerebrospinal axis.

Nociceptor: A nerve for receiving and transmitting painful stimuli.

Nonconductor: Any substance that does not transmit heat, sound, or electricity or that conducts it with difficulty. Strictly speaking, there is no perfect nonconductor. On the application of a sufficiently high voltage, current may be caused to flow through materials usually spoken of as nonconductors. Syn: Insulator.

Noxious: Harmful.

Oncotic pressure, colloidal: The total influence of the protein on the osmotic activity of plasma water.

Opiate receptor: Specific sites on cell surfaces that interact in a highly selective fashion with opiate drugs. These receptors mediate the major known pharmacologic actions of opiates and the physiologic functions of the enodgenous opiate-like substance, endorphins, and enkephalins, q.v.

Oscilloscope: An instrument for making visible the presence, nature, and form of oscillations or irregularities of an electric current.

Osmotic pressure: 1. Pressure that develops when two solutions of different concentrations are separated by a semipermeable membrane. 2. Pressure that would develop if a solution were enclosed in a membrane impermeable to all solutes present and surrounded by pure solvent. Osmotic pressure varies with concentration of the solution and with temperature increase. Animal cells have an osmotic pressure approximately equal to that of the circulating fluid, the blood. Solutions exerting this osmotic pressure are said to be isotonic or isomotic; stronger solutions that cause cells to shrink are hypertonic; weaker solutions that cause cells to swell are hypotonic.

Osteoblast: Any cell of mesodermal origin that is concerned with the formation of bone.

Pain rating scale: Most commonly used for pain assessment.

Pattern theory: The pattern or coding of sensory information is the key element. It involves the temporal and spatial sequencing of action potentials in the periphery.

This theory negates the idea of a specific pain receptor, but rather considers the intense stimulation of nonspecific receptors as the adequate stimulus for eliciting pain sensation.

Pearl-chain formation: A nonthermal effect of diathermy that is produced when micro-organisms, unicellular organisms, fat globules in milk, or red blood cells in serum become oriented in chain formation parallel to the lines of force in the electromagnetic field.

Peripheral vascular disease: An imprecise term indicating diseases of the arteries and veins of the extremities, especially those conditions that interfere with adequate flow of blood to or from the extremities, such as atherosclerosis with narrowing of the arterial lumen.

Permanent cells: Cells that cannot reproduce themselves after birth.

Phagocytosis: Ingestion and digestion of bacteria and particles by phagocytes.

Phonophoresis: Driving of medication into tissue by ultrasound.

Piezoelectric crystal: A transducer that converts electrical energy into sound energy, and vice versa. (Examples: Quartz, barium titanate, lead zirconate titanate.)

Piezoelectric effect: The vibration of a crystal as a result of receiving electrical current.

    p.e., Direct: The generation of an electric voltage across a crystal when the crystal is compressed. This effect is used for converting ultrasound into an electrical signal that replicates the sound pattern.

    p.e., Reverse (indirect): The contraction or expansion of a crystal in response to a voltage applied across its face. This effect is used to generate ultrasound at any desired frequency.

Photon: A light quantum or unit of energy of a light ray or other form of radiant energy. Generally considered to be a discrete particle with zero mass, no electric charge, and of indefinitely long life.

Presynaptic inhibition: This process does not involve any direct inhibitory effect upon the postsynaptic membrane, but instead causes a reduction in the release of transmitter substance at the presynaptic terminal of the excitatory synapse.

Prostaglandins: Abbr: PG. A large group of biologically active, carbon-20, unsaturated fatty acids that represent some of the metabolites of arachidonic acid. The PGs, all of which are short-lived in the circulation, have a wide assortment of biologic effects that are not mediated by plasma, but they act as local intercellular or intracellular modulators of the biochemical activity of the tissues in which they are formed. Thus, they are classed as autocoids rather than as hormones.

Pulse-average intensity: The maximal intensity of a pulsed sound beam during the "on" phase. Also known as the temporal peak intensity.

Pus: Liquid product of inflammation composed of albuminous substances, a thin fluid, and leukocytes; generally yellow in color. If red, it suggests rupture of small vessels. If blue or green, it indicates presence of *Pseudomonas aeruginosa.*

Radiation: 1. Process by which energy is propagated through space or matter. 2. Emission of rays in all directions from a common center.

    r., Electromagnetic: Rays that travel at the speed of light. They exhibit both magnetic and electrical properties.

    r., Infrared: Invisible heat rays beyond the red end of the spectrum. Near or short infrared extends from 7200 to 14,000 angstroms (AU); far or long infrared extends from 15,000 to 120,000 AU.

    r., Ionizing: Radiation that either directly or indirectly induces ionization of radiation-absorbing material used for diagnostic or therapeutic purposes.

Radiculitis: Inflammation of spinal-nerve roots, accompanied by pain and hyperesthesia.

Rarefaction: Process of decreasing density and weight, as of air.

Reactive hyperemia: The increased presence of blood in an area after restoration of blood flow following a decreased supply.

Referred pain: Pain seeming to arise in an area other than its origin.

Reflection: The throwing back of a ray of radiant energy from a surface not penetrated.

Refraction: Deflection from a straight path, as of light rays as they pass through media of different densities; the change of direction of a ray when it passes from one medium to another of a different density.

Reliability: Suggests consistent dependability of judgment, character, performance, or result.

Resistance: Opposition to, or the ability to oppose, anything, such as the power of a fluid to retard that which is passing through it; of the air; or opposition of the body to passage of an electric current.

Reticulin: An albuminoid or scleroprotein substance in the connective tissue framework of reticular tissue.

Serotonin: A chemical present in platelets. Serotonin is a potent vasoconstrictor. It is thought to be involved in neural mechanisms important in sleep and sensory perception.

Skin graft: Using the skin from another part of the body, or from a donor, to repair a defect or trauma of the skin.

Solenoid: A coil of insulated wire in which a magnetic force is created in the long axis of the coil when an electric current flows through the wire.

Somatotopic: Concerning the correspondence between a particular part of the body and a particular area of the brain.

Spasm: An involuntary sudden movement or convulsive muscular contraction. Spasms may be clonic (characterized by alternative contraction and relaxation) or tonic (sustained). They may involve either visceral (smooth) muscle or skeletal (striated) muscle. When contractions are strong and painful, they are called cramps. The effect depends upon the part affected.

Spasticity: Increased tone or contractions of muscles causing stiff and awkward movements; the results of upper motor neuron lesion.

Spatial average intensity: The average intensity of ultrasound as measured by dividing the total power output (in watts) of the ultrasound applicator by the effective radiating area (in cm^2) of the applicator face.

Spatial peak intensity: The greatest intensity of ultrasound anywhere within the beam.

Specific gravity: Weight of a substance compared with an equal volume of water. For solid and liquid materials, water is used as a standard and considered to have a specific gravity of one (1,000). For gases, the weight per unit volume is compared with dry air at a specified temperature.

Specific heat: The number of calories required to raise the temperature of 1 g of a substance 1°C, or the number of BTU's per pound per degree Fahrenheit.

Specificity theory of pain: Proposed that a specific pain system existed. There is receptor specialization for each sensation (heat, cold, touch, pain).

Sprain: Trauma to a joint that causes pain and disability depending upon degree of injury to ligaments. In severe sprain, ligaments may be completely torn.

Statis ulcer: See: Decubitus ulcer.

Stimulated emission: An issuance or discharge; the sending forth or discharge, such as of an atomic particle, exhalation, or of a light or heat wave.

Strain: Trauma to the muscle or the musculotendinous unit from violent contraction or excessive forcible stretch. May be associated with failure of synergistic action of muscles.

Subliminal: Below the threshold of sensation; too weak to arouse sensation or muscular contraction.

Substance P: An 11-amino acid peptide that is believed to be important as a neurotransmitter in the pain-fiber system. This substance may also be important in eliciting local tissue reactions resembling inflammation.

Substantia gelatinosa: Gray matter of the cord surrounding central canal and capping head of posterior horns of spinal cord.

Syncope: A transient loss of consciousness due to inadequate blood flow to the brain. Fainting.

Temporal average intensity: The intensity of pulsed ultrasound obtained by averaging the intensity during both the "on" and "off" periods.

Temporal peak intensity: See: Pulse average intensity.

Tendinitis: Inflammation of a tendon.

Thermography: In medicine, the use of a device that detects and records the heat present in very small areas of the part being studied. When these multiple readings are accumulated, the relatively hot and cold spots on the body surface are revealed. The technique has been used to study blood flow to limbs and to detect cancer of the breast.

Thermostat: An automatic device for regulating the temperature.

Thrombophlebitis: Inflammation of a vein in conjunction with the formation of a thrombus. Usually occurs in an extremity, most frequently a leg.

Transducer: Device that converts one form of energy to another. Used in medical electronics to receive the energy produced by sound or pressure and relay it as an electrical impulse to another transducer, which can either convert the energy back into its original form or make a record of it on a recording device.

Transformer: A stationary induction apparatus to change electrical energy at one voltage and current to electrical energy at another voltage and current through the medium of magnetic energy, without mechanical motion.

   t., Step-down: Transformer that changes electricity to a lower voltage.

   t., Step-up: Transformer that changes electricity to a higher voltage.

Transudate: The fluid that passes through a membrane, especially that which passes through capillary walls. Compared to an exudate, q.v., a transudate has fewer cellular elements and is of a lower specific gravity.

Trigger point: Any place on the body that when stimulated causes a sudden pain in a specific area, especially a type of pain previously felt spontaneously at the same location.

Ultrasound: Inaudible sound in the frequency range of approximately 20,000 to 10 billion (10^9) cycles per second (hertz). Ultrasound has different velocities in tissues that differ in density and elasticity from others. Use of ultrasound for diagnostic and therapeutic purposes requires special equipment.

Urticaria: A vascular reaction of the skin characterized by the eruption of pale evanescent wheals, which are associated with severe itching.

   u., Cold: Cold-induced urticarial eruption, which may progress to angioedema.

Vasoconstriction: Decrease in the caliper of blood vessels.

Vasodilation: Increase in the caliper of blood vessels.

Viscosity: Resistance offered by a fluid to change of form or relative position of its particles due to attraction of molecules to each other.

Wavelength: The distance between the beginning and end of a single wave cycle, usually measures from the top of one wave to the top of the next one.

APPENDIX 1

Temperature Conversions for Fahrenheit and Centigrade

To convert Centigrade to Fahrenheit: $\frac{9}{5}C + 32$

°C	°F	°C	°F
46	114.8	22	71.6
45	113.0	21	69.8
44	111.2	20	68.0
43	109.4	19	66.2
42	107.6	18	64.4
41	105.8	17	62.6
40	104.0	16	60.8
39	102.2	15	59.0
38	100.4	14	57.2
37	98.6	13	55.4
36	96.8	12	53.6
35	95.0	11	51.8
34	93.2	10	50.0
33	91.4	9	48.2
32	89.6	8	46.4
31	87.8	7	44.6
30	86.0	6	42.8
29	84.2	5	41.0
28	82.4	4	39.2
27	80.6	3	37.4
26	78.8	2	35.6
25	77.0	1	33.8
24	75.2	0	32.0
23	73.4		

To convert Fahrenheit to Centigrade: $\frac{5}{9}$ (F − 32)

°F	°C	°F	°C
120	48.9	76	24.4
119	48.3	75	23.9
118	47.8	74	23.3
117	47.2	73	22.7
116	46.7	72	22.2
115	46.1	71	21.7
114	45.6	70	21.1
113	45.0	69	20.6
112	44.4	68	20.0
111	43.9	67	19.4
110	43.3	66	18.9
109	42.8	65	18.3
108	42.2	64	17.8
107	41.7	63	17.2
106	41.1	62	16.7
105	40.5	61	16.1
104	40.0	60	15.5
103	39.4	59	15.0
102	38.8	58	14.4
101	38.3	57	13.9
100	37.8	56	13.3
99	37.2	55	12.8
98	36.7	54	12.2
97	36.1	53	11.7
96	35.5	52	11.1
95	35.0	51	10.6
94	34.4	50	10.0
93	33.9	49	9.4
92	33.3	48	8.9
91	32.8	47	8.3
90	32.2	46	7.8
89	31.7	45	7.2
88	31.1	44	6.6
87	30.6	43	6.1
86	30.0	42	5.6
85	29.4	41	5.0
84	28.9	40	4.4
83	28.3	39	3.9
82	27.8	38	3.3
81	27.2	37	2.8
80	26.7	36	2.2
79	26.1	35	1.7
78	25.6	34	1.1
77	25.0	33	0.6
		32	0

INDEX

A page number in *italics* indicates a figure. A "t" following a page number indicates a table.

289

Pattern theory, of pain, 20, *20*, 281–282
PEMFs. *See* Pulsed electromagnetic field(s)
Periarticular tissue(s), ultrasound and, 145
Peripheral vascular disease, 123, 282
Phagocytosis
    definition of, 282
    laser effect on, 207–208
Phonophoresis
    for athletic injuries, 252–254, *254*, *255*
    for medication delivery, 152–153, 161, *254*, 282
    for plantar fascitis, 254
Piezoelectric effect(s)
    definition of, 282
    of ultrasound, 141–142, *142*
Plantar fasciitis, phonophoresis for, 254
Plantar warts, ultrasound for, 155–156
Plasma extravasation, ultrasound effect on, 154
Polyarthritis, 259. *See also* Osteoarthritis;
        Rheumatoid arthritis
Pool therapy
    equipment and safety in, 129
    patient selection for, 128
    temperature in, 129
    water forces in
        bouyancy, 109–110, 128
        hydrostatic pressure, 110, 127
        specific gravity, 110, 128
        viscosity, 110, 127–128
Positioning
    for thermal treatment, of rheumatic disease, 259
    for ultrasound therapy, 161–162, *162*, *163*
Povidone—iodine solution, 123–124
Power
    distribution of, 48–50, *49*
    output of, in diathermy, 60, 182–184, *183*
Pregnant women
    diathermy and, 195
    laser and, 213
    ultrasound and, 162
Pressure algometer
    in pain assessment, 233–235, *234*
        threshold and, 223–224
        tolerance, 234
Proposal, in clinical research, 225
Psoriasis, ultraviolet heating for, 216
Pulsed electromagnetic field(s), (PEMFs)
    application of, 187
    creation of, *182*, 182–183
    instrumentation and application methods in, 187
    mode of action of, 184
    power output and heat production from,
        182–183, *183*, 187
    radiofrequency radiation in, 181–182
Pulsing pattern, of ultrasound, 139–140, *140*

R

RA. *See* Rheumatoid arthritis
Radiation
    definition and types of, 282
    in diathermy
        effects of, 46, *46*
        from exposure, 195–196
        microwave, 180–181
        pulsed electromagnetic, 181–182
    infrared, 100, 240

    in water, 111
    in thermography, 240
Range of motion (ROM)
    goniometry and, 235–236
    heat and stretch treatment for, 102–103
    in osteoarthritis, heat and, 257
    in rheumatic disease, 259, 271
    in rheumatoid arthritis
        Fluidotherapy and, 264
        heat versus cold therapy and, 266
Raynaud's phenomenon, 84–85
Referred pain
    definition of, 33, 283
    theories of
        convergence-facilitation, 33
        convergence-projection, 33
        trigger points in, 33–34
Reflex sympathetic dystrophy, ultrasound for, 151
Refraction
    definition of, 283
    of microwaves, 181
Reliability, in research method, 224
Research
    clinical evaluation in
        functional test in, 239–240
        instrumentation for, 231–232
        muscle performance and, 238–239
        pain assessment and, 232–233
        of range of motion, 235–236
        related procedures in, 240
        volumetric, *236*, 236–237
    principles of
        hypothesis for, 223–224
        information collection for, 223
        methodology for, 224–225
        planning and preparation for, 222
        proposal for, 225
        question in, 222
        results dissemination in, 225
    study types in
        comparative design and, 226–231, *228*, *230*
        single-case, 225–226
        single-group, 226
Rheumatic disease(s)
    clinic versus homecare in, 260, *261*, *262*
    considerations in
        for physical therapy, 258
        for thermal treatment, 259–261
    polyarticular arthritis
        categories of, 262–263
        characteristics of, 262t
        osteoarthritis, 266–268
        rheumatoid, 262t, 263–266
        treatment goals in, 261–262
    thermal treatment of, 259–261
    treatment of
        application techniques and, 271
        clinical and laboratory tests, 271, 272t
        concurrent medication and, 268, 270
        disease stage and, 268
        factors influencing, 268, 270–271
        natural disease course and, 268
        pain and, 270t, 270–271
        patient feelings and, 271
        range of motion in, 271